# Master Techniques
## IN CATARACT AND REFRACTIVE SURGERY

EDITED BY

## F. Hampton Roy, MD, FACS

CLINICAL ASSOCIATE PROFESSOR OF OPHTHALMOLOGY
UNIVERSITY OF ARKANSAS FOR MEDICAL SCIENCES

MEDICAL DIRECTOR
HAMPTON ROY EYE CENTER
LITTLE ROCK, ARK

AND

## Carlos Walter Arzabe, MD

DIRECTOR
HOSPITAL DEL OJO
SANTA CRUZ, BOLIVIA

*An innovative information, education, and management company*
6900 Grove Road • Thorofare, NJ 08086

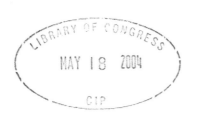
The procedures and practices described in this book should be implemented in a manner consistent with the professional standards set for the circumstances that apply in each specific situation. Every effort has been made to confirm the accuracy of the information presented and to correctly relate generally accepted practices. The author, editor, and publisher cannot accept responsibility for errors or exclusions or for the outcome of the application of the material presented herein. There is no expressed or implied warranty of this book or information imparted by it.

Care has been taken to ensure that drug selection and dosages are in accordance with currently accepted/recommended practice. Due to continuing research, changes in government policy and regulations, and various effects of drug reactions and interactions, it is recommended that the reader review all materials and literature provided for each drug, especially those that are new or not frequently used.

Any review or mention of specific companies or products is not intended as an endorsement by the author or publisher.

The work SLACK Incorporated publishes is peer reviewed. Prior to publication, recognized leaders in the field, educators, and clinicians provide important feedback on the concepts and content that we publish. We welcome feedback on this work.

Library of Congress Cataloging-in-Publication Data
Master techniques in cataract and refractive surgery / edited by F. Hampton Roy and Carlos Walter Arzabe.
p. ; cm.
Includes bibliographical references and index.
ISBN 1-55642-696-8 (hard cover)
1. Cataract--Surgery.
[DNLM: 1. Cataract Extraction--methods. 2. Refractive Errors--surgery. 3. Corneal Diseases--surgery. WW 260 M423 2004] I. Roy, Frederick Hampton. II. Arzabe, Carlos W.
RE451.M348 2004
6177'42059--dc22
2003027796

Printed in the United States of America.

Published by:     SLACK Incorporated
6900 Grove Road
Thorofare, NJ 08086 USA
Telephone: 856-848-1000
Fax: 856-853-5991
www.slackbooks.com

Contact SLACK Incorporated for more information about other books in this field or about the availability of our books from distributors outside the United States.

For further information on CCC, check CCC Online at the following address: http://www.copyright.com.

Last digit is print number: 10   9   8   7   6   5   4   3   2   1

# DEDICATION

Drs. Roy and Arzabe dedicate this book to the forward-thinking authors who have written its excellent chapters.

# CONTENTS

*Dedication* . . . . . . . . . . . . . . . . . . . . . . . . . . . . . . . . . . . . . . . . . . . . . . . . . . . . . . . . . *iii*
*Acknowledgments* . . . . . . . . . . . . . . . . . . . . . . . . . . . . . . . . . . . . . . . . . . . . . . . . . . . *vii*
*About the Editors* . . . . . . . . . . . . . . . . . . . . . . . . . . . . . . . . . . . . . . . . . . . . . . . . . . . . . *ix*
*Contributing Authors* . . . . . . . . . . . . . . . . . . . . . . . . . . . . . . . . . . . . . . . . . . . . . . . . . . *xi*
*Introduction* . . . . . . . . . . . . . . . . . . . . . . . . . . . . . . . . . . . . . . . . . . . . . . . . . . . . . . . . *xiii*
    F. Hampton Roy, MD, FACS and Carlos Walter Arzabe, MD

SECTION 1    CATARACT SURGERY . . . . . . . . . . . . . . . . . . . . . . . 1

Chapter 1    Surgical Management of Aniridia . . . . . . . . . . . . . . . . . . . . . . . . 3
    Scott E. Burk, MD, PhD and Robert H. Osher, MD

Chapter 2    Bioptics in Cataract Surgery . . . . . . . . . . . . . . . . . . . . . . . . . . . 11
    R. Gale Martin, MD

Chapter 3    Congenital Cataract . . . . . . . . . . . . . . . . . . . . . . . . . . . . . . . . 23
    Howard V. Gimbel, MD, MPH, FRCSC, FACS; Brian M. DeBroff, MD, FACS; and Jennifer A. Dunbar, MD

Chapter 4    Cataract With Zonular Dialyses . . . . . . . . . . . . . . . . . . . . . . . . 35
    Scott E. Burk, MD, PhD and Robert J. Cionni, MD

Chapter 5    Cataract With Dislocated and Subluxated Lenses . . . . . . . . . . . . . . 43
    Steve Charles, MD

Chapter 6    Cataract With Corneal Astigmatism . . . . . . . . . . . . . . . . . . . . . . 47
    Harry B. Grabow, MD

Chapter 7    Cataract With Uveitis . . . . . . . . . . . . . . . . . . . . . . . . . . . . . . . 63
    Gustavo Barbosa Abreu, MD

Chapter 8    Dislocation and Decentration of Intraocular Lenses . . . . . . . . . . . . 73
    Lisa Brothers Arbisser, MD

Chapter 9    Intraocular Lens Exchange . . . . . . . . . . . . . . . . . . . . . . . . . . . 85
    Francisco Contreras, MD and Cecilia Contreras, MD

Chapter 10    Laser Cataract Extraction . . . . . . . . . . . . . . . . . . . . . . . . . . . 89
    Jack M. Dodick, MD and Iman Ali Pahlavi, MD

Chapter 11    Lensectomy With Accommodating Lens . . . . . . . . . . . . . . . . . . . 93
    Roberto Zaldivar, MD; Susana Oscherow, MD; and Virginia Piezzi, MD

Chapter 12    Lensectomy With Multifocal Lens . . . . . . . . . . . . . . . . . . . . . . 101
    I. Howard Fine, MD; Richard S. Hoffman, MD; and Mark Packer, MD

Chapter 13    Phacolytic Phacomorphic Glaucomas . . . . . . . . . . . . . . . . . . . 109
    S. Fabian Lerner, MD

Chapter 14    Cataract Surgery in Pseudoexfoliation Syndrome . . . . . . . . . . . . . 113
    William J. Rand, MD; Gabriel E. Velázquez, MD; and Barry A. Schechter, MD

Chapter 15    Piggyback Intraocular Lens Implantation . . . . . . . . . . . . . . . . . . 133
    James P. Gills, MD and Myra Cherchio, COMT

Chapter 16    Surgical Implantation of Telescopic Intraocular Lenses . . . . . . . . . . 139
    Christina Canakis, MD and Gholam A. Peyman, MD

SECTION 2 REFRACTIVE SURGERY . . . . . . . . . . . . . . . . . 149

Chapter 1 Astigmatism: LASIK, LASEK, and PRK . . . . . . . . . . . 151
*Noel A. Alpins, FRACO, FRCOphth, FACS and Carolyn M. Terry, BOptom*

Chapter 2 Reducing Astigmatism . . . . . . . . . . . . . . . . . . . . 161
*R. Bruce Wallace III, MD, FACS*

Chapter 3 Toric Intraocular Lenses . . . . . . . . . . . . . . . . . . . 165
*Stephen Bylsma, MD*

Chapter 4 Hyperopia and Myopia Treatment After Radial Keratotomy . . . . . 171
*Joao Alberto Holanda de Freitas, MD and Paulo de Tarso da Silva Alvim, MD*

Chapter 5 Phakic Lenses and LASIK . . . . . . . . . . . . . . . . . . 177
*Luis F. Restrepo, MD*

Chapter 6 Hyperopia and Conductive Thermokeratoplasty . . . . . . . . . 181
*José A.P. Gomes, MD and Daniela Endriss, MD*

Chapter 7 Hyperopia: LASIK, LASEK, and PRK . . . . . . . . . . . . . 187
*Robin F. Beran, MD, FACS*

Chapter 8 Hyperopia: Treatment With Accommodative Esotropia and/or Nystagmus . . 207
*Hugo Daniel Nano Jr, MD*

Chapter 9 Phakic Lens Implantation in Myopia and Hyperopia . . . . . . . 211
*Daljit Singh, MS, DSc*

Chapter 10 Phakic Refractive Lenses . . . . . . . . . . . . . . . . . . 227
*Alexander Hatsis, MD, FACS and George Rozakis, MD, FACS*

Chapter 11 Intacs: Breaking the Prolate and Refractive Reversal Barrier . . . . . 237
*JE "Jay" McDonald II, MD; Allyson Mertins, OD; and David Deitz, Research Assistant*

Chapter 12 Myopia: PRK, LASIK, and LASEK . . . . . . . . . . . . . . 245
*Patricia Sierra Wilkinson, MD; David R. Hardten, MD; Richard L. Lindstrom, MD;*
*and Elizabeth A. Davis, MD*

Chapter 13 Presbyopia: Cataract Surgery With
Implantation of the 1 CU Accomodative Lens . . . . . . . . . . 261
*Michael Küchle, MD; Nguyen X. Nguyen, MD; Achim Langenbucher, PhD; and Berthold Seitz, MD*

Chapter 14 Presbyopic Lens Exchange . . . . . . . . . . . . . . . . . 267
*Kevin L. Waltz, OD, MD and R. Bruce Wallace III, MD, FACS*

Chapter 15 Surgical Reversal of Presbyopia . . . . . . . . . . . . . . . 273
*Gene W. Zdenek, MD*

*Index* . . . . . . . . . . . . . . . . . . . . . . . . . . . . . . . . . 289

# ACKNOWLEDGMENTS

We would like to acknowledge the assistance of Renee Tindall and Angie Brown in the production of this book. Without their dedication and persistence, this book could not have been published.

F. Hampton Roy, MD, FACS
LITTLE ROCK, ARK

The Bolivian Ophthalmological Society and I would like to express our gratitude to Dr. Roy for his teaching and collaboration with this country over the past 3 decades.

Carlos Walter Arzabe, MD
SANTA CRUZ, BOLIVIA

# ABOUT THE EDITORS

F. Hampton Roy, MD, FACS, has a private practice in Little Rock, Ark. He is the author of 120 articles and 33 books, and is Medical Director of the World Eye Foundation. Dr. Roy has worked in Peru, Bolivia, China, and India to improve current information systems. He is Clinical Associate Professor of Ophthalmology at University of Arkansas for Medical Sciences.

Carlos Walter Arzabe, MD, practices medicine in Santa Cruz, Bolivia. Dr. Arzabe is a former Research Fellow of Harvard University Eye Research Institute from Boston and Schepens Retina Associates. He has written in several world ophthalmic journals and books, and in the past few years has published with the Pan American Association of Ophthalmology a diabetic retinopathy manual. Most recently, with the support of the World Eye Foundation and Dr. Roy's guidance, teaching, and editing, he published a glaucoma manual (written in Spanish), which has been distributed for free in 16 countries. In 1996 he was the winner of the world contest, the Ten Outstanding Young Persons of the World Award, in the category of Medical Innovations, by the Junior Chamber International, Inc.

Both doctors practice general ophthalmology with an emphasis on cataract and refractive surgery.

Because one editor is from Little Rock, Ark and one editor is from Santa Cruz, Bolivia, this book has an international flavor that will certainly please the readers.

# CONTRIBUTING AUTHORS

GUSTAVO BARBOSA ABREU, MD
Penido Burnier Eye Institute
Campinas, Brazil

NOEL A. ALPINS, FRACO, FRCOPHTH, FACS
New Vision Clinics
Cheltenham, Australia

LISA BROTHERS ARBISSER, MD
Eye Surgeons Associates, PC
Spring Park Surgery Center
Davenport, Iowa

ROBIN F. BERAN, MD, FACS
Mt. Carmel East Hospital
Columbus, Ohio

SCOTT E. BURK, MD, PhD
Cincinnati Eye Institute
Cincinnati, Ohio

STEPHEN BYLSMA, MD
Associate Clinical Instructor
Department of Ophthalmology—UCLA
Santa Clara, Calif

CHRISTINA CANAKIS, MD
Department of Vitreoretinal Diseases and Surgery
Ophthalmochirougiki Eye Center
Athens, Greece
Formerly Clinical Vitreoretinal Fellow
Tulane University School of Medicine
New Orleans, La

STEVE CHARLES, MD
Clinical Professor
University of Tennessee Health Science Center
Memphis, Tenn

MYRA CHERCHIO, COMT
Director, Clinical Research
St. Luke's Cataract & Laser Institute
Tarpon Springs, Fla

ROBERT J. CIONNI, MD
Cincinnati Eye Institute
Cincinnati, Ohio

CECILIA CONTRERAS, MD
Clinica Ricardo Palua
Lima, Peru

FRANCISCO CONTRERAS, MD
Clinica Ricardo Palua
Lima, Peru

ELIZABETH A. DAVIS, MD
Minnesota Eye Consultants
Minneapolis, Minn

BRIAN M. DeBROFF, MD, FACS
Assistant Professor of Ophthalmology and Visual Science
Program Director and Vice Chairman
Department of Ophthalmology and Visual Science
Yale University School of Medicine
New Haven, Conn

DAVID DEITZ, RESEARCH ASSISTANT
McDonald Eye Associates
Fayetteville, Ark

JOAO ALBERTO HOLANDA DE FREITAS, MD
Director
Clinica de olhos Holanda de Freitas
Professor and Chairman
Pontificia Universidade Catolica de Sao Paulo (PUC-SP)
Campinas, Brazil

PAULO DE TARSO DA SILVA ALVIM, MD
Pontificia Universidade Catolica de Sao Paulo (PUC-SP)
Campinas, Brazil

JACK M. DODICK, MD
Manhattan Eye, Ear, & Throat Hospital
New York City, NY

JENNIFER A. DUNBAR, MD
Assistant Professor of Ophthalmology
Department of Ophthalmology
Loma Linda University
Loma Linda, Calif

DANIELA ENDRISS, MD
Observer Fellow
Cornea and External Eye Disease Service
Federal University of Sao Paulo
Sao Paulo, Brazil

I. HOWARD FINE, MD
Professor of Ophthalmology
Casey Eye Institute
Oregon Health and Science University
Eugene, Ore

JAMES P. GILLS, MD
St. Luke's Cataract & Laser Institute
Tarpon Springs, Fla

HOWARD V. GIMBEL, MD, MPH, FRCSC, FACS
Gimbel Eye Centre
Calgary, Alberta, Canada
Professor and Chairman, Dept. of Ophthalmology
Loma Linda University
Loma Linda, Calif
Clinical Professor, Dept. Of Ophthalmology
University of California
San Francisco, Calif

JOSÉ A.P. GOMES, MD
Associate Professor
Cornea and External Eye Disease Service
Federal University of Sao Paulo
Sao Paulo, Brazil

HARRY B. GRABOW, MD
Clinical Assistant Professor
University of South Florida
Founder and Medical Director
Sarasota Cataract & Laser Institute,
Center for Advanced Eye Surgery
Sarasota, Fla

DAVID R. HARDTEN, MD
Minnesota Eye Consultants
Minneapolis, Minn

ALEXANDER HATSIS, MD, FACS
Instructor
Nassau Co Medical Center
Rockville Center, NY

RICHARD S. HOFFMAN, MD
Clinical Instructor of Ophthalmology
Casey Eye Institute
Oregon Health and Science University
Eugene, Ore

MICHAEL KÜCHLE, MD
Department of Ophthalmology
and University Eye Hospital
University Erlangen-Nürnberg
Erlangen, Germany

ACHIM LANGENBUCHER, PhD
Department of Ophthalmology
and University Eye Hospital
University Erlangen-Nürnberg
Erlangen, Germany

S. FABIAN LERNER, MD
Buenos Aires, Argentina

RICHARD L. LINDSTROM, MD
Minnesota Eye Consultants
Minneapolis, Minn

R. GALE MARTIN, MD
Carolina Eye Association
Southern Pines, NC

J.E. "JAY" MCDONALD II, MD
McDonald Eye Associates
Fayetteville, Ark

ALLYSON MERTINS, OD
McDonald Eye Associates
Fayetteville, Ark

HUGO DANIEL NANO JR, MD
Instituto De Ojos
Buenos Aires, Argentina

NGUYEN X. NGUYEN, MD
Department of Ophthalmology
and University Eye Hospital
University Erlangen-Nürnberg
Erlangen, Germany

SUSANA OSCHEROW, MD
Instituto Zaldivar
Mendoza, Argentina

ROBERT H. OSHER, MD
Cincinnati Eye Institute
Cincinnati, Ohio

MARK PACKER, MD
Clinical Assistant Professor of Ophthalmology
Casey Eye Institute
Oregon Health and Science University
Eugene, Ore

IMAN ALI PAHLAVI, MD
Manhattan Eye, Ear, & Throat Hospital
New York City, NY

GHOLAM A. PEYMAN, MD
Department of Ophthalmology
Tulane Medical School
New Orleans, La

VIRGINIA PIEZZI, MD
Instituto Zaldivar
Mendoza, Argentina

WILLIAM J. RAND, MD
Rand Eye Institute
Pompano Beach, Fla

LUIS F. RESTREPO, MD
Refractive Surgeon
Pereira, Colombia

GEORGE ROZAKIS, MD, FACS
Northeastern Eye Center
North Olmstead, Ohio

BARRY A. SCHECHTER, MD
Rand Eye Institute
Pompano Beach, Fla

BERTHOLD SEITZ, MD
Department of Ophthalmology
and University Eye Hospital
University Erlangen-Nürnberg
Erlangen, Germany

DALJIT SINGH, MS, DSc
Daljit Singh Eye Hospital
Armisar, India

CAROLYN M. TERRY, BOptom
New Vision Clinics
Cheltenham, Australia

GABRIEL E. VELÁZQUEZ, MD
Rand Eye Institute
Pompano Beach, Fla

R. BRUCE WALLACE III, MD, FACS
Wallace Eye Surgery
Alexandria, La

KEVIN L. WALTZ, OD, MD
Eye Surgeons of Indiana
Indianapolis, Ind

PATRICIA SIERRA WILKINSON, MD
Minnesota Eye Consultants
Minneapolis, Minn

ROBERTO ZALDIVAR, MD
Instituto Zaldivar
Mendoza, Argentina

GENE W. ZDENEK, MD
Zdenek Eye Institute
Reseda, Calif

# INTRODUCTION

What would warrant a book on cataract and refractive surgery?

Cataract surgery is hundreds of years old. This book is a testament to the many forward-thinking ophthalmologists; it provides the latest thoughts on the thorniest problems such as the decentered natural lens and cataract with uveitis. It also covers new techniques such as ocular telescopes and the accommodating intraocular lens.

Pure refractive surgery is a field in its infancy. It is a field barely 25 years old. Respected ophthalmic surgeons have made this a progressive, viable subspecialty.

As editors we have attempted to invite "master" surgeons to demonstrate the most progressive cataract and refractive surgery techniques. Neither of us have written a chapter because this might have interfered with the editorial process.

Most of our authors are from North and South America. Thank you for your interest in this exciting, dynamic field.

F. Hampton Roy, MD, FACS
LITTLE ROCK, ARK

Carlos Walter Arzabe, MD
SANTA CRUZ, BOLIVIA

# SECTION 1
## CATARACT SURGERY

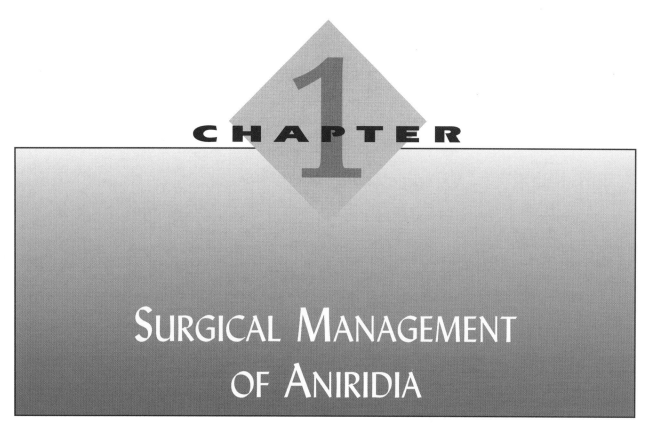

# CHAPTER 1

# SURGICAL MANAGEMENT OF ANIRIDIA

*Scott E. Burk, MD, PhD and Robert H. Osher, MD*

## INTRODUCTION

Iris absence—whether partial or complete, traumatic or congenital—poses a significant challenge to the cataract surgeon because he or she must either eliminate or reduce the tremendous glare disability caused by the lack of an effective iris diaphragm. Fortunately, artificial iris devices offer a safe alternative for those patients who previously had no viable options for iris reconstruction.

## ANATOMY AND PHYSIOLOGY

There are many causes of iris deficiency, both congenital and acquired. Congenital causes of iris deficiency include aniridia, anterior segment dysgenesis, coloboma, and ocular albinism. Congenital aniridia is the most common of these inherited iris deficiencies seen in our clinic and represents about 40% of all of our cases of iris deficiency. Overall, however, the condition is relatively rare affecting approximately 1 in every 100,000 births.[1] Congenital aniridia is characterized by a hypoplastic or rudimentary iris, and is often accompanied by abnormalities in the cornea, anterior chamber angle, lens, retina, and optic nerve.[2,3]

Acquired iris deficiency is most commonly the result of trauma and represents about 35% of our cases of iris deficiency. Traumatic iris deficiency is also frequently associated with ocular abnormalities including corneal scarring, zonular dialysis, ruptured capsule, angle recession, and even retinal damage. Acquired iris deficiency may also result from conditions that reduce the effectiveness of the iris diaphragm, such as, irido-corneal-endothelial (ICE) syndrome, herpetic iris atrophy, and traumatic mydriasis.

The management of these patients is often quite challenging due to their underlying ocular problems. A great variety of factors may contribute to poor visual acuity in these patients; however, they all share a common complaint of disabling glare or photophobia. Although there may be various definitions of "glare" and many factors that contribute to a person's perception of "glare," a fundamental optical origin of glare is the lack of a complete iris diaphragm.[2,3]

The primary function of the iris is to act as a diaphragm regulating the amount of light entering the eye. Because light enters through the entire area of the pupillary aperture, enlargement of the pupil diameter (diameter = 2r) results in an exponential increase in the area through which light enters the eye (area = $\pi r^2$). Stated simply, the area through which light enters an aniridic eye with a 12-mm aperture

$(r^2 = 36)$ is 4 fold greater than the amount of light entering an eye with a 6-mm pupil $(r^2 = 9)$. In addition to reducing the amount of light entering the eye, the iris diaphragm promotes depth of focus and serves to limit spherical and chromatic aberrations related to the edge of the lens.

# PREOPERATIVE EVALUATION

Whether the iris insufficiency is congenital or acquired, a comprehensive preoperative examination will help the surgeon better anticipate the challenges to be dealt with in the operating room. An assessment of the best-corrected visual acuity (BCVA) for near and distance should be determined. In addition to the routine preoperative assessment, the surgeon should characterize and draw the iris defect describing the amount and location of residual or rudimentary iris. A thorough characterization of the anatomy of the patient's anterior chamber angle is necessary. The capsular and zonular integrity should be assessed and any degree of phacodonesis should be documented. Co-existing ocular pathology should be noted and the patient made clearly aware of his or her visual limitations in order to avoid unrealistic expectations.

Informed consent should be modified. The patient should be specifically counseled about the benefits and limitations of the prosthetic iris devices. Patients must also be made aware that the prosthetic iris devices are not yet approved by the US Food and Drug Administration (FDA).

# PROSTHETIC IRIS DEVICES

The first prosthetic iris implantation, an anterior chamber lens, was performed in the United Kingdom by Mr. Peter Choyce in 1956. Another English surgeon, Mr. John Pearce is credited with implanting an iris diaphragm in the posterior chamber in the 1970's. In 1994, Dr. Ranier Sundmacher and coworkers from Germany reported implantation of a single-piece black iris diaphragm intraocular lens (IOL) for correction of aniridia.[4-5] Kenneth Rosenthal, MD, reported the first American case of small incision prosthetic iris implantation at the Welch Cataract Congress in 1996. Since then there have been other reports describing the use of the single-piece black iris diaphragm IOL, and we have published our experience with both the single-piece iris diaphragm IOL as well as endocapsular prosthetic iris devices.[6-10]

To date the majority of our experience has been with prosthetic iris devices produced by the Morcher Company in Germany. However, Ophtec, a company based in the Netherlands, also produces prosthetic iris devices and has recently begun clinical trials seeking FDA approval.

When contemplating the use of a prosthetic iris device, the surgeon must first define the clinical situation, determine that iris suturing techniques would not be sufficient, and then choose the appropriate device based on the relevant anatomy. Currently there are 2 main categories of prosthetic iris implants available, each with specific indications.

The single-piece devices include the black diaphragm IOL from Morcher (Figure 1-1) and brown-, green-, or blue-colored diaphragm IOLs from Ophtec. They each provide a full iris diaphragm and IOL that can be placed in the ciliary sulcus fixated either by capsular support or by transscleral sutures. A significant drawback of the single-piece iris diaphragm IOL is that a relatively large incision size is required—resulting in prolonged healing, increased astigmatism, and an increased risk of intraoperative hemorrhage. In addition, Sundmacher noted mild persistent intraocular inflammation, and worsening of preexisting glaucoma after implantation of the Morcher single-piece black diaphragm IOL.[8] Nonetheless, a single-piece iris diaphragm IOL is the implant of choice when capsular support is inadequate or absent.

Endocapsular devices represent the other main category of prosthetic iris devices that are currently available. The Morcher endocapsular ring with iris diaphragm was developed by Volker Rasch, MD, while the Ophtec Iris Prosthetic System (IPS) was designed by Heino Hermeking, MD. Because these prosthetic iris devices do not have an optical portion, they can be inserted through a relatively small incision. This approach offers the advantages of a full iris diaphragm and a separate optical system, each of which may be inserted through a sutureless small incision.

Morcher offers 2 styles of endocapsular rings used as iris prostheses. One ring with a single fin (Type 96G) is used for sectoral iris loss (Figure 1-2) and 2 separate rings with multiple fins that interdigitate (Type 50C) are used to create a full iris diaphragm (Figure 1-3). The multiple fin endocapsular rings produce an iris diaphragm with a pupil size of approximately 6.0 mm, which reduces the excess light entering the eye by approximately 75%, yet provides an aperture compatible with excellent fundus viewing.

The IPS consists of single elements and double elements used alone or in combination to treat iris defects ranging from sectoral to complete. The IPS also uses a fixation ring that acts to stabilize multiple elements within the capsular bag and counteract late contraction of the capsular bag. The Ophtec devices are designed to produce a pupil diameter of either 4 or 3 mm, which should reduce the excess light entering the eye by approximately 89% to 94% (Figure 1-4).

The optimal pupil size has yet to be determined and must balance the need for reducing the excess light entering the eye with the ability to view the peripheral retina.

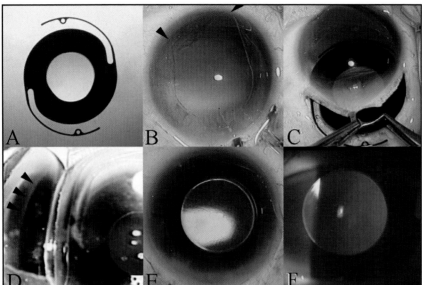

**Figure 1-1.** Morcher type 67G single-piece iris diaphragm IOL. (A) The 67G IOL with iris diaphragm has an optic diameter of 5.0 mm, centered in a black diaphragm 10 mm in diameter. Note that the haptics have eyelets for suture placement, and span 12.5 mm. (B) This photograph highlights the anterior capsular fragility seen in congenital aniridia. Note 2 separate extensions of the capsulorrhexis (arrows). (C) The wound must be enlarged to accommodate the 10-mm diameter of the single-piece iris diaphragm IOL. (D) Intraoperative gonioscopy is used to confirm ciliary sulcus placement under the iris stump (arrows). (E) Surgeon's view after implantation. (F) Retroillumination slit lamp examination demonstrates the opacity of the iris diaphragm.

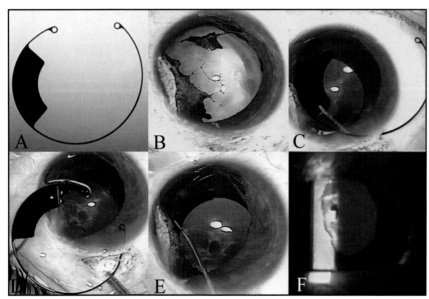

**Figure 1-2.** Morcher 96G single-fin endocapsular ring. (A) The 96G endocapsular ring has 1 fin spanning 3 clock hours and an overall diameter of 11 mm. (B) Clinical photograph demonstrating an eye posttrauma with a mature white cataract and loss of 6 clock hours of iris tissue. (C) The first 96G ring is placed into the capsular bag through a small incision. (D) In this case a second 96G ring is inserted into the capsular bag and brought into alignment forming a hemi-iris diaphragm. (E) Surgeon's view completing the alignment. (F) Retroillumination slit lamp examination demonstrates the iris diaphragm.

# INDICATIONS AND CONTRAINDICATIONS

Patients with either functional or anatomic iris deficiency who have severe glare disability derive the most benefit from implantation of a prosthetic iris. However, because implantation of the prosthetic device requires either capsular or suture support, we have limited our use of these devices to adult patients who are aphakic or who have a visually significant cataract.

The endocapsular ring and IPS devices are designed for endocapsular placement. When capsular support is absent or insufficient, a single-piece device is indicated.

# SURGICAL TECHNIQUES

## Anesthesia

A long-acting retrobulbar anesthetic is preferred due to the complicated nature of these cases. Elevated intraorbital pressure should be minimized.

**Figure 1-3.** Morcher 50C multiple-fin endocapsular ring. (A) The 50C endo-capsular ring has multiple fins and an overall diameter of 10 mm. (B) The first 50C ring is placed into the capsular bag through a small incision. (C, D) The second 50C ring is inserted into the capsular bag and brought into alignment so that the fins inter-digitate, forming a full iris dia-phragm. (E) Surgeon's view after implantation. (F) Retroillumination slit lamp examination demonstrates the iris diaphragm.

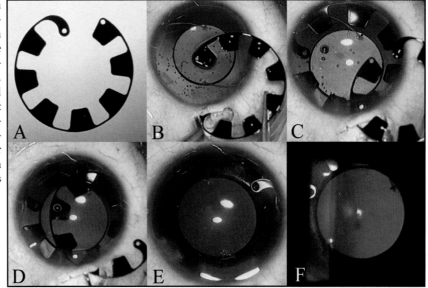

**Figure 1-4.** IPS. (A) Drawing of an IPS double element inside the capsular bag along with an endocapsular tension ring and an IOL. (B) Drawing of the second IPS double element inside the capsular bag aligned to produce a com-plete iris diaphragm. (C) Intraoperative implantation of the first IPS double element. (D) The second IPS double element is inserted into the capsular bag and aligned 180 degrees opposite orientation to the first to create a full iris diaphragm. (E) Implantation of a central stabilizing ring. (F) Surgeon's view after implantation. (Illustrations provided courtesy of OPHTEC USA, Boca Raton, Fla and Heino Herm-eking, MD, University of Witten Herdecke, Germany. Surgical images provided courtesy of Michael E. Snyder, MD, Cincinnati Eye Institute.)

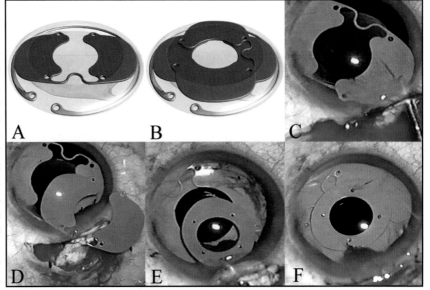

## Procedure

The exact surgical procedure will vary from patient to patient depending on the clinical situation and the device(s) chosen. The surgeon is wise to approach any case of iris defi-ciency with knowledge and caution. A thorough preopera-tive evaluation can help minimize intraoperative surprises, and with a repertoire of anterior segment reconstruction techniques and devices, the surgeon is prepared to undertake iris-deficient cases.

The incision is generally made in a meridian to facilitate phacoemulsification or secondary lens implantation. We generally operate temporally utilizing a near-clear cornea approach for the endocapsular devices. A scleral tunnel fol-lowed by a shelved scleral incision is constructed for the larg-er, single-piece devices. Occasionally, the single-piece device is placed through the open sky when the patient is undergo-ing a concurrent corneal transplant.

Capsulorrhexis can vary depending on the etiology of iris deficiency. Eyes with traumatic iris loss may have preexisting

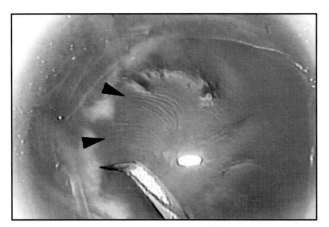

**Figure 1-5.** Rivulets in the anterior capsule produced during the capsulorrhexis in a patient with congenital aniridia and correlated the fragile intraoperative behavior of the anterior capsule, with severe thinning.

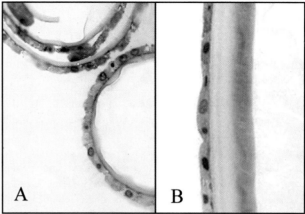

**Figure 1-6. (A)** Anterior capsule from a patient with congenital aniridia (200X). Note the thin anterior capsule and curling nature, as compared to (B), the anterior capsule from a patient without aniridia (200X).

defects in the capsular bag. The surgeon has 2 options to manage a preexisting capsular tear: either completely incorporate the tear within the capsulorrhexis (thereby excising the defect), or create the capsulorrhexis in an area remote to the location of the defect, avoiding it altogether. Frequently the fibrosis around a preexisting capsular defect will be sufficient to keep the defect from enlarging.

The capsulorrhexis in patients with congenital aniridia deserves special attention. Our initial experience with prosthetic iris implantation for aniridia led to a clinical observation that some aniridics have abnormal anterior capsules that behave in an unusually fragile manner during cataract surgery (Figure 1-5).[9,10] To explain the etiology of this clinical observation, we submitted several specimens for histopathological analysis.

We examined the anterior capsules from 5 eyes of 4 patients with aniridia (Figure 1-6). Although our sample size was quite small, there appeared to be 2 groups of aniridic patients—those with extremely thin anterior capsules that behaved in a clinically "fragile" manner, and those with normal anterior capsular thickness that behaved normally. Interestingly, it was the anterior capsules from the young patients that consistently measured less than 8 µm in thickness, while the anterior capsules from the older patients measured 17.56 µm on average and were similar to non-aniridic controls (average 17.84 µm).[11]

Although the exact etiology of capsular thinning has yet to be discovered, an awareness of the fragility of anterior capsules is very important so that great care can be taken to avoid tearing the capsule. This is extremely important when the surgeon is planning to implant a prosthetic iris device into the capsular bag. Both the Morcher 50C multi-finned overlapping rings and the Sector 96 device require an intact

capsular bag. Therefore, a torn anterior capsule can markedly alter the surgical plan. We recommend several strategies for performing the capsulorrhexis in the aniridic eye. These include using a highly retentive viscoelastic agent, injecting indocyanine green or trypan blue to stain the capsule, making the capsulorrhexis slightly smaller, and carefully avoiding any contact with the anterior capsule by an instrument during the procedure.

Once the capsulorrhexis is complete, hydrodissection is performed gently but thoroughly followed by slow motion phacoemulsification.[7] After final removal of the lens material the eye is refilled with viscoelastic, and the prosthetic iris and IOL of choice are implanted. The Morcher endocapsular devices can be inserted through a 3.2- to 3.5-mm incision. The Ophtec iris prosthetic system requires an incision size of approximately 5 mm. Allowing a little extra room in the incision reduces the risk of fracturing the device while facilitating the maneuvering necessary to place the device(s) into the capsular bag. The surgeon should note, however, when using multiple or multipiece devices, that the capsular bag can become somewhat crowded and great care must be taken not to damage the fragile anterior capsule of patients with congenital aniridia.

The single-piece devices may be sutured to the ciliary sulcus using Gortex or 9.0 prolene and the knots are either rotated in or buried under a scleral flap depending on the suturing technique employed. If the surgeon has chosen to implant the single-piece device in the ciliary sulcus without suture fixation, it is important to confirm correct haptic placement by intraoperative gonioscopy. This will prevent irritation of the trabecular meshwork, which may result in low-grade persistent inflammation and worsening glaucoma.

# COMPLICATIONS
# AND MANAGEMENT

## Intraoperative Complications

Caution should be exercised when implanting the Morcher devices as they are somewhat brittle and susceptible to fracture. Indeed, early in our learning curve we fractured 3 prosthetic iris devices in 2 cases. Two 50C rings were fractured during attempted implantation in 1 eye and a 96G ring was fractured while loading an injector (the Geuder [Germany] "shooter" device). Additionally, as we noted previously, the anterior capsules of eyes with congenital aniridia were often quite fragile. This capsular fragility prevented the completion of the capsulorrhexis in 1 case and contributed to anterior capsular tears in 5 other cases.

## Postoperative Complications

Hypotony developed in 2 eyes, both of which had 10-mm incisions to accommodate a Morcher single-piece black diaphragm IOL implant. The hypotony was transient in 1 eye due to deliberate "loose" suturing of the wound to preempt a postoperative IOP spike in an eye with preexisting glaucoma. The second case of hypotony occurred in a patient who slept without his eye shield on the second postoperative night, and developed a wound leak that required surgical repair.

Postoperatively cystoid macular edema (CME), which was refractory to medical treatment, developed in 1 eye with severe trauma and required a pars plana vitrectomy with membrane peeling. Following pars plana vitrectomy this patient developed a retinal detachment, which was repaired by additional vitreoretinal surgery. The surgeon noted that the prosthetic iris did not interfere with his ability to examine the peripheral fundus.

# OUTCOMES

The following outcomes data are derived from our ongoing study of the Morcher prosthetic iris devices. Although we have some experience at the Cincinnati Eye Institute with the Ophtec devices, which appear promising, we do not have sufficient data to comment meaningfully on the outcomes following implantation of these devices.

All patients who presented to the cataract service at the Cincinnati Eye Institute with functional or anatomic iris loss were considered for entry into our study. Inclusion criteria were: a subjective perception of moderate to severe glare either fully or partially related to the iris deficiency, the ability to understand and sign an Institutional Review Board approved informed consent form, and a willingness to participate in the clinical trial.

The initial study group consisted of 50 patients (58 eyes) and was comprised of 21 women and 29 men with an average age of 44 years (range 19 to 80). Twenty-eight of the iris deficiencies were of congenital origin (24 aniridia, 3 albino, and 1 coloboma). Twenty-five of the iris defects were traumatic in nature, and 5 of these iris defects resulted from ophthalmic surgery, including 2 eyes that had undergone partial scleroiridogoniocyclectomy treatment for iris melanoma. Five additional eyes in the study had severe iris atrophy: 2 related to herpetic uveitis, 1 chemical burn, 1 ICE syndrome and 1 eye with traumatic mydriasis. The majority (40 out of 58) of the devices implanted were the endocapsular ring prosthetic iris devices, while the remaining 18 out of 58 were single-piece prosthetic iris IOLs.

We monitored the surgical ease of insertion of the prosthetic iris devices, intraoperative and postoperative complications, anatomic results, as well as the change in visual acuity and glare disability. To evaluate the subjective degree of glare disability, patients were asked to report their level of difficulty in bright light or high-contrast settings. Using a 4-point scale (none = 0, mild = 1, moderate = 2, and severe = 3), patients graded their preoperative and postoperative glare disability. When applicable, patients were asked to grade their preoperative glare disability as that which they experienced with the iris deficiency prior to development of their cataract.

Snellen visual acuity was determined using a Baylor Visual Acuity Tester (B-VAT) (Medtronic-Solan Surgical Products, Jacksonville, Fla).[13] Snellen visual acuity was converted to a line score to record the number of lines gained or lost postoperatively.

## Surgery

The surgery was often technically challenging due to the ocular abnormalities associated with trauma, uveitis, and congenital aniridia. Corneal scarring, related to trauma or congenital aniridia, often limited visualization. Preexisting capsular defects, either frank rupture after trauma or extreme fragility in the congenital aniridics, contributed to the complexity of these cases.

Overall the surgeons were satisfied with the ease of implanting of the prosthetic iris devices. The endocapsular ring style prosthetic iris devices (50C and 96G) were preferred for their endocapsular fixation and insertion through a small incision. However, we learned early in our surgical experience that gentle surgical technique is essential because the black polymethyl methacrylate (PMMA) material is brittle and susceptible to fracture. Additionally, placement of 2 devices and an IOL into the capsular bag results in some crowding that may cause difficulty when aligning the fins.

To date, the patients have been followed postoperatively for an average of 15 months, range (1 to 45 months). The implants have remained well centered and stable in all but 1 eye. This eye initially presented after severe trauma with an equatorial capsular tear, vitreous hemorrhage, and pha-coantigenic glaucoma. This patient underwent multiple vit-reoretinal surgeries for macular edema retinal detachment and epiretinal membrane. The patient also underwent a corneal transplant, which unfortunately failed. Following multiple surgeries, the multiple-fin prosthetic iris implants and IOL appear to have dislocated slightly anterior. This patient is currently scheduled for a repeat penetrating ker-atoplasty and exchange of the endocapsular prosthetic iris rings/IOL for a single-piece prosthetic iris/IOL that will be sutured to the ciliary sulcus.

## Visual Acuity

Visual acuity improved in 36 of 58 eyes (62%) averaging 3.7 lines for the entire group (Table 1-1). Subgroup analysis demonstrated that the eyes with congenital iris deficiencies gained an average of 2.7 lines, while the eyes with traumatic or surgical iris loss gained an average of 4.4 lines of Snellen visual acuity. The 5 eyes with iris atrophy, averaged an improvement of 6.0 lines of Snellen visual acuity. Three eyes with traumatic aniridia, aphakia, and sensory exotropia demonstrated a significant improvement of visual acuity and gradual reversal of the exotropia after implantation of a sin-gle-piece iris diaphragm IOL. Only 2 eyes in the study lost 2 lines of visual acuity, and only 1 eye lost 3 lines of visual acuity. One patient with congenital aniridia, aphakia, and corneal surface disease accounts for 2 of these eyes. Preoperatively the patient was wearing rigid gas permeable (RGP) contact lenses, which helped overcome some of his corneal surface irregularity. However, he was becoming intolerant to the contact lenses and was happy with his reduction in glare after implantation of single-piece pros-thetic iris devices despite his small loss of visual acuity.

## Glare

Glare disability was assessed by directly questioning patients and recording their subjective appraisal of their pre-operative and postoperative impairment in bright lights and high contrast settings. The average preoperative glare dis-ability reported for the entire group was 2.8 using the fol-lowing scale: none = 0, mild = 1, moderate = 2, and severe = 3. Glare disability was improved in 46 of the 48 eyes (96%) for which we attained a response to our survey, resulting in an overall average postoperative glare score of 1.0 (Table 1-2).

Subgroup analysis demonstrated that subjective glare dis-ability was reduced from an average of 2.6 preoperatively to 1.3 postoperatively in eyes with congenital iris deficiencies. The average glare disability reduction was equally impressive in eyes with traumatic iris loss (2.7 to 0.7), and in the group of eyes with iris atrophy (3.0 to 1.0).

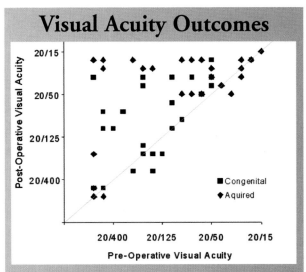

The preoperative visual acuity is plotted horizontally while the final postoperative visual acuity is plotted vertically. The diagonal line represents the level at which the preoperative and postopera-tive visual acuities are equal. The postoperative visual acuity improved for all points plotted above the diagonal.

**TABLE 1-1**

## Glaucoma

Coexisting glaucoma was a frequent problem. Over 43% (25 of 58) of all eyes had a preexisting diagnosis of glaucoma requiring medication or surgery. Glaucoma control wors-ened in 4 eyes during the follow up period. Three of these eyes received a single-piece iris diaphragm IOL in the ciliary sulcus, while the fourth eye underwent implantation of the 50C multiple fin iris rings with a foldable acrylic IOL. It is unclear if any causal relationship exists between implanta-tion of the prosthetic iris devices and worsening of glaucoma control, even though 1 of these 4 cases did have prolonged (3 months) low-grade inflammation that may have con-tributed to the worsening glaucoma. Many of these eyes are prone to develop glaucoma as a result of their underlying dis-ease or injury. Our rates of both prolonged inflammation and the development of glaucoma are much lower than reported previously.[8,10] We attribute these results to the fact that the majority of devices in this study were implanted within the capsular bag, avoiding irritation to the ciliary body. In addition, the single-piece iris diaphragm IOL was usually sutured to the scleral wall minimizing any intermit-tent contact that it might have with the trabecular mesh-work.

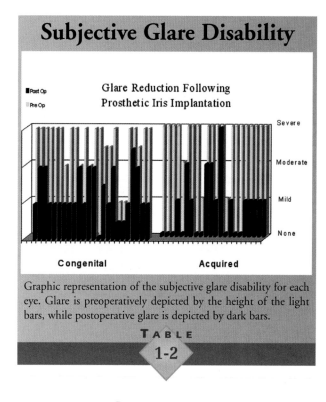

**Subjective Glare Disability**

■ Post Op
▪ Pre Op

### Glare Reduction Following Prosthetic Iris Implantation

Severe

Moderate

Mild

None

**Congenital**　　　　**Acquired**

Graphic representation of the subjective glare disability for each eye. Glare is preoperatively depicted by the height of the light bars, while postoperative glare is depicted by dark bars.

**T A B L E**

**1-2**

## CONCLUSION

Operating on a traumatized or congenitally aniridic eye presents special challenges, and implantation of an artificial iris device appears to be a safe and effective method for reducing the subjective perception of glare resulting from iris deficiency. Prosthetic iris devices provide a novel way to rehabilitate these symptomatic eyes for which there was previously no alternative.

## REFERENCES

1. Shaw M, Falls H, Neel J. Congenital aniridia. *Am J Hum Genet.* 1960;12:389.

2. Hittner H. Aniridia. In: Ritch R, Shields M, Krupin T, eds. *The glaucomas.* St. Louis: CV Mosby; 1989;873-879.

3. Nelson LB, Spaeth GL, Nowinski T, et al. Aniridia: a review. *Surv Ophthalmol.* 1984;28:621.

4. Reihnhard T, Sundmacher R, Althaus C. Irisblenden-IOL bei traumatischer aniridie. *Klin Monatsbl Augenheilkd.* 1994;205: 196-200.

5. Sundmacher R, Reihnhard T, Althaus C. Black diaphragm intraocular lens for correction of aniridia. *Ophthalmic Surg Lasers.* 1994;25:180-185.

6. Tanzer DJ, Smith RE. Black iris-diaphragm intraocular lens for aniridia and aphakia. *J Cataract Refract Surg.* 1999;25: 1548-1551.

7. Thompson CG, Fawzy K, Bryce IG, Noble BA. Implantation of a black diaphragm intraocular lens for traumatic aniridia. *J Cataract Refract Surg.* 1999;25:808-813.

8. Reinhard T, Engelhardt S, Sundmacher R. Black diaphragm aniridia intraocular lens for congenital aniridia: long term follow-up. *J Cataract Refract Surg.* 2000;26:375-381.

9. Osher RH, Burk SE. Cataract surgery combined with implantation of an artificial iris. *J Cataract Refract Surg.* 1999;25:1540-1547.

10. Burk SE, Da Mata AP, Snyder ME, Cionni RJ, Cohen JS, Osher RH. Prosthetic iris implantation for congenital, traumatic, or functional iris deficiencies. *J Cataract Refract Surg.* 2001;27(11):1732-40.

11. Schneider S, Osher RH, Burk SE, Lutz TB, Montione, R. Thinning of the anterior capsule: a new finding associated with congenital aniridia. *J Cataract Refract Surg.* 2003;29:645-51.

12. Osher RH. Slow motion phacoemulsification approach (Letter). *J Cataract Refract Surg.* 1993;19:667.

13. Zanoni D, Rosenbaum AL. A new method for evaluating visual acuity. *J Pediatr Ophthalmol Strabismus.* 1991;28:255-260.

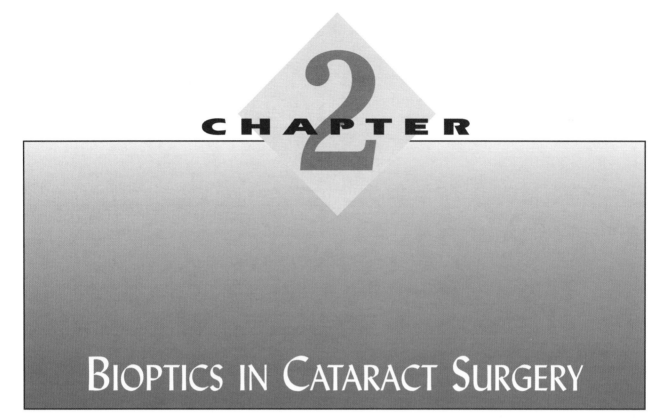

# CHAPTER 2

# BIOPTICS IN CATARACT SURGERY

*R. Gale Martin, MD*

Bioptics is the combined use of any 2 refractive systems to correct myopia or hyperopia. Myopia is defined as an overpowered eye in which parallel light rays from distant objects are brought to focus in front of the retina. Hyperopia is defined as a condition in which the eye is underpowered. Thus light rays coming from a distant object strike the retina before coming to sharp focus; true focus is said to be "behind the retina." Astigmatism is the condition where parallel rays of light from an external source converge or diverge unequally in different meridians. The obvious objective is to get the light rays to focus at a point on the retina (Figures 2-1, 2-2, and 2-3).

Myopia and hyperopia can be corrected with an IOL power designed to create emmetropia or reduce myopia or hyperopia to the desired level. Other lenticular options include phakic IOLs, astigmatism IOLs, and piggyback IOLs. These lenses are designed for implantation in the posterior capsular bag (Table 2-1).

Corneal options for bioptics include corneal relaxing incisions (CRI), anterior limbal relaxing incisions (ALRI), laser-assisted epithelial keratomileusis (LASEK), photorefractive keratectomy (PRK), radial keratotomy (RK), laser thermal keratoplasty (LTK), conductive keratoplasty (CK), thermal keratoplasty (TK), and intracorneal rings (ICRs).[1-13]

This chapter will include corneal incision nomograms and techniques for the correction of astigmatism post cataract surgery, the results of a randomized prospective

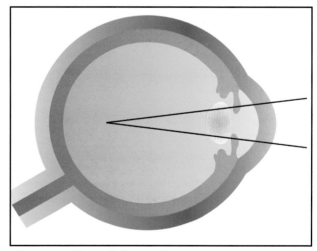

**Figure 2-1.** Distant light rays focus anterior to the retina.

study comparing ALRIs to the original STAAR toric IOLs, and a brief discussion corneal procedures in pseudophakic patients.

In the early 1970s, Richard Troutman, MD, introduced CRIs and wedge resections to correct astigmatism. Initially, incisions were made at the limbus. These results were limited, especially in young people, so incisions were placed farther into the cornea, at times creating optical zones as small

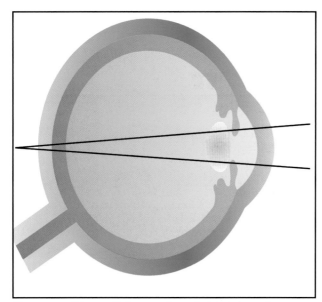

**Figure 2-2.** Distant light rays focus behind the retina.

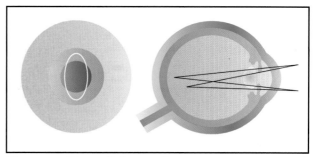

**Figure 2-3.** Distant light rays diverge or converge unequally in different meridians.

## Intraocular Lens Powers From Various Manufacturers

| IOL | Minimum | Maximum |
|-----|---------|---------|
| STAAR* | -4.00 | +4.00 |
| Storz * | -18.00 | -1.00 |
| Alcon | +5.00 | +34.00 |
| Array | +16.00 | +24.00 |
| Sensar | +10.00 | +30.00 |
| STAAR | +9.50 | +34.00 |
| Storz | Plano | +45.00 |

\* Lowest range of IOLS

**TABLE 2-1**

as 5 mm. This caused glare and optical aberrations, resulting in the consensus that the smallest optical zone with a favorable risk-benefit ratio was 8 mm.[14]

# ANTERIOR CORNEAL RELAXING INCISIONS

Our most commonly used technique for correcting astigmatism in refractive cataract or refractive lensectomy patient is anterior corneal relaxing incisions, based on the Nasal Corneal Relaxing Nomogram (Table 2-2). The amount of astigmatism to be corrected is based on the central 2 mm of EyeSys corneal topographical astigmatism. If the patient is phakic or pseudophakic, the amount of correction is determined by the *refractive cylinder*. If the prepseudophakic patient is young or has extremely high levels of astigmatism, either a toric IOL is combined with CRIs or an excimer laser corneal refractive procedure is performed when the postoperative refraction is stable (Figures 2-4 and 2-5).

The anterior limbal nomogram was based on patients aged 70 to 79 years because the majority of my patients were cataract patients. I chose the nasal anterior limbus because most of the visually distorting astigmatism in this age group is against the rule. Though the incisions are created in a circumferential pattern, the amount is measured in cord lengths. An advantage of this technique compared with corneal degrees is that surgeons can use calipers instead of purchasing new measuring instruments.

For each age decade below 70, 1 mm is added to the cord length for the desired correction. The length of the incision is also varied depending on the location of the astigmatism.

I do not adjust the nomogram for nasal incisions. For temporal incisions, 2 mm are added; for vertical incisions, 1 mm is added; for oblique temporal incisions, 1.5 mm are added; for nasal oblique incisions, 0.5 mm is added (Figure 2-6). Generally, I do not correct against-the-rule astigmatism <+0.50 D or with-the-rule astigmatism <+1.00 D.

If 1 incision does not correct the astigmatism, I add a second ALRI. If the first one was placed nasally, the sutureless temporal corneal incision must not be cut. Bisecting the temporal corneal incision often creates wound leaks. In these cases, I use a 2-step temporal, ALRI on axis with the plus axis of astigmatism. I use the cord length to fit the nomogram. The second incision usually yields about half of the correction of the first incision. If more correction is needed, either a toric IOL is implanted or a corneal relaxing incision is made at the 8-mm optical zone. This nomogram is presented in Table 2-3.

# Martin's Nasal Anterior Limbal Corneal Relaxing Incision Nomogram

| Age (years) | 1 D | 2 D | 3 D | 4 D | 5 D |
|---|---|---|---|---|---|
| 20 to 29 | 8 mm | 9 mm* | 10 mm* | 11 mm* | 12 mm* |
| 30 to 39 | 7 mm | 8 mm | 9 mm* | 10 mm* | 11 mm* |
| 40 to 49 | 6 mm | 7 mm | 8 mm | 9 mm* | 10 mm* |
| 50 to 59 | 5 mm | 6 mm | 7 mm | 8 mm | 9 mm* |
| 60 to 69 | 4 mm | 5 mm | 6 mm | 7 mm | 8 mm |
| 70 + | 3 mm | 4 mm | 5 mm | 6 mm | 7 mm |

(mm in Cord Length)

(*) Do not exceed a 6-mm nasal ALRI or 8-mm superior, inferior, or temporal ALRI.
❖ Subtract 40 μm from most shallow pachymetric reading.
❖ If vertical, add 1 mm.
❖ If temporal, add 2 mm.
❖ If oblique and nasal, add 0.5 mm.
❖ If oblique and temporal, add 1.5 mm.
❖ If 1 incision does not adequately correct astigmatism, add second ALRI.
❖ If second incision is required, calculate the length based on achieving one-half of the correction from the first incision.
❖ Extended surgical incision is calculated using the ALRI nomogram.
❖ If more correction is needed, use 8-mm OZ CRI nomogram.
Note: This is a starting point for you to develop your own nomogram.

**TABLE 2-2**

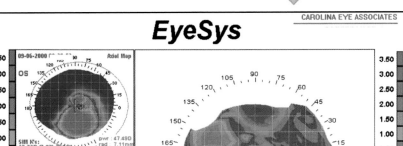
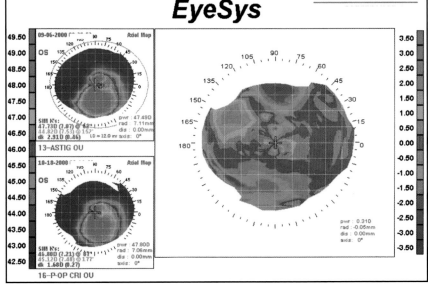

**Figure 2-4.** 61-year-old patient with 7.5-mm ALRI at 86 degrees.

I attempt to correct all of the against-the-rule astigmatism; occasionally, if patients want depth of focus, I induce approximately 1.00 D of with-the-rule astigmatism. On the other hand, I try not to overcorrect with-the-rule astigmatism. Some patients prefer to have about 1.00 D with-the-rule astigmatism, and many tend to get multifocal corneas, as discussed by Dr. James Gills and others. Therefore, I tend to overcorrect against-the-rule astigmatism and undercorrect with-the-rule astigmatism.

## MEASUREMENT

I rely primarily on the central 2 mm of topographical corneal astigmatism as measured by the EyeSys corneal topographical system in prepseudophakic patients. It is important to compare the patient's old refraction(s) and present K-readings to help confirm the topography. Second, before any keratometric or topographical analysis is made, other tests

**Figure 2-5.** A 76-year-old patient with 3.50-D central 2-mm topographical astigmatism 3.25-mm nasal ALRI; +3.50-D toric IOL at 180 degrees.

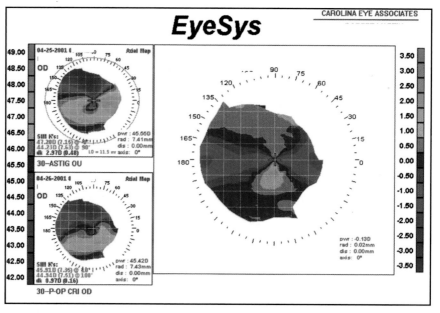

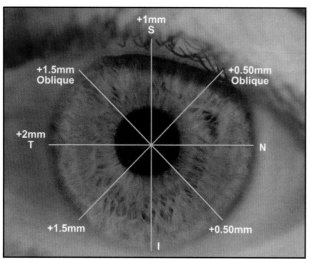

**Figure 2-6.** Millimeters in cord length added to nasal ALRI nomogram for other astigmatic meridians.

# Martin's 8-mm ALRI Nomogram for Astigmatism

| Age (Years) | Correction |
| --- | --- |
| 20 to 29 | 0.40 |
| 30 to 39 | 0.45 |
| 40 to 49 | 0.55 |
| 50 to 59 | 0.60 |
| 60 to 69 | 0.65 |
| 70 to 79 | 0.70 |

(Correction in diopters per mm.)

❖ Optical zone at 8 mm.
❖ Cuts at 100% intraoperative pachymetric reading at the site(s) of incision(s).
❖ Cuts three 2 mm; cuts are arcuate. Do not exceed 60 degrees at any OZ.
❖ Second series of cuts at OZ 9 or 10 (cord length 4.5 to 5 mm or 60 degrees) gives 1/3 of the amount of correction obtained at OZ 8.
❖ DO NOT exceed 4-mm cut at OZ 8.
❖ Avoid cuts OZ 5.
❖ A series of cuts anterior limbal with a cord length of 5mm should add about 1/3 more correction. If the steep area exceeds 45 degrees, add Canrobert "C" procedure (2 or more arcuates on the bisector meridians). 15 degrees toward steep meridian.

**TABLE 2-3**

including A-scans and tensions by applanation should be avoided. Patients should blink until the tear film covers the cornea. If the surface is distorted, consider using artificial tears, having the patients blink, and repeating the test. If topography is not reproducible, surgical astigmatism correction should not be performed until the postoperative refraction is stable. At that time the refractive cylinder can be used to correct the astigmatism, per the nomogram listed in Table 2-2. In the postoperative pseudophake or in phakic eyes, corneal topography and keratometric readings play secondary or confirmatory roles in determining astigmatism. I almost never rely solely on keratometric readings in phakic or pseudophakic patients to determine the amount of astigmatism to be corrected.

## PREOPERATIVE MARKING

There are 3 options for marking with the patient at the slit lamp: at the 180-degree and 90-degree meridians, at the

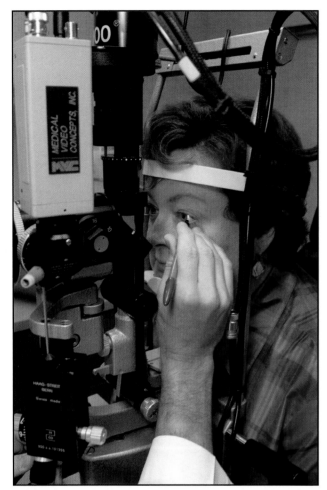

**Figure 2-7.** A surgical marking pen used at slit lamp to mark the corneal limbus.

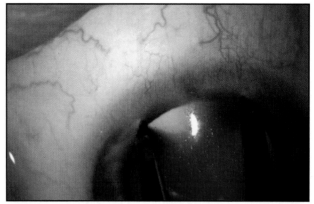

**Figure 2-8.** Caliper straddling plus axis of astigmatism.

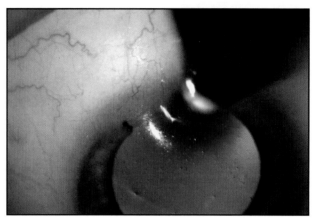

**Figure 2-9.** Multiple pachymetric readings are taken along the anterior limbus.

plus axis of astigmatism, or a combination of the two. We have enough experience so that we usually mark the plus axis of astigmatism. If only the vertical and horizontal meridians are marked at the slit lamp, then a degree marker such as a Mendez ring can be used in surgery to determine the appropriate surgical astigmatic axis. Before all markings, we apply proparacaine hydrochloride (lidocaine 4% and sensorcaine 0.75%, 1:1). To assure proper head position, it is very important to take into account that the anatomical center of the visual axis is not in the center of the pupil. Frequently, a 90-degree mark is shifted nasally because the visual axis is in the nasal pupil. Determining the appropriate visual axis rather than the anatomical center of the pupil is very important to improve the accurate placing of astigmatic keratotomies (Figure 2-7).

# SURGICAL TECHNIQUE

After being marked, the patient is prepped and draped. We perform almost all cases under topical anesthesia. If the plus axis of astigmatism has not been marked, then we use the Mendez ring to determine the appropriate plus axis astigmatism. After the plus axis of astigmatism has been identified, I use a caliper with the cord length determined by the nomogram. I place the caliper straddling the plus axis of astigmatism at the anterior limbus (Figure 2-8) and take intraoperative pachymetric readings across the cord length (Figure 2-9). If the cord length is long and there are significant differences in depth, then we may use a second micrometer diamond knife setting to treat the deeper section of the cornea (Figure 2-10). Across a 4-mm cord length, it is not uncommon to find pachymetric depth variances of 40 to 50 μm.

All diamonds are set at 500 μm at the micronscope by an experienced technician to ensure the accuracy (Figure 2-11).

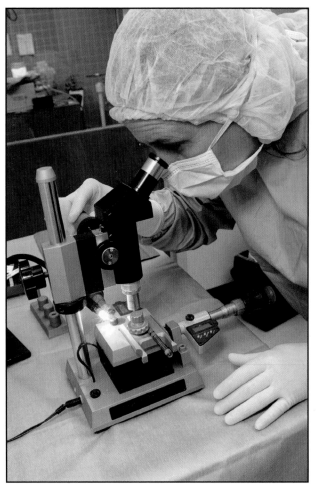

**Figure 2-10.** Arcuate cuts made in anterior limbus.

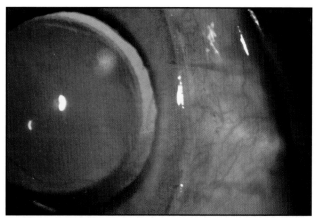

**Figure 2-11.** Technician adjusts micron diamond knife setting.

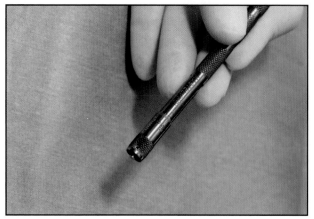

**Figure 2-12.** Technician examines micron diamond for quality and sets it at 500 microns.

The knives are transported to the operating room suite in a sterile diamond knife carrying case. The technician then adjusts the micrometer diamond knife setting so that it equals 40 μm more shallow than the most shallow pachymetric measurement. I create an incision immediately anterior to the anterior limbus. For cases with more astigmatism than my nomogram manages, I move the incision 0.5 mm more central.

## EQUIPMENT PREPARATION

Micronscopes, calipers, and pachymetric equipment are critical and are serviced and maintained so that they measure accurately. We use the micronscopes on each case prior to prepping and draping to assure that the diamond is not chipped and that the footplates are smooth, without burrs or protein build-up. After examination, the technician sets the micron diamond blade at 500 μm in a sterile setting and the micrometer diamond is placed in a sterile protective case to be transported to the operative suite (Figure 2-12).

I adamantly oppose using "permanently" set diamonds or metal blades. It is well known that settings vary from manufacturer to manufacturer, from case to case, and over time from regular use. In my experience, 1, 2, or 3 blade settings do not fit all eyes. I believe that the blades should be checked along with all other instruments the surgeon uses on each case to ensure that the depth is appropriate for that particular case. Any nomogram is a starting point that should provide immediate good results that will improve over time as the surgeon adjusts his or her nomogram based on clinical experience.

## PREOPERATIVE CONDITIONS

Preoperative evaluation and treatment are often necessary to achieve the best outcomes. For example, patients with poor personal hygiene have a greater risk of infection. In many of these cases it may be wise to avoid additional incisions due to their increased risk for infection. Patients with blepharitis must be treated before surgery. It is important to

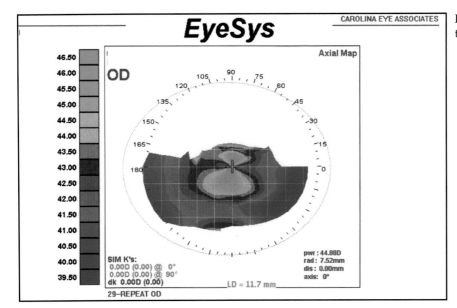

**Figure 2-13.** 5.00 D of astigmatism in the central 2 mm of the topography.

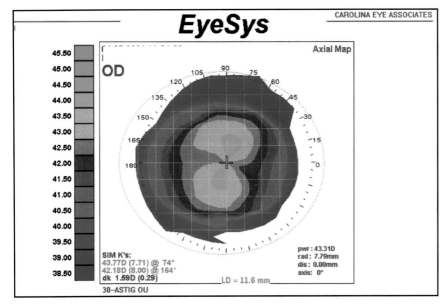

**Figure 2-14.** 1.50 D of astigmatism in the central 2 mm of the topography.

remember that patients with dry eyes often have abnormal keratometric and topographical imaging. The following preoperative and postoperative topography of dry eye patients show the dramatic changes that occur after the dry eye is treated. Resolution of their dry eye condition allowed a much more accurate refractive surgical technique. The following case is a 55-year-old female with cataracts and dry eyes. Her Schirmer test was 16 mm and 6 mm respectively in the right and left eyes. Tear break-up time was instantaneous OU. The patient was treated with punctal plugs, HydroEye (Science Based Health, Carson City, Nev) 2 by mouth BID and lubrication. The central 2 mm of topographical astigmatism was reduced from 5.00 D to 1.50 D in the right eye and from 5.00 D to 2.50 D in the left eye. As you can see, CRI surgery based on the initial "dry eye" topography would have given an overcorrection. The patient

ended up with 20/25+ UCVA postoperation OU (Figures 2-13, 2-14, 2-15, and 2-16).

Patients who present with the above dry eye pattern topography or a very irregular topographical pattern should not be treated because this pattern is almost always abnormal. We treat these patients with increased hydration, increased humidity, artificial tears, HydroEye, and punctual plugs until corneal topography is stable.

Corneal lesions such as pterygia, Salzmann's nodular degeneration, and epithelial basement disease almost always distort the corneal image. For example, horizontal pterygia give plus axis vertical astigmatism. I almost always remove the pterygium before correcting corneal astigmatism if the pterygium is inducing astigmatism.

Correcting astigmatism coexisting with pterygia is, in my opinion, unwise. The pterygium should be removed and the

**Figure 2-15.** 5.00 D of astigmatism in the central 2 mm of the topography.

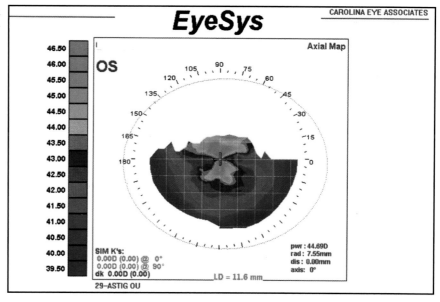

**Figure 2-16.** 2.50 D of astigmatism in the central 2 mm of the topography.

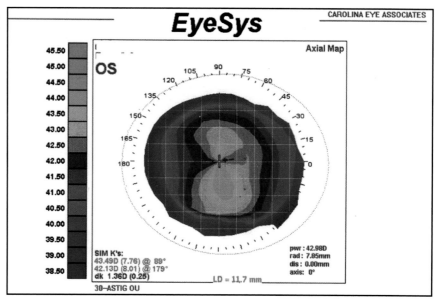

cornea stabilized before any corneal refractive surgery. This holds true when implanting a toric IOL or using other refractive techniques.

Patients with other conditions such as epithelial basement membrane disease, corneal degenerations, or dystrophies are at risk for image distortions and misinterpretations and abrasions or perforations at surgery. Some anterior corneal disorders such as epithelial basement membrane disease or Salzmann's nodular degeneration may be treated with epitheliectomy or superficial keratectomy before performing cataract or refractive corneal surgery. After the cornea stabilizes, keratometry and topographical analysis must be repeated. These measurements will almost always be significantly different.

Previous corneal surgery, including penetrating keratoplasty or refractive corneal surgery such as LTK or CK can

cause overcorrections. In these cases, I reduce the nomogram by a half. I also use an intraoperative corneoscope ring or keratometer to avoid overcorrections even when using half the nomogram. Furthermore, when possible I perform an immediate postoperative refraction to determine if more surgery is needed.

I do not recommend performing ALRI in grafts to correct induced astigmatism; I prefer CRIs placed just inside the donor-host recipient wound. Small amounts of astigmatic keratoplasty can give corrections 2 to 3 times the amount predicted by nomograms. Again, much less correction, perhaps one-half as much, is needed to avoid undesirable overcorrections. An intraoperative corneoscope or keratometer is helpful in these cases. It is best to remove the lid speculum to avoid corneal distortion and misinterpretation.

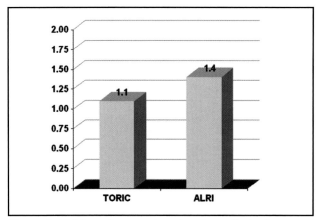

**Figure 2-17.** Mean decrease in refractive cylinder between toric IOL and ALRI.

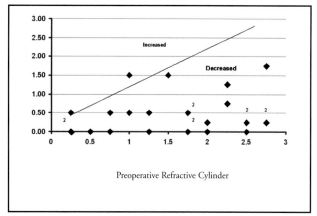

Preoperative Refractive Cylinder

**Figure 2-18.** Preoperative versus postoperative refractive cylinder in the TIOL.

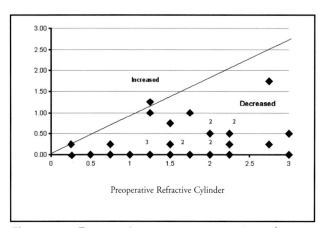

Preoperative Refractive Cylinder

**Figure 2-19.** Preoperative versus postoperative refractive cylinder in the ALRI.

# TORIC IOLS

We were part of a randomized prospective study that compared toric IOLs with anterior limbal corneal relaxing incisions for pre-existing corneal astigmatism. As an initial investigator for FDA approval for the STAAR Surgical (Monrovia, Calif) UV-Absorbing Collamer toric implantable contact lens (TICL) for myopia and astigmatism, I felt it was important to compare this STAAR TICL with its competitive technique, the anterior limbal corneal relaxing incision. This clinical trial involved 60 patients randomized to receive either the STAAR toric IOL or an anterior limbal corneal relaxing incision to correct pre-existing corneal astigmatism. Healthy eyes with 1.00 to 3.50 D of corneal astigmatism, correctable with an implant having a spherical power range of +17.00 to 24.00 D (the lenses initially available), were included. We excluded patients whose white-to-white measurements were greater than 11.75 mm.

The surgical technique was a clear, self-sealing, temporal corneal incision measuring 2.65 to 3 mm. The cases randomized to receive the toric IOL received model AA4203T if they had a cylinder of +1.00 to +2.50 D and model AA4203TF for cylinder of greater than 2.50 to 3.50 D. At 2 to 4 months, follow-up was 100% for the toric IOLs and 97% for the anterior corneal relaxing incision patients. Preoperative mean refractive cylinder for the toric IOLs was 1.50 D and 1.70 D for the ALRI patients. The mean refractive cylinder at the last postoperative visit was 0.39 for the toric IOL patients and 0.35 for the anterior limbal corneal relaxing incision patients. The mean decrease in refractive cylinder was 1.10 D for the toric IOL compared with 1.40 D for the anterior limbal CRI patients (Figure 2-17). All cases except 1 had significant decrease in their refractive cylinder (Figure 2-18) and the same is true for the anterior limbal corneal relaxing incision (Figure 2-19). The mean decrease in keratometric cylinder for the toric group was surprising at only 0.01 D. Essentially no astigmatism was induced with the corneal incision. As expected, the anterior limbal CRI group had decreases in refractive and keratometric cylinder. The mean induced refractive cylinder in the toric cases was 1.60 D and in the ALRI cases was 1.50 D.

# COMPLICATIONS

Three of 30 toric IOL cases had an axis rotation more than 30 degrees. These implants were shifted at slit lamp under topical anesthesia 10 to 14 days postoperative with a 30-gauge needle. The investigators discovered that trying to rotate the lens early in the postoperative period was ineffective because it shifted back to its original position. At 10 days the capsule begins to fibrose slightly, this allows the lens to remain where it is rotated. Eighty-three percent saw 20/40 or better uncorrected, but 14% of the toric IOL patients saw

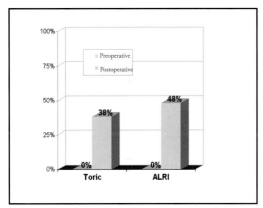

**Figure 2-20.** Uncorrected vision 20/25 or better in the TIOL versus the ALRI.

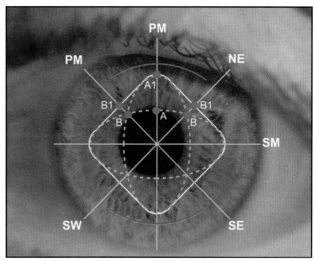

**Figure 2-21.** Cause of keratopyramis.

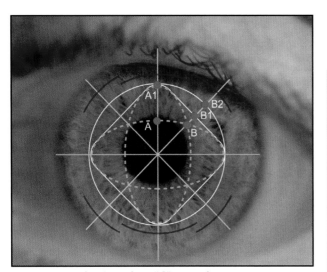

**Figure 2-22.** The Canrobert "C" procedure.

## Canrobert "C" Procedure Nomogram for Astigmatism

| D | 2D | 3D | 4D | 5D | 6D* |
|---|----|----|----|----|-----|
| OZ (mm) | 7.5/8.5 | 7.0/8.0 | 6.5/7.5 | 6.0/7.0 | 6.0/7.0 |
| Arc Length | 45/22.5 | 60/22.5 | 60/30 | 60/30 | 60/45 |

Figure for patients less than 40 years old.
Patients older than 40 years, increase optical zone by 0.5 mm.

*Please note that on 6-D "C" incisions, the 45° incision shifts 15° toward steep meridian.

**TABLE 2-4**

20/20 or better uncorrected compared with 28% of the ALRI patients. Best-corrected visual acuity (BCVA) was 20/25 or better for 38% of the toric patients compared with 48% of the ALRI patients (Figure 2-20).

In 1999, when the study was completed, only 2 toric IOL powers were available: the STAAR model AA4203T corrected about 1.35 D and the STAAR model 4203TF, which corrected 2.35 D. CRIs, however, can correct a wide range of refractive errors. Since this study was completed, there have been a number of changes in the lenses, including an increase the length of the toric IOL to 10.8 mm. Now that this lens is not placed in eyes with a white-to-white longer than 11.75 mm, the malposition rate has fallen to approximately 1%. We expect future improvements to in the lens, including a stickier lens material such as collamer or acrylic lens material. Lenses made of these materials have an extremely low tendency to rotate.

One of the complications of astigmatic keratotomy is the "keratopyramis phenomenon" described by Dr. Canrobert Oliveira.[15] This is especially evident in moderate- to high-corneal astigmatism cases. The phenomenon is associated with a shifting of the plus axis of astigmatism to either side of the relaxing incision. It can usually be resolved by non-connecting C-incisions 1-mm posterior and beside the CRI or anterior corneal relaxing incision (Figures 2-21, 2-22, and Table 2-4).

## BIOPTICS

Bioptics is defined as a second, complementary refractive procedure and includes a variety of techniques. Excimer laser correction for residual refractive errors can be performed with laser-assisted in-situ keratomileusis (LASIK), LASEK, or PRK following initial surgical procedures, including refractive lensectomy, refractive cataract surgery, and corneal transplantation. Some surgeons create a LASIK flap before cataract surgery or refractive lensectomy. Following the procedure, when the refraction has stabilized, the flap can be elevated and most residual refractive error corrected. The drawback is that this is a secondary LASIK flap manipulation with an increased epithelial ingrowth rate of about 5%. I prefer to create the flap when the surgical wound and refractive error are stabilized. I discourage this in sutured incisions and/or incisions larger than 4 mm.

Dr. Leonardo Akaishi pioneered using toric or nontoric STAAR implantable contact lenses (phakic posterior chamber IOL) to correct residual refractive errors following cataract surgery and IOL implantation in the bag. This technique is highly effective and can be done under topical anesthesia through a small sutureless corneal incision. These implantable contact lenses are stable and rarely rotate after they are positioned in the ciliary sulcus on the anterior surface of an IOL. We have not seen rotation of these lenses in more than 200 procedures for myopic correction.

## CORNEAL REFRACTIVE PROCEDURES

The most common bioptic corneal refractive procedures are LASIK and PRK. Before any bioptic corneal incision is created after the first operation, the refractive error and surgical incision must be stable and the patient must be well informed of the reasonable surgical options and risks. Also, the risk:benefit ratio should be favorable.

## LASER-ASSISTED IN-SITU KERATOMILEUSIS

In my hands, LASIK is safe as early as 1 month after the initial surgery. We perform a thorough preoperative examination and informed consent, insert temporary punctal plugs, and begin HydroEye, 1 capsule PO BID for at least the first month before surgery. After prepping but no draping, a Moria plated speculum is used to retract the lids. I use a modified CB Moria microkeratome to create the flap with a superior hinge. The flap is folded internal surface to internal so that if the laser does ablate the hinge, it will strike the edge of the epithelium on the flap.

I use my personalized nomogram and constantly adjust my nomogram based on monthly postoperative refractions. We continually upgrade our nomograms by following our patients using the Holladay software for analyzing outcomes.

I reposition the flap with minimal irrigation and use a Johnson flap compressor to squeeze excess fluid from the interface. I dry the edges with a wet Merocel sponge and instill levofloxacin (Quixin, Santen, Japan). Patients are informed to keep their eyes closed until the slit lamp examination 30 to 60 minutes after surgery. The eye is shielded and the patient is discharged and instructed to rest until the next day.

The routine postoperative regimen is a shield for the first week; one HydroEye capsule PO BID for at least 1 month; levofloxacin, 1 drop TID for 4 days; fluorometholone (FML, Allergan, Irvine, Calif) or loteprednol (Lotemax, Bausch & Lomb, Rochester, NY) TID for 4 days; and frequent lubrication with preservative-free artificial tears.

## SURFACE ABLATION

I rarely perform PRK or LASEK for a variety of reasons, one of which is that the modified manual CB Moria microkeratome provides flap thickness ranging from 80 to 120 µm. The flap depth varies with the speed of the turn. When chosen, PRK requires the same evaluation and informed consent as LASIK. I use the Amoils (Innovative Excimer Solutions, Canada) corneal brush to remove the epithelium, then ablate using the personalized nomogram. I place a high-water bandage contact lens along with Quixin and shield the eye. The patient is given pain medication and returns the following day.

## LASER-ASSISTED EPITHELIAL KERATOMILEUSIS

Although it has not earned widespread support, LASEK continues to gain popularity among refractive surgeons. There are several different methods of removing the epithelium before ablation, then replacing it after the refractive correction is made. Some surgeons peel the epithelium back after first loosening its attachments with a diluted alcohol solution. Another technique uses a device that captures the epithelium in a rolled pattern. At the end of the laser treatment, the epithelium is unfurled back over the treated corneal bed, straightened, and a bandage contact lens is applied.

## RADIAL KERATOTOMY, LASER THERMAL KERATOPLASTY, CONDUCTIVE KERATOPLASTY, AND INTRACORNEAL RINGS

Once well-known and popular worldwide, RK has become far less common. We now know that the procedure can cause progressive hyperopia and tends to destabilize the cornea more than other more modern refractive techniques. Today it is rarely performed.

Some surgeons have reported varying degrees of success with laser TK for undercorrected hyperopic pseudophakes or overcorrected myopic pseudophakes.

Conductive TK is a newer technique which, in addition to being less expensive than other procedures, has the advantage of allowing the surgeon to place the TK needle on the flat axis and adjust astigmatism.

ICRs are another option to correct residual myopia, but its relatively high cost and lengthy operating time have made this a rarely used bioptics technique following lens extraction with IOL implantation.

I think the public is underinformed about the capabilities of refractive procedures following other anterior segment surgeries; I believe the ophthalmic community has a duty to educate our patients that many of the refractive errors created following cataract surgery, corneal transplantation, retinal detachment, and glaucoma procedures can be corrected. Residual refractive errors can be treated with excimer laser procedures, astigmatic keratotomy, piggyback IOLs, and phakic IOLs. This knowledge might lead to a large market of patients wanting to improve their functional vision, even if the procedure were not reimbursable.

## *Postoperative Regimen for Anterior Limbal Corneal Relaxing Incisions or Corneal Relaxing Incisions*

- ❖ Quixin 1 drop to operated eye TID for 10 days and stop.
- ❖ Pred Forte QID for 7 days, BID for 7 days and stop.
- ❖ Frequent lubrication with preservative-free artificial tears.

If combined case with cataract extraction and lens implant and either corneal relaxing incision or anterior limbal relaxing incisions:

- ❖ Quixin TID for 10 days and stop
- ❖ Pred Forte QID for 2 weeks, t.i.d. for a week, BID for a week, QID for a week and then stop.
- ❖ Preservative-free artificial tears
- ❖ (We avoid prostaglandin inhibitors with corneal incisions)

# REFERENCES

1. Alio JL, de la Hoz F, Ruiz-Moreno JM, Salem TF. Cataract surgery in highly myopic eyes corrected by phakic anterior chamber angle-supported lenses. *J Cataract Refract Surg.* 2000;26(9):1303-11.

2. Artola A, Ayala MJ, Claramonte P, Perez-Santonja JJ, Alio JL. Photorefractive keratectomy for residual myopia after cataract surgery. *J Cataract Refract Surg.* 1999;25(11):1456-60.

3. Donoso R, Rodriguez A. Piggyback implantation using the AMO array multifocal intraocular lens. *J Cataract Refract Surg.* 2001;27(9):1506-10.

4. Gills JP, Van der Karr MA. Correcting high astigmatism with piggyback toric intraocular lens implantation. *J Cataract Refract Surg.* 2002;28(3):547-9.

5. Inoue T, Maeda N, Sasaki K, et al. Factors that influence the surgical effects of astigmatic keratotomy after cataract surgery. *Ophthalmology.* 2001;108(7):1269-74.

6. Mierdel P, Kaemmerer M, Krinke HE, Seiler T. Effects of photorefractive keratectomy and cataract surgery on ocular optical errors of higher order. *Graefes Arch Clin Exp Ophthalmol.* 1999;237(9):725-9.

7. Muller-Jensen K, Fischer P, Siepe U. Limbal relaxing incisions to correct astigmatism in clear corneal cataract surgery. *J Refract Surg.* 1999;15(5):586-9.

8. Patterson A, Kaye SB, O'Donnell NP. Comprehensive method of analyzing the results of photoastigmatic refractive keratectomy for the treatment of post-cataract myopic anisometropia. *J Cataract Refract Surg.* 2000;26(2):229-36.

9. Artola A, Ayala MJ, Claramonte P, Perez-Santonja JJ, Alio JL. Photorefractive keratectomy for residual myopia after cataract surgery. *J Cataract Refract Surg.* 1999;25(11):1456-60.

10. Muller-Jensen K, Fischer P, Siepe U. Limbal relaxing incisions to correct astigmatism in clear corneal cataract surgery. *J Refract Surg.* 1999;15(5):586-9.

11. Oshika T, Yoshitomi F, Fukuyama M, et al. Radial keratotomy to treat myopic refractive error after cataract surgery. *J Cataract Refract Surg.* 1999;25(1):50-5.

12. Oshika T, Shimazaki J, Yoshitomi F, et al. Arcuate keratotomy to treat corneal astigmatism after cataract surgery: a prospective evaluation of predictability and effectiveness. *Ophthalmology.* 1998;105(11):2012-6.

13. Budak K, Friedman NJ, Koch DD. Limbal relaxing incisions with cataract surgery. *J Cataract Refract Surg.* 1998;24(4):503-8.

14. Troutman RC, Buzard KA. *Corneal Astigmatism: Etiology, Prevention and Management.* St. Louis, MO: CV Mosby; 1992.

15. Canrobert Oliveira R. *The keratopyramis phenomenum and the Canrobert "C" procedure.* Presented at the International Society of Refractive Keratoplasty 1993 Pre-American Academy of Ophthalmology meeting. Chicago, IL. November 12-13, 1993.

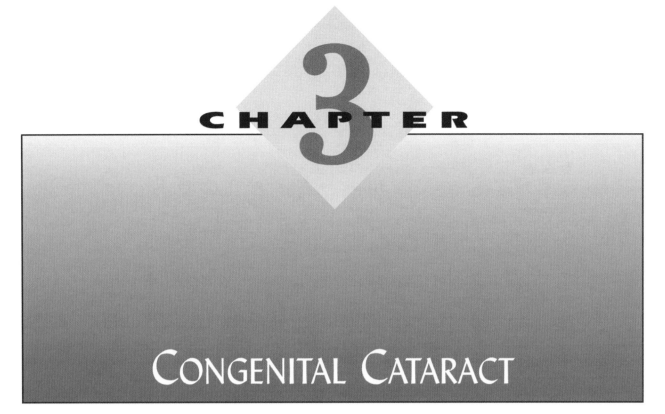

# CHAPTER 3

# CONGENITAL CATARACT

*Howard V. Gimbel, MD, MPH, FRCSC, FACS;*
*Brian M. DeBroff, MD, FACS; and Jennifer A. Dunbar, MD*

## INTRODUCTION

Congenital cataracts offer a complex set of challenges to the ophthalmologist, which requires an understanding of children and the pediatric eye and dexterity in anterior segment surgery. The surgical decision-making process, surgical technique, and complications of surgery differ from the adult procedure.

Aspects of pediatric cataract surgery requiring special preoperative care include the difficulty of examining infants and children and the possibility of underlying systemic disease. The distinct tissue characteristics of the pediatric eye require special intraoperative techniques; structures are smaller, and there is greater elasticity of the tissue, particularly the sclera and the lens capsule, making capsulotomy more challenging. There is often more posterior vitreous pressure as compared with adults and the vitreous is more formed than adults. Congenital cataracts may involve the capsule itself with an attenuated posterior capsule, such as in posterior lentiglobus, or even preexisting defects in the posterior capsule. Dense fibrotic or vascular attachments predispose to vitreous hemorrhage, such as in persistent hyperplastic primary vitreous (PHPV). Pediatric patients are more prone to severe postoperative inflammation, secondary cataract membranes, and glau-

coma. Choice of IOL power is made difficult by the changing size and refractive power of the child's eye.

Equally important to the actual surgery is meticulous preoperative and postoperative care. A team approach may involve the child's pediatrician or a geneticist in the evaluation for associated systemic disease, and a pediatric ophthalmologist to assist in postoperative refraction, contact lens fitting, and management of associated amblyopia and strabismus.

Fortunately, because of advances in technique such as continuous curvilinear capsulorrhexis (CCC), posterior continuous curvilinear capsulorrhexis (PCCC), and posterior optic capture, and technologies such as high-viscosity viscoelastics, pharmacologically treated IOLs, and automated vitrectomy, the surgical management of pediatric cataracts is safer and more effective than ever before.

## PREOPERATIVE EVALUATION

Careful preoperative assessment is especially important in children. Because many children with cataracts are preverbal or preliterate, determining the visual significance of the cataract may be difficult. While some cataracts, such as anterior polar cataracts, are rarely visually significant, any cataract causing amblyopia that is not responding to treatment should be treated surgically. The elements of the physical examination are similar to those in the adult; however, the method of obtaining the information may be different in children.

## Determining Visual Significance of Cataracts

Assessing the visual significance of cataracts involves determining both the visual acuity and the obscuration of the visual axis.

Determining the visual acuity in children age newborn to 3 months involves the assessment of fix and follow behavior, or photophobic response. After the onset of binocularity at age 3 to 5 months, the maintaining of fixation is compared between the 2 eyes to assess for amblyopia. In the absence of strabismus, a 10.00-D prism is placed base down to check for refixation movement on each eye, and compared between the 2 eyes.[1] Preferential looking and spatial sweep visual evoked potentials are additional methods available for the evaluation of preverbal infants and toddlers.[2] Children ages 3 and older should be able to perform some form of optotype testing, such as Allen Figures or the H, O, T, and V letter test (HOTV). Developmentally normal children over the age of 6 years can be tested by their ability to read Snellen figures.

The obscuration of the visual axis should be determined by evaluating the effect of the size and density of the opacity on the red reflex both with and without pupillary dilation. Some patients with small lenticular opacities may require a trial of amblyopia therapy prior to determining the necessity of surgery. For example, some children with unilateral cataracts respond to amblyopia therapy consisting of chronic dilation to see around the cataract and patching of the contralateral eye.[3,4] Some surgeons use 3 mm as a rule of thumb for determining if the size of the opacity is visually significant in a preverbal child. Others use the retinoscopic reflex. If retinoscopy cannot be performed around the opacity, then it is likely to be visually significant.[5] Merin and colleagues suggest that the density, rather than the size of the opacity, portends to a poor visual prognosis.[6] Dilation with a cycloplegic agent should be performed with retinoscopy to assess refractive error. If a small opacity is accompanied by significant anisometropia, other capsular irregularities, or irregular astigmatism, these optical aberrations may be as amblyogenic as the lenticular opacity itself.

## Physical Examination

An examination under sedation or general anesthesia should be performed for pediatric patients in whom adequate preoperative physical examination cannot be obtained in the office.

Many cataracts disrupt binocularity at an early age and cause strabismus.[7] Strabismus should be evaluated preoperatively with cover testing wherever possible, although in cases of vision loss, Hirschberg or Krimsky light reflex tests may

be more appropriate. The rotations should be checked with ductions and versions, or vestibulo-ocular response.

Evaluation of the pupils for afferent pupillary defect will help to assess the possibility of posterior retinal or optic nerve malformations, which may affect the final visual prognosis.

The anterior segment evaluation should involve inspection for microphthalmia, as well as measurement of the corneal diameter with calipers. Slit lamp examination may be performed with a portable slit lamp in infants and toddlers, while many children ages 2 and older are able to sit at a slit lamp. The nature of the cataract should be determined with the slit lamp, such as anterior polar, nuclear, lamellar, or posterior lentiglobus. Smaller eyes with prominent ciliary processes may have persistent hyperplastic primary vitreous.

Biometry involving A-scan and keratometry is useful for determining intraocular lens power. In addition, preoperative keratometry values may be helpful for the fitting of contact lenses postoperatively in infants who will be left aphakic. Axial lengths may be followed to assess progressive axial myopia and/or aphakic glaucoma. In older children, these may be performed preoperatively in the clinic; however, in many infants and young children these are best performed under general anesthesia just prior to cataract surgery.

Intraocular pressure (IOP) should be measured to follow for the possibility of glaucoma. When determined under anesthesia, the pressure should be taken during masked induction as measurement too early in anesthesia may elevate IOP. Similarly, deep anesthesia may artificially lower IOP. Preoperative gonioscopy provides a baseline from which to follow the angle for developmental anomalies or the possibility of synechiae and aphakic or pseudophakic glaucoma in the future.

Evaluation of the posterior segment includes indirect ophthalmoscopy wherever possible. Often the posterior pole structures may be visualized around the opacity. When this is not possible, B-scan ultrasonography should be performed.

## Preoperative Evaluation for Systemic Disease

Preoperative assessment should include appropriate history and laboratory evaluation to determine the possibility of underlying systemic disease. The differential diagnosis of bilateral cataracts includes genetic conditions, most commonly autosomal dominant hereditary cataracts, Down syndrome, or Lowe's syndrome. Infectious causes include intrauterine infection with toxoplasmosis, rubella, cytomegalovirus, or *herpes simplex* virus. Metabolic causes include galactosemia and galactokinase deficiency.

Many unilateral cataracts require no additional work-up; however, bilateral cataracts should receive consideration for systemic workup. In a large series of pediatric cataract patients, Lambert describes 50% of bilateral patients receiving a systemic diagnosis providing an etiology for the cataracts.[8] Past medical history should include careful questioning regarding other family members with childhood cataracts to rule out autosomal dominantly inherited cataracts. The mother should be questioned regarding maternal fevers or infection during pregnancy. History of developmental delay or growth retardation should be addressed.

A history of failure to thrive may indicate a metabolic or genetic abnormality. Laboratory evaluation may include serum titers of IgG and IgM for toxoplasmosis, rubella, cytomegalovirus, and *h. simplex* virus. Urine for reducing substances, RBC galactokinase or urine amino acids, calcium, and phosphorus may also assist in the diagnosis. Examination of family members may reveal subtle lenticular opacities indicating a hereditary form of cataracts. Mothers and sisters of males with Lowe's syndrome may have tiny cataracts that aid in the diagnosis. Dysmorphic features suggest that referral to a geneticist may be in order for syndromes such as Down syndrome or Hallermann Streiff syndrome.

A pediatrician should be consulted for all children to assess their suitability to undergo general anesthesia.

# INDICATIONS, CONTRAINDICATIONS, AND TIMING OF SURGERY

## *Indications and Contraindications*

Surgery is indicated for all visually significant cataracts in children. Small lens opacities causing amblyopia; not responding to treatment; or causing amblyogenic optical aberrations such as anisometropia, irregular astigmatism, or capsular irregularities should also be removed.

Relative contraindications include systemic conditions rendering the risk of general anesthesia greater than the risk of vision loss and active uveitis.

## *Timing of Surgery*

Timing of cataract extraction depends on the age of the patient, visual significance of the cataract, and laterality of the cataract. Emphasis is placed on prompt removal of the amblyogenic lens and commencement of optical and patching therapy for amblyopia.

Traditionally, unilateral cataracts in visually immature children have portended a poor prognosis because of amblyopia.[9] Early surgery followed by amblyopia therapy can provide good visual results. Surgery should be performed within the first few weeks of life, or as soon as the cataract is diagnosed, to allow amblyopia therapy to commence before the end of the critical period for visual development. Bilateral cataracts may allow for a slightly longer critical period because the visual deprivation is symmetric between the 2 eyes. Nevertheless, if bilateral cataracts are not removed in a timely manner, nystagmus and permanent bilateral deprivation amblyopia may develop.

For congenital cataracts that are diagnosed after the critical period, surgery may still provide a successful visual outcome. Some unilateral cataracts, especially those with posterior lenticonus, may be progressive. This would allow for a period of early normal visual development prior to the worsening of the opacity and would suggest the possibility of good visual results.[10] Studies where surgery was performed in the first 4 to 6 months of life also showed improved vision.[11,12] This is confirmed by the work of Wright et al, who report some patients with either unilateral or bilateral cataracts receiving surgery after 10 months of age still achieved good visual acuity.[13]

# SURGICAL TECHNIQUE

Surgical techniques have evolved to address the unique challenges of pediatric cataract surgery, such as decreased scleral rigidity, increased posterior pressure, and elasticity of the anterior and posterior capsule. In addition, surgical techniques focus on decreasing the incidence of the most important complication of pediatric cataract surgery: secondary cataract.

Two 4-0 silk traction sutures are placed, one at the superior rectus and one at the inferior rectus. These are used to proptose and manipulate the position of the globe. Some physicians use a corneal ring in neonates to support the highly collapsable infant globe. A limbal peritomy is performed and a 2-mm scratch incision is made at the 12-o'clock position 2- to 3-mm from the limbus. A scleral tunnel is made through to clear cornea. A paracentesis is made at the 2-o'clock position and high-viscosity viscoelastic such as Healon 5 or Healon GV (Pfizer, New York, NY) is instilled into the anterior chamber. When the globe is formed, the anterior chamber is entered through the scleral tunnel using a keratome.

## *Methods for Performing Anterior Capsulorrhexis*

Traditionally, even under the best of conditions, capsulorrhexis has been technically challenging in children because of the elasticity of pediatric tissues and increased posterior pressure. Radial tears were frequent. In the case of white cataracts, or liquified cataracts, control of the anterior capsule was even more difficult because of decreased visibility. Can-opener capsulorrhexis was commonly used. Wilson et al described a technique for mechanized vitrector capsulotomy.[14] The advent of high-viscosity viscoelastics such as Healon GV and Healon 5 has made CCC in children less difficult. The use of dyes such as indocyanine green (ICG) and trypan blue has improved visibility and further improved control of the anterior capsule during CCC. New

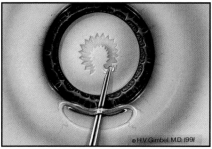

**Figure 3-1.** A bent 27-gauge needle or cystotome is used to create a can opener capsulotomy. (Reprinted with permission from *J Cataract Refract Surg*, 19, Gimbel HV, Willerscheidt AB, What to do with limited view: the intumescent cataract, 659, Copyright [1993], with permission from The American Society of Cataract and Refractive Surgery and the European Society of Cataract and Refractive Surgery.)

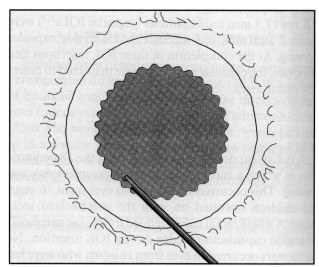

**Figure 3-2.** The vitrector is used to create an anterior capsular opening.

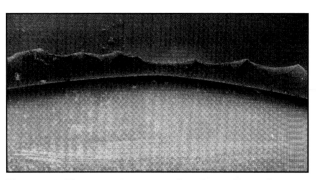

**Figure 3-3.** Electron microscopy showing a discontinuous capsular edge following vitrector capsulotomy. (Reprinted with permission from *J Cataract Refract Surg*, 25, Andeo LK, Wilson ME, Apple DJ, Elastic properties and scanning electron microscopic appearance of manual continuous curvilinear capsulorrhexis and vitrectorhexis in an animal model of pediatric cataract, 537-538, Copyright [1999], with permission from The American Society of Cataract and Refractive Surgery and the European Society of Cataract and Refractive Surgery.)

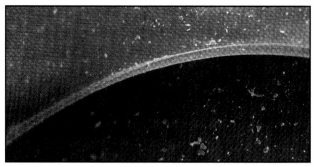

**Figure 3-4.** Electron microscopy showing continuous capsular edge following CCC. (Reprinted with permission from *J Cataract Refract Surg*, 25, Andeo LK, Wilson ME, Apple DJ, Elastic properties and scanning electron microscopic appearance of manual continuous curvilinear capsulorrhexis and vitrectorhexis in an animal model of pediatric cataract, 537-538, Copyright [1999], with permission from The American Society of Cataract and Refractive Surgery and the European Society of Cataract and Refractive Surgery.)

technologies such as diathermy and the fugo blade may offer additional means to safely perform capsulotomies in difficult pediatric cases.[15,16]

### CAN-OPENER CAPSULORRHEXIS

After the instillation of viscoelastic, a cystotome is used to create small nicks in the capsule to form a can-opener capsulorrhexis. The capsular openings are then joined using the cystotome (Figure 3-1).

The elasticity of the pediatric capsule may make this difficult; therefore, the anterior vitrector is used to remove any capsular tags or remnants. In cases of white or liquified cataracts where visibility of the capsule is difficult, the vitrector could be used to complete, modify, or enlarge the capsular opening.

### VITRECTOR CAPSULORRHEXIS

After the instillation of viscoelastic, an anterior vitrector is placed with the port directed downward toward the cap-

sule. The aspiration of the instrument is activated and the anterior capsule is engaged in the vitrector port.

The cutting function of the vitrector is then activated to create an opening in the anterior capsule. The vitrector is then used to enlarge the opening as desired (Figure 3-2).[17]

The elasticity of the pediatric capsule allows the serrated capsular edge to roll under and to create a round appearance, although at a microscopic level, it still appears discontinuous (Figures 3-3 and 3-4).[18]

### CONTINUOUS CURVILINEAR CAPSULORRHEXIS

#### *Indocyanine Green*

In cases of poor capsular visibility such as white, opaque cataracts, ICG, or trypan blue may assist in visualization of the capsulorrhexis.[19] ICG use has been described in pediatric patients.[20] A small lake of balanced salt solution (BSS) is

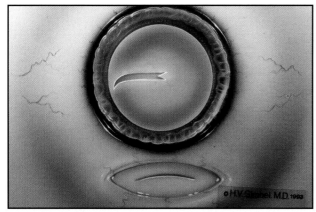

**Figure 3-5.** The initial 2-mm capsular tear is located at the 3 o'clock position.

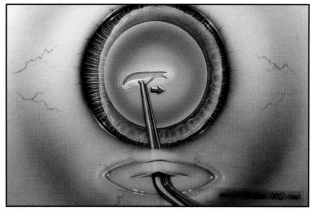

**Figure 3-6.** Forceps are used to grasp the flap and tear superiorly towards the 12 o'clock position.

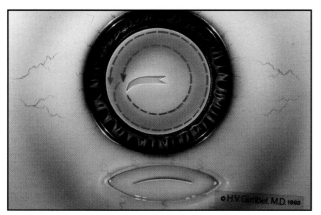

**Figure 3-7.** The tear is then directed 360 degrees.

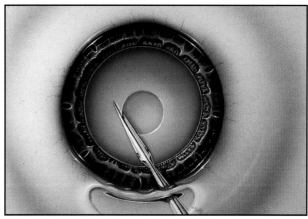

**Figure 3-8.** Vannas scissors are used to create a second snip if initiating the capsulorrhexis is difficult.

instilled beneath the Healon GV or Healon 5 using a blunt 23-gauge cannula. The diameter and positioning of the BSS is geared to the size and positioning desired for the CCC. A syringe of dye is then prepared with a filter attached. A blunt cannula is used to add the dye to the pool of BSS. The tip of the cannula is used to gently distribute the dye throughout the BSS lake, stroking the capsular surface to stain the capsule in the location and diameter desired for the CCC. The viscoelastic acts as a barrier to protect the corneal endothelium from the dye. The dye is then removed by aspirating it through the cannula. If necessary, any viscoelastic that has been stained by dye is also removed or displaced to provide a clear view of the capsule.

CCC provides the advantage of the controlled creation of a stable, smooth-edged anterior capsular opening.[21,22] A 27-gauge needle with the tip bent or a cystotome is used to create a 2-mm anterior capsular tear at the 3-o'clock position (Figure 3-5).

Utrata forceps are used to grasp the capsule and direct the tear first superiorly toward the 12-o'clock position. (Figure 3-6).

The tear is then continued counterclockwise 360 degrees (Figure 3-7). The direction of pull may require greater tan-

gential force than in adults and more frequent regrasping with the forceps may be needed because of the capsule elasticity and tendency for radial extension. The elasticity of the capsule often causes the capsulorrhexis opening to end up larger than intended. A shearing motion directed tangentially to the progressing tear often prevents too large of an opening or an extension peripherally.

The elasticity of the capsule may make beginning the capsulorrhexis difficult. After puncturing the lens with the cystotome, if the elasticity of the capsule prevents beginning a flap tear, use of Vannas scissors in a modification of the 2-stage capsulorrhexis may enhance the surgeon's ability to begin or enlarge the capsulorrhexis.[23] This technique employs Vannas scissors to create a second snip in the initial capsular opening created by the cystotome or 27-gauge needle. It is important to close the blade of the scissors only partially to avoid creating a nick in the capsule at the end of the second snip. This initiates a controlled linear tear to enable additional manipulation of the capsulorrhexis (Figure 3-8).

Tissue displacement by the viscoelastic may affect the CCC centration and/or size. The space-occupying viscoelastic may inferiorly decenter the iris opening or the lens itself, making central placement of the CCC difficult. These decentrations must be taken into account when the placement for the CCC is chosen. The size of the capsular opening should be 4 to 6 mm. Because of the stretching of ocular tissues by the highly viscous Healon GV or Healon 5, the size of the capsular opening may be overestimated. The size and placement of the CCC should be adjusted according to the surgeon's judgment of the amount of tissue displacement by the viscoelastic.

## Removal of the Lens

Historically, because of the unique difficulties associated with soft pediatric cataracts, optical iridectomy, discission, and linear extraction were advocated. In 1960 Scheie popularized aspiration of pediatric and soft cataracts.[24,25] Modifications of this aspiration technique made possible by technological advances continue to be used to the present day.

Recent technology makes several methods of aspiration possible. Either an ocutome, an infusion/aspiration (I/A) handpiece, a blunt cannula on a syringe, or a phacoemulsification handpiece may be used depending on the nature of the cataract, although because of the soft nature of the cataract ultrasound is rarely needed.[26] Having a variety of techniques available allows for the creative response to the multitude of intraoperative conditions in pediatric patients.

Vitrectomy instruments may be optimal in cases where the cataract is associated with fibrotic membranes for which a cutting tool is needed in addition to aspiration. At times an microvitreoretinal (MVR) blade is necessary to dissect dense fibrotic membranes into ribbons small enough to be engaged by the vitrector mouthpiece. In addition, some pediatric cataracts may have an attenuated or absent posterior capsule. In these cases, having immediate vitrectomy capabilities available may aid in the controlled removal of lens material associated with vitreous prolapse through the posterior capsule opening without its loss into the vitreous. Use of the I/A handpiece or blunt cannula on a syringe may be optimal in cases where small and angled ports are necessary to remove cortex. Use of the phacoemulsification handpiece may be helpful in cases where the lens has hard, calcified portions or subcapsular plaques.[27]

## Management of the Posterior Capsule

Postoperative opacification of the posterior capsule is common in children. It is the most important complication of pediatric cataracts because even a technically successful surgery may eventually be functionally unsuccessful if the visual axis does not remain clear for long-term amblyopia therapy. Many authors advocate a planned primary posterior capsular opening at the time of initial cataract surgery for all children under 6 years of age.[28,29] Vitrectomy instrumentation has been used for this purpose; however, with recent advances in viscoelastics, PCCC has been described.[30]

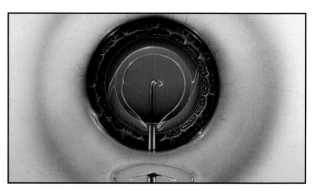

**Figure 3-9.** Creation of the posterior capsular opening. (Reprinted with permission from *J Cataract Refract Surg*, 20, Gimbel HV, DeBroff BM, Posterior capsulorrhexis with optic capture: maintaining a clear visual axis after pediatric cataract surgery, 659, Copyright [1994], with permission from The American Society of Cataract and Refractive Surgery and the European Society of Cataract and Refractive Surgery.)

### VITRECTOMY POSTERIOR CAPSULOTOMY

The posterior capsule may be removed from an anterior or posterior approach. For the anterior approach: After removal of the lens material, the ocutome is once again placed port side downward over the posterior capsule. The aspiration function is activated and the posterior capsule engaged. The cutting function is then activated and the posterior capsule penetrated. A thorough anterior vitrectomy is then performed through the posterior capsular opening to remove the vitreous face, and any scaffolding for fibrosis. The posterior capsule may be removed by a pars plana approach as well.

### POSTERIOR CONTINUOUS CURVILINEAR CAPSULORRHEXIS

PCCC provides the advantage of a smooth edge and controlled posterior capsular opening.[31] The integrity of this smooth capsular opening makes posterior optic capture of the IOL possible.[30,32,33] The advent of high-viscosity viscoelastic agents such as Healon GV or Healon 5 has made PCCC more technically facile in children by decreasing posterior vitreous pressure.

After removal of the lens material, high-viscosity viscoelastic such as Healon GV or Healon 5 is instilled both in front of and into the capsular bag. A cystotome or barbed, disposable 27-gauge needle is used to create an opening in the posterior capsule (Figure 3-9).

Healon GV or Healon 5 on a blunt 30-gauge cannula is then instilled behind the posterior capsule to create a plane between the posterior capsule and the vitreous face (Figure 3-10).

Failure to thus separate the posterior capsule and the vitreous face may result in rupture of the vitreous face and the uncontrolled extrusion of vitreous forward.

The needle is then used to hook, lift, and tear the capsule to create a triangular opening and capsular flap (Figure 3-11).

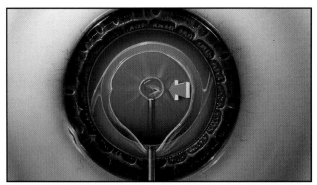

**Figure 3-10.** Injection of viscoelastic behind the posterior capsule. (Reprinted with permission from *J Cataract Refract Surg*, 20, Gimbel HV, DeBroff BM, Posterior capsulorrhexis with optic capture: maintaining a clear visual axis after pediatric cataract surgery, 659, Copyright [1994], with permission from The American Society of Cataract and Refractive Surgery and the European Society of Cataract and Refractive Surgery.)

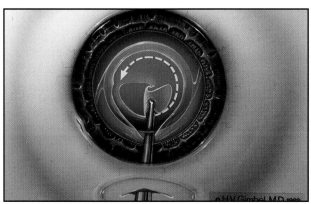

**Figure 3-12.** Capsular forceps are used to direct the posterior capsulotomy superiorly. Injection of viscoelastic behind the posterior capsule. (Reprinted with permission from *J Cataract Refract Surg*, 20, Gimbel HV, DeBroff BM, Posterior capsulorrhexis with optic capture: maintaining a clear visual axis after pediatric cataract surgery, 659, Copyright [1994], with permission from The American Society of Cataract and Refractive Surgery and the European Society of Cataract and Refractive Surgery.)

The elastic nature of the pediatric posterior capsule may make beginning the tear difficult. If no direct tear line is available, using Vannas or retinal scissors to create a controlled beginning for the tear may be necessary.[23] Utrata forceps are then used to create the rhexis. The tear is first directed radially toward 3 o'clock, then superiorly (Figure 3-12). It is then directed counterclockwise 360 degrees.

Dye may be used to stain the posterior capsule.[20] If restaining of the capsule is done after the posterior capsule has been opened, then the vitreous face may also stain. This may not resolve with time. The ICG-stained vitreous may serve as a partial opacity that may be amblyogenic if an adequate anterior vitrectomy is not performed.

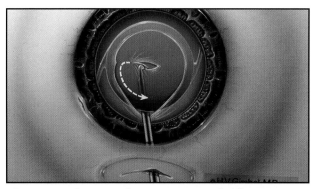

**Figure 3-11.** Creation of a posterior capsular flap. Injection of viscoelastic behind the posterior capsule. (Reprinted with permission from *J Cataract Refract Surg*, 20, Gimbel HV, DeBroff BM, Posterior capsulorrhexis with optic capture: maintaining a clear visual axis after pediatric cataract surgery, 659, Copyright [1994], with permission from The American Society of Cataract and Refractive Surgery and the European Society of Cataract and Refractive Surgery.)

## New Technologies

### DIFFICULT POSTERIOR CAPSULE SITUATIONS

At times a tough fibrous membrane may be incorporated into the posterior capsule. This may not respond to removal with the vitrector, especially if there is a smooth edge to the membrane that will not engage in the vitrector port. Slowing the cut rate allows greater time for the capsular membrane to engage within the vitrector, and may sometimes aid in removal of the membrane. If this is not successful, then using an MVR blade to section the membrane into thin strips the width of the vitrector port may allow the membrane to engage and be removed by the vitrector.[34]

In cases of PHPV, a fibrovascular stalk may be incorporated into the membrane. Various techniques have been described for its removal, including partial posterior capsulotomy, allowing the remaining capsule to pull the stalk out of the visual axis, and intraocular diathermy to control bleeding from the stalk (which may create a vitreous hemorrhage that could be amblyogenic).

In some cases, portions of the posterior capsule may be attenuated or even absent. The surgeon should have a high clinical index of suspicion in cases of posterior lenticonus, or in cases where there is partial dissolving of the cataract, debris in the anterior vitreous. The surgeon should proceed with great caution when removing the lenticular material so as not to inadvertently cause uncontrolled traction on the vitreous while in the lens aspiration mode. At times, anterior vitrectomy is necessary prior to removing the residual cortical material that remains in the capsular ring.

## Anterior Vitrectomy

After opening the posterior capsule, the vitrector port is inserted below the posterior capsule. An anterior vitrectomy

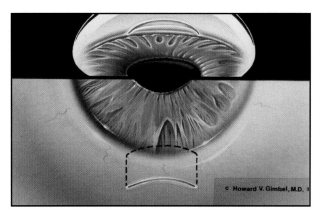

**Figure 3-13.** Intraoperative gonioscopy reveals gape of the internal portion of the wound. (Reprinted with permission from *J Cataract Refract Surg*, 20, Gimbel HV, Sun R, DeBroff BM, Recognition and management of internal wound gape, 122-123, Copyright [1997], with permission from The American Society of Cataract and Refractive Surgery and the European Society of Cataract and Refractive Surgery.)

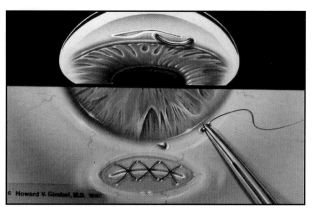

**Figure 3-14.** Securing the internal lip of the wound with 10-0 nylon suture. (Reprinted with permission from *J Cataract Refract Surg*, 20, Gimbel HV, Sun R, DeBroff BM, Recognition and management of internal wound gape, 122-123, Copyright [1997], with permission from The American Society of Cataract and Refractive Surgery and the European Society of Cataract and Refractive Surgery.)

is performed to remove a core of vitreous from the visual axis. Even if a posterior capsulotomy is performed, the vitreous face may act as a scaffold for the formation of secondary cataracts.[35] Special attention is placed at the 12-o'clock position. The shape and motion of the anterior and posterior capsular openings allow an estimation of the completeness of vitrectomy. A peaked capsular rim suggests an incomplete vitrectomy. The vitrector is then removed and a cyclodialysis spatula is inserted through the paracentesis port and used to sweep the anterior chamber for vitreous. A Weck Cell vitrectomy is then performed at the wound to test for vitreous. If the question of residual vitreous to the wound remains, then Miochol (CIBA Vision, Duluth, Ga) or Miostat (Alcon, Fort Worth, Tex) may be instilled into the anterior chamber. A peaked pupil suggests that vitreous may remain. Some research suggests that vitreous to the wound predisposes to retinal detachment later in life.[36]

### Techniques in Neonates

In children within the first few weeks of life, or in microphthalmic eyes, a 2-port technique may be the least traumatic method in the small eye. A 20-gauge MVR blade is used to create 2 paracentesis openings at the 10-o'clock and 2-o'clock limbus. A 20-gauge chamber maintainer with BSS is placed in one, and the vitrector port without the irrigating sheath in the second.

After opening the anterior capsule, aspiration of the lenticular material and anterior vitrectomy are then performed. Aspiration may be achieved using the 20-gauge vitrectomy handpiece with the irrigation sheath removed, or using a cannula on a syringe. This method makes capsulorrhexis techniques extremely difficult because of the small size of the paracentesis openings.

### Closing the Wound

Pediatric cataract and paracentesis wounds should be sutured. The elasticity of pediatric tissues predisposes for wound leaks, which may lead to hypotony or endophthalmitis. The most commonly used suture is 10-0 nylon with advantages including its ease of use. Disadvantages include the possible need for removal under general anesthesia at a later date. 8-0 or 9-0 Vicryl (Ethicon, Piscataway, NJ) has been shown to minimize complications such as corneal scarring and irritation. It has the additional advantage of not requiring removal at a later date.[37]

The elasticity of pediatric tissues predisposes them to fish mouthing at the internal portion of the wound.[38] Intraoperative gonioscopy may reveal this failure to oppose the internal portion of the wound (Figure 3-13). This may contribute to postoperative astigmatism.

This may require suturing with a single 10-0 nylon stitch. Repeat gonioscopy reveals closure of the internal portion of the wound (Figure 3-14).

### Subconjunctival Injection

Subconjunctival injections of dexamethasone sodium phosphate and betamethasone (Celestone Soluspan, Schering Corp, Kenilworth, NJ) and cephalosporin are often given in infants and children because of their propensity to rub the eye and the possibility of difficulty of instilling postoperative medications.[26]

### Postoperative Care

The eye should then be dressed with atropine ointment or drops and a steroid and antibiotic ointment, patch, and shield. Follow-up is to be in 1 day. Preliminary postoperative refraction can be done within a few days of surgery so that in the appropriate cases aphakic contact lenses or other opti-

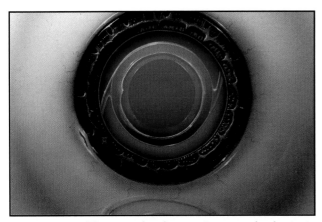

**Figure 3-15.** The completed posterior capsulorrhexis is smaller than the anterior capsular opening but large enough to capture the IOL. (Reprinted with permission from *J Cataract Refract Surg*, 20, Gimbel HV, DeBroff BM, Posterior capsulorrhexis with optic capture: maintaining a clear visual axis after pediatric cataract surgery, 659, Copyright [1994], with permission from The American Society of Cataract and Refractive Surgery and the European Society of Cataract and Refractive Surgery.)

cal correction and patching therapy for amblyopia may be initiated at the earliest possible date, preferably within a week after surgery. Topical steroid and atropine is continued for several weeks following surgery to decrease postoperative inflammation, and reduce posterior synechiae. The child is then followed approximately every 3 weeks for amblyopia therapy, and the fit and refractive power of the aphakic lenses or other optical correction. Bifocals may be needed for near vision.

# INTRAOCULAR LENSES

IOL in children has been described since the 1950s when Choyce first used an anterior chamber lens and Binkhorst used an iris-fixated lens.[39,40] Difficulties in fitting and maintaining aphakic contact lenses in children and the resulting vision loss from amblyopia make IOL implantation an attractive option. However, complications such as fibrinous uveitis, posterior synechiae, IOL deposits, and IOL erosion caused early skepticism.[41,42] Therefore, IOLs were initially utilized for unilateral cataract patients at higher risk for amblyopia and vision loss.[43] Reports of long-term success and improvements in IOL design and surgical techniques have made even successful bilateral IOL implantation possible.[44-48]

## Patient Selection

The use of IOLs in infants under 6 months of age continue to show a higher complication rate than in older children.[49] However, improvements in IOLs and techniques have made IOLs standard in children 2 years of age and

older.[50] As experience with IOLs accumulates, successful implantation is achieved in younger and younger children.

## Choice of Intraocular Lens

PMMA IOLs have the longest track record in children. Foldable acrylic lenses can be inserted through a 3.5-mm incision, and have been shown to be biocompatible in pediatric eyes, and are increasingly favored.[51] They may have lower posterior capsule opacification rates,[52] and have also successfully been employed using a posterior optic capture technique.[53] IOLs with heparin surface coating may minimize inflammatory lens deposits.[54] Optics with larger diameters from 5.5 to 6.5 mm depending on IOL type may decrease iris capture in children, who have a propensity to larger dilation than adults.

## Choice of IOL Power

The small size and changing power of the pediatric eye continue to challenge the selection of IOL power. IOL power calculation formulae may be less accurate in small pediatric eyes.[55,56] During the first weeks and months of life, keratometry rapidly changes over several diopters.[57-59] Therefore, use of an average K value may be most useful if an IOL is to be implanted in these very young infants. Many authors show an age-dependent myopic shift in children with IOL implants.[60,61] However, others suggest that pseudophakic patients show less myopic shift than aphakic patients.[62,63]

SRK, SRKII, SRKT, Hoffer Q, and Holladay formulae have all been successfully applied in children.[55,56,64,65] Many authors suggest that in children under 6 years of age, the IOL power be chosen to provide for some degree of hypermetropia based on the expected myopic shift for that child's age.[64,66] Optical correction with spectacles or contact lenses can be added and then appropriately adjusted to compensate for the myopic shift over the ensuing years.[67] Others suggest that IOL power be chosen for emmetropia to facilitate immediate amblyopia therapy. Optical correction throughout the years, or even refractive surgery could be employed in adulthood for any long-term myopic shift. The difficulty in predicting myopic shift in any individual patient suggest that IOL power be selected on an patient by patient basis.[68]

## Posterior Optic Capture

Posterior optic capture is a technique recently described to manage posterior capsular opacification and secondary cataract in children undergoing IOL implantation.[30,32,33,69,70] In addition, there is some suggestion that this technique may decrease the incidence of aphakic glaucoma by creating a barrier between the anterior chamber and vitreous cavity.[64]

After CCC and lens removal, posterior optic capture is initiated after IOL implantation in the bag. Optic size of 6 mm or less is important to allow for an appropriately small posterior capsular opening. PCCC as described above is per-

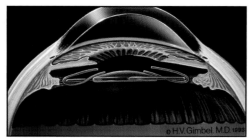

**Figure 3-16.** The optic is captured posteriorly by the posterior capsule while the haptics remain anterior. (Reprinted with permission from *J Cataract Refract Surg*, 20, Gimbel HV, DeBroff BM, Posterior capsulorrhexis with optic capture: maintaining a clear visual axis after pediatric cataract surgery, 659, Copyright [1994], with permission from The American Society of Cataract and Refractive Surgery and the European Society of Cataract and Refractive Surgery.)

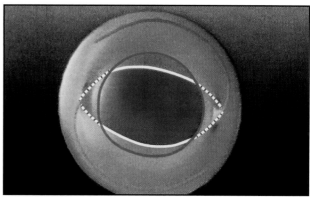

**Figure 3-17.** Schematic of posterior capture of the optic. (Reprinted with permission from *J Cataract Refract Surg*, 20, Gimbel HV, DeBroff BM, Posterior continuous curvilinear capsulorrhexis and optic capture of the intraocular lens to prevent secondary opacification in pediatric cataract surgery, 654, Copyright [1997], with permission from The American Society of Cataract and Refractive Surgery and the European Society of Cataract and Refractive Surgery.)

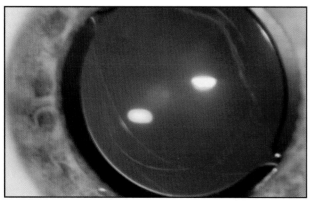

**Figure 3-18.** Photograph of posterior capture of the optic. (Reprinted with permission from *J Cataract Refract Surg*, 20, Gimbel HV, DeBroff BM, Posterior continuous curvilinear capsulorrhexis and optic capture of the intraocular lens to prevent secondary opacification in pediatric cataract surgery, 654, Copyright [1997], with permission from The American Society of Cataract and Refractive Surgery and the European Society of Cataract and Refractive Surgery.)

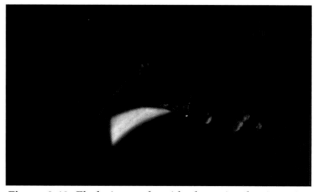

**Figure 3-19.** Elschnig pearls with clear visual axis maintained by captured optic. (Reprinted with permission from *J Cataract Refract Surg*, 20, Gimbel HV, DeBroff BM, Posterior continuous curvilinear capsulorrhexis and optic capture of the intraocular lens to prevent secondary opacification in pediatric cataract surgery, 654, Copyright [1997], with permission from The American Society of Cataract and Refractive Surgery and the European Society of Cataract and Refractive Surgery.)

formed underneath the IOL. It is sized smaller than the CCC to allow capture of the optic but large enough to allow the optic to pass through (Figure 3-15).

Viscoelastic is instilled through the PCCC as needed throughout to prevent anterior displacement of the vitreous face.

Scissors may be needed to lyse adhesions between the vitreous face and posterior capsule. Vitrectomy is used only if vitreous prolapses through the PCCC.

The scleral wound is sutured, but viscoelastic is allowed to remain anterior and posterior to the IOL. A spatula or cannula is then used to slip the optic under the PCCC, first inferiorly, then superiorly to achieve posterior capture of the optic.

The optic is thus captured anterior to the vitreous face by the posterior capsule (Figures 3-16, 3-17, and 3-18).

Viscoelastic material is left between the IOL and the vitreous face, but is carefully aspirated from the anterior chamber while BSS is irrigated to ensure that anterior prolapse of the IOL and vitreous face do not occur. As time passes, although Elschnig pearls form, these are prevented from obscuring the visual axis by emptying into the anterior chamber anterior to the captured optic. The tight seal of the anterior and posterior capsule at the optic haptic junction prevents migration of the pearls onto the vitreous face. A slim optic haptic junction may be key to this sealing factor (Figure 3-19).

# References

1. Wright KW, Walonker F, Edelman P. 10-diopter fixation test for amblyopia. *Arch Ophthalmol.* 1981;99:1242.

2. Cates CA, Simon JW, Jenkins PL, et al. Preferential looking as a guide for amblyopia therapy in monocular infantile cataracts. *J Pediatr Ophthalmol Strabismus.* 1987;24:56.

3. Costenbader F, Albert D. Conservatism in the management of congenital cataracts. *Am J Ophthalmol.* 1957;58:426.

4. Drummond GT, Hinz BJ. Management of monocular cataract with long-term dilation in children. *Can J Ophthalmol.* 1994;29:227.

5. Nelson LB. Diagnosis and management of cataracts in infancy and childhood. *Ophthalmic Surg.* 1984;15:688.

6. Merin S, Crawford J. Assessment of incomplete cataract. *Can J Ophthalmol.* 1972;7:56.

7. France TD, Frank JW. The association of strabismus and aphakia in children. *J Pediatr Ophthalmol Strabismus.* 1984;21:221.

8. Lambert SR, Amaya LG, Taylor D. Detection and treatment of infantile cataracts. *Int Ophthalmol Clin.* 1989;29:51.

9. Helveston EM, Saunders RA, Ellis FD. Unilateral cataracts in children. *Ophthalmic Surg.* 1980;11:102.

10. Crouch ER Jr, Parks M. Management of posterior lenticonus complicated by unilateral cataract. *Am J Ophthalmol.* 1978;85:503.

11. Robb RM, Mayer DL, Moore BD. Results of early treatment of unilateral congenital cataracts. *J Pediatr Ophthalmol Strabismus.* 1987;24:178.

12. Cheng KP, Hiles DA, Biglan AW, et al. Visual results after early surgical treatment of unilateral congenital cataracts. *Ophthalmology.* 1991;98:903.

13. Wright KW, Christensen LE, Noguchi BA. Results of late surgery for presumed congenital cataracts. *Am J Ophthalmol.* 1992;114:409.

14. Wilson ME, Bluestein EC, Wang XH, et al. Comparison of mechanized anterior capsulectomy and manual continuous capsulorrhexis in pediatric eyes. *J Cataract Refract Surg.* 1994;20:602.

15. Hausmann N, Richard G. Investigations on diathermy for anterior capsulotomy. *Invest Ophthalmol Vis Sci.* 1991;32:2155.

16. Singh D. Use of the fugo blade in complicated cases. *J Cataract Refract Surg.* 2002;28:573.

17. Wilson ME, Saunders RA, Roberts EL, et al. Mechanized anterior capsulectomy as an alternative to manual capsulorrhexis in children undergoing intraocular lens implantation. *J Pediatr Ophthalmol Strabismus.* 1996;33:237.

18. Andreo LK, Wilson ME, Apple DJ. Elastic properties and scanning electron microscopic appearance of manual continuous curvilinear capsulorrhexis and vitrectorhexis in an animal model of pediatric cataract. *J Cataract Refract Surg.* 1999;25:534.

19. Pandey SK, Werner L, Escobar-Gomez M, et al. Dye-enhanced cataract surgery. Part 1: anterior capsule staining for capsulorrhexis in advanced/white cataract. *J Cataract Refract Surg.* 2000;26:1052.

20. Wakabayashi T, Yamamoto N. Posterior capsule staining and posterior continuous curvilinear capsulorrhexis in congenital cataract. *J Cataract Refract Surg.* 2002;28:2042.

21. Gimbel HV, Neuhann T. Development, advantages, and methods of the continuous circular capsulorrhexis technique. *J Cataract Refract Surg.* 1990;16:31.

22. Andreo LK, Wilson ME, Jr, Apt L. Elastic properties and scanning electron microscopic appearance of manual continuous curvilinear capsulorrhexis and vitrectorhexis in an animal model of pediatric cataract. *J Cataract Refract Surg.* 1999;25:534.

23. Gimbel H. Two-stage capsulorrhexis for endocapsular phacoemulsification. *J Cataract Refract Surg.* 1990;16:246.

24. Scheie HG. Aspiration of congenital or soft cataracts: a new technique. *Am J Ophthalmol.* 1960;50:1048.

25. Hiles DA, Parks M. Management of infantile cataracts. *Am J Ophthalmol.* 1967;63:10.

26. Sinskey RM, Karel F, Dal Ri E. Management of cataracts in children. *J Cataract Refract Surg.* 1989;15:196.

27. Hiles DA, Wallar PH. Phacoemulsification versus aspiration in infantile cataract surgery. *Ophthalmic Surg.* 1974;5:13.

28. Buckley EG, Klombers LA, Seaber JH, et al. Management of the posterior capsule during pediatric intraocular lens implantation. *Am J Ophthalmol.* 1993;115:722.

29. Jensen AA, Basti S, Greenwald MJ, et al. When may the posterior capsule be preserved in pediatric intraocular lens surgery? *Ophthalmology.* 2002;109:324.

30. Gimbel HV. Posterior capsulorrhexis with optic capture in pediatric cataract and intraocular lens surgery. *Ophthalmology.* 1996;103:1871.

31. Castaneda VE, Legler UFC, Tsai JC, et al. Posterior continuous curvilinear capsulorrhexis. *Ophthalmology.* 1992;99:45.

32. Gimbel HV. Posterior continuous curvilinear capsulorrhexis and optic capture of the intraocular lens to prevent secondary opacification in pediatric cataract surgery. *J Cataract Refract Surg.* 1997;23(Suppl 1):652.

33. Gimbel HV, DeBroff BM. Posterior capsulorrhexis with optic capture: maintaining a clear visual axis after pediatric cataract surgery. *J Cataract Refract Surg.* 1994;20:658.

34. Paysse EA, McCreery KM, Coats DK. Surgical management of the lens and retrolenticular fibrotic membranes associated with persistent fetal vasculature. *J Cataract Refract Surg.* 2002;28:816.

35. Morgan KS, Karciouglu KA. Secondary cataracts in infants after lensectomies. *J Pediatr Ophthalmol Strabismus.* 1987;24:45.

36. Toyofuku H, Hirose T, Schepens CL. Retinal detachment following congenital cataract surgery. *Arch Ophthalmol.* 1980;98:669.

37. Lavrich JB, Goldberg DS, Nelson LB. Suture use in pediatric cataract surgery: a survey. *Ophthalmic Surg.* 1993;24:554.

38. Gimbel HV, Sun R, DeBroff BM. Recognition and management of internal wound gape. *J Cataract Refract Surg.* 1995;21:121.

39. Choyce DP. Correction of uni-ocular aphakia by means of anterior chamber acrylic implants. *Trans Ophthalmol Soc U K.* 1958;78:459.

40. Binkhorst CD. Iris-clip and irido-capsular lens implants (pseudophakoi). *Br J Ophthalmol.* 1967;51:767.

41. Hiles DA. Peripheral iris erosions associated with pediatric intraocular lens implants. *J Am Intraocul Implant Soc.* 1979;5:210.

42. Hiles DA, Watson BA. Complications of implant surgery in children. *J Am Intraocul Implant Soc.* 1979;5:24.

43. Burke JP, Willshaw HE, Young TL. Intraocular lens implants for uniocular cataracts in childhood. *Br J Ophthalmol.* 1989;73:860.

44. Sinskey RM, Stoppel JO, Amin P. Long-term results of intraocular lens implantation in pediatric patients. *J Cataract Refract Surg.* 1993;19:405.

45. Gimbel HV, Basti S, Ferensowicz M, et al. Results of bilateral cataract extraction with posterior chamber intraocular lens implantation in children. *Ophthalmol.* 1997;104:1737.

46. Gimbel HV, Ferensowicz M, Raanan M, et al. Implantation in children. *J Pediatr Ophthalmol Strabismus.* 1993;30:69.

47. Peterseim MW, Wilson ME. Bilateral intraocular lens implantation in the pediatric population. *Ophthalmology.* 2000;107:1261.

48. O'Keefe M, Mulvihill A, Yeoh PL. Visual outcome and complications of bilateral intraocular lens implantation in children. *J Cataract Refract Surg.* 2000;26:1758.

49. Plager DA, Yang S, Neely DE, et al. Complications in the first year following cataract surgery with and without IOL in infants and older children. *J AAPOS.* 2002;6:9.

50. Ellis FJ. Management of pediatric cataract and lens opacities. *Curr Opin Ophthalmol.* 2002;13:33.

51. Wilson ME, Elliott L, Johnson B, et al. Acrysof acrylic intraocular lens implantation in children: clinical indications of biocompatibility. *J AAPOS.* 2001;5:377.

52. Yun B, Shi Y. Pediatric phacoemulsification with acrysof intraocular lens implantation. *Chung Hua Yen Ko Tsa Chih.* 2001;37:111.

53. Argento C, Badoza D, Ugrin C. Optic capture of the acrysof intraocular lens in pediatric cataract surgery. *J Cataract Refract Surg.* 2001;27:1638.

54. Basti S, Aasuri MK, Reddy MK, et al. Heparin-surface-modified intraocular lenses in pediatric cataract surgery: Prospective randomized study. *J Cataract Refract Surg.* 1999;25:782.

55. Kora Y, Kinohira Y, Inatomi M, et al. Intraocular lens power calculation and refractive change in pediatric cases. *Nippon Ganka Gakkai Zasshi.* 2002;106:273.

56. Andreo LK, Wilson ME, Saunders RA. Predictive value of regression and theoretical IOL formulas in pediatric intraocular lens implantation. *J Pediatr Ophthalmol Strabismus.* 1997;34:240.

57. Inagaki Y. The rapid change of corneal curvature in the neonatal period and infancy. *Arch Ophthalmol* 1986;104:1026.

58. Asbell PA, Chiang B, Somers ME, et al. Keratometry in children. *CLAO J.* 1990;16:99.

59. Pollard ZF. Keratometry readings in infants. *J Pediatr Ophthalmol Strabismus.* 1982;19:169.

60. Crouch ER, Crouch ER Jr, Pressman SH. Prospective analysis of pediatric pseudophakia: myopic shift and postoperative outcomes. *J AAPOS.* 2002;6:277.

61. Plager DA, Kipfer H, Sprunger DT, et al. Refractive change in pediatric pseudophakia: 6-year follow-up. *J Cataract Refract Surg.* 2002;28:810.

62. McClatchey SK, Dahan E, Maselli E, et al. A comparison of the rate of refractive growth in pediatric aphakic and pseudophakic eyes. *Ophthalmology.* 2000;107:118.

63. Superstein R, Archer SM, Del Monte MA. Minimal myopic shift in pseudophakic versus aphakic pediatric cataract patients. *J AAPOS.* 2002;6:271.

64. McClatchey SK. Intraocular lens calculator for childhood cataract. *J Cataract Refract Surg.* 1998;24:1125.

65. Zwaan J, Mullaney PB, Awad A, et al. Pediatric intraocular lens implantation. Surgical results and complications in more than 300 patients. *Ophthalmology.* 1998;105:112.

66. Dahan E, Drusedau MU. Choice of lens and dioptric power in pediatric pseudophakia. *J Cataract Refract Surg.* 1997;23 Suppl 1:618.

67. Dahan E. Intraocular lens implantation in children. *Curr Opin Ophthalmol.* 2000;11:51.

68. Enyedi LB, Peterseim MW, Freedman SF, et al. Refractive changes after pediatric intraocular lens implantation. *Am J Ophthalmol.* 1998;126:772.

69. Raina UK, Gupta V, Arora R, et al. Posterior continuous curvilinear capsulorrhexis with and without optic capture of the posterior chamber intraocular lens in the absence of vitrectomy. *J Pediatr Ophthalmol Strabismus.* 2002;39:278.

70. Metori Y, Kageyama T, Aramaki T, et al. Pediatric cataract surgery with posterior capsulorrhexis and optic capture of the intraocular lens. *Nippon Ganka Gakkai Zasshi.* 2000;104:91.

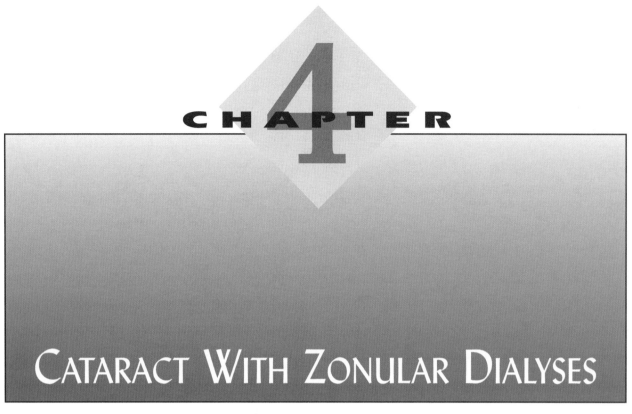

# CHAPTER 4

# CATARACT WITH ZONULAR DIALYSES

*Scott E. Burk, MD, PhD and Robert J. Cionni, MD*

## INTRODUCTION

Weakened or missing zonules present a serious challenge to the cataract surgeon. Zonular compromise, be it congenital, iatrogenic, due to trauma, or disease, complicates every step of lens surgery from the capsulotomy to final removal of the viscoelastic. It makes both intraoperative complications such as vitreous loss and nucleus subluxation, and postoperative complications such as decentration of the IOL more likely. Historically, surgical removal of the subluxated lens has been undertaken with great caution because of numerous reports of complications and poor visual outcomes.[1-3] Until recently, the surgical management of a malpositioned lens in the face of significant zonular compromise had been limited to iridectomy, laser iridotomy, or intracapsular extraction.[4] However, new devices and techniques that minimize the stress on the compromised zonules during and after surgery have been shown to decrease the risk of complications in these challenging patients.[5,6]

## ANATOMY AND PHYSIOLOGY

The lens is suspended just behind the iris plane by a 3-D system of radially arranged fibers called zonules. These diaphanous fibers arise from the ciliary body epithelium and attach to the lens capsule near the equator. The zonules fixate the lens behind the iris, centered within the pupil. The zonules transmit the motion of the ciliary body to the lens allowing accommodation. Each zonule measures 5 to 30 μm in diameter and is composed of bundles of microfibrils. Biochemical analysis has revealed that the zonules are composed of fibrillin, the protein product of the gene linked to Marfan syndrome.

Marfan syndrome, as well as several other hereditary disorders such as homocystinuria, Weil-Marchesani syndrome, hyperlysinemia, and sulfite oxidase deficiency may be manifest in the eye as zonular insufficiency, resulting in lens subluxation (Figure 4-1). Zonular insufficiency may also commonly occur as a result of uveitis, hypermature cataracts, and pseudoexfoliation syndrome, but the most common cause of zonular insufficiency is trauma.

## PREOPERATIVE EVALUATION

Whether the zonular insufficiency is hereditary, or acquired, a comprehensive preoperative examination will help the surgeon better anticipate the challenges to be dealt with in the operating room. An assessment of the BCVA for near and distance should be determined, keeping in mind that the patient may see best with an aphakic correction if

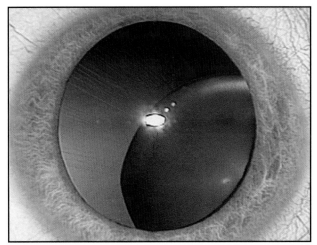

**Figure 4-1.** A congenitally subluxed lens in a young boy with Marfan syndrome.

the lens is markedly subluxed. In addition to the routine preoperative assessment, the surgeon should characterize and draw the zonular defect describing the weakness in terms of degrees of loss, location of the defect, and presence or absence of vitreous within the anterior segment. Any degree of phacodonesis should be noted, keeping in mind that phacodonesis is more noticeable prior to dilation, which stabilizes the ciliary body and iris, and may dampen lens movement.

The surgeon should be particularly wary of the inferiorly subluxated lens, which often indicates 360 degrees of very significant zonular insufficiency combined with the effect of gravity. When significant generalized zonular weakness is present a pars plana lensectomy should be considered because it is unlikely that the surgeon will be able to remove the lens and maintain the capsular bag for posterior chamber intraocular lens (PCIOL) support.

The presence or absence of additional ocular pathology must be taken into consideration and the patient counseled accordingly.

Many patients with Marfan syndrome have significant systemic problems, which increase the risk of death or morbidity. These patients need to be evaluated by their primary medical doctor or cardiologist prior to surgery. Patients taking anticoagulant medicine for heart, vessel, and/or valvular abnormalities, need to be counseled in detail concerning the implications of discontinuing anticoagulants versus undergoing surgery while anticoagulated.

Informed consent should be modified from the routine cataract. The patient should be specifically informed about the possibility of either a sutured posterior chamber intraocular lens or a capsular tension ring. The patient must also be made aware that the modified CTR is not yet FDA approved.

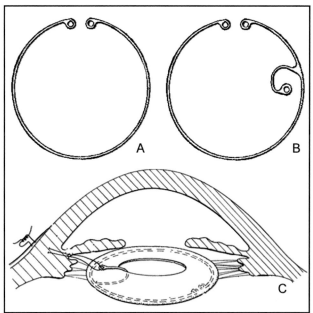

**Figure 4-2.** Diagram demonstrating the (A) CTR (B) Cionni modified CTR and (C) illustrating how the modified CTR can be sutured through the ciliary sulcus to the scleral wall without violating the integrity of the capsular bag.

## CAPSULAR TENSION RINGS

The introduction of small incision surgery and vitreous cutting devices has dramatically improved our ability to manage zonular weakness, and pars plana vitrectomy/lensectomy with aphakic contact lens wear, or anterior chamber intraocular lens (ACIOL), remains a common surgical practice. The development of materials and techniques to allow suture fixation of a PCIOL to the ciliary sulcus provide surgeons with another popular option that has even been advocated for children.[7] Iris fixation IOLs have also gained in popularity.[8,9] Recently, CTRs have given us the ability to perform small incision phacoemulsification with in-the-bag implantation of a PCIOL.[5]

In 1991 Dr. Hara introduced the CTR (Figure 4-2A) and in 1993, Dr. Witschel and Dr. Legler demonstrated that the CTR could provide both intraoperative and postoperative stabilization of the capsular bag and IOL in patients with zonular dialysis.[10,11] Since its introduction, the CTR has revolutionized our approach to zonular dialyses, and many surgeons have come to depend on the CTR for their patients with zonular compromise. These PMMA rings can be inserted into the capsular bag at any point after the capsulorrhexis has been completed and remain within the bag postoperatively.[5] The effect is a dramatic expansion and stabilization of the capsular bag.

Although the CTR has helped surgeons manage patients having a moderate loss of zonular support, eyes with profound zonular compromise, or lens subluxation, may still not obtain adequate stabilization or centration despite CTR placement. Additionally, long-term stability of the bag and IOL is uncertain in eyes with progressive zonular loss, as in patients with pseudoexfoliation or Marfan syndrome. We have seen several cases of complete posterior dislocation of the IOL within the capsular bag, which occurred years following the original cataract surgery. We are also aware of cases where a CTR was implanted initially, yet progressive zonular weakening eventually resulted in complete dislocation of the capsular bag, PCIOL, and CTR complex postoperatively. With this in mind, several surgeons devised techniques for suturing the CTR to the scleral wall for better support and centration. Dr. Robert Osher demonstrated the technique of suturing the CTR to the scleral wall by straddling the CTR with a 10.0 Prolene suture, double-armed with CIF-4 needles.[12] This technique may work well, yet involves passing needles through the peripheral capsular bag, risking rupture of the bag. Dr. Vladimir Pfeifer preferred to fashion a small peripheral capsulorrhexis through which a similar passage of suture could be made.[13] Both techniques provide a solution for eyes with severe zonular insufficiency, however both violate the integrity of the peripheral capsular bag.

The modified CTR (MCTR), designed by Dr. Robert Cionni, incorporates a unique fixation hook to provide scleral fixation without violating the integrity of the capsular bag (Figure 4-2B).[6] The MCTR is manufactured by Morcher GmbH in Stuttgart, Germany. Like the original capsular tension ring, it consists of an open, flexible PMMA filament. However, the MCTR has a fixation hook that loops anteriorly and in a second plane wrapping around the capsulorrhexis edge. At the free end of the hook is an eyelet through which a suture can be passed for scleral fixation (Figure 4-2C). Currently, there are 3 MCTR models that vary in the fixation hook position and number.

# INDICATIONS AND CONTRAINDICATIONS

Progressive subluxation of the crystalline lens will commonly induce large refractive errors and anisometropia. Additionally, movement of the dislocated lens can cause an intermittent phakic or aphakic visual axis leading to marked visual disturbances. Such disturbances in a child undergoing visual development will often result in amblyopia. Thus, it is important to intervene to prevent amblyopia in young children with significant lenticular subluxation. However, not all subluxed lenses require surgery. Many of these lenses remain centered long enough to allow the child to develop normal vision well beyond the amblyogenic years. If the lens is not threatening to dislocate posteriorly or anteriorly and, if an

accurate refraction can be obtained, observation is warranted along with amblyopia treatment. Nonetheless, if there is significant and progressive dislocation or if amblyopia cannot be effectively treated with conventional means such as glasses, contact lenses, and/or patching, lens extraction may be the best option.

For older children and adults, lens extraction should be considered if there is poor visual acuity attributed to the subluxated lens which is not amenable to spectacle correction, or if the lens is threatening to dislocate anteriorly or posteriorly.

# SURGICAL TECHNIQUES

## *Anesthesia*

A long-acting retrobulbar anesthetic is preferred due to the complicated nature of these cases. Elevated intraorbital pressure should be minimized.

## *Procedure*

When starting the procedure, the surgeon should attempt to make the incision away from the area of zonular weakness. This will help reduce the stress placed on the existing zonules during phacoemulsification. Unfortunately, many of these patients have generalized zonular weakness, in which case the incision should be placed in the quadrant to which the lens has subluxed, since the zonules in the opposite quadrant have proven to be the weakest. Nevertheless, the surgeon should not compromise his or her surgical abilities by operating in a meridian that is uncomfortable.

The surgeon should always work through the smallest incision possible without compromising his or her ability to perform the necessary maneuvers. Doing so will minimize fluid egress through the incision and therefore will help to limit anterior chamber collapses. Make the initial anterior chamber entry just large enough to insert the viscoelastic cannula and place a generous amount of a highly retentive viscoelastic over the area of zonular dialysis to tamponade vitreous and to maintain a deep, non-collapsing anterior chamber.

The capsulorrhexis should be initiated in an area remote from the dialysis in order to employ the stronger remaining zonules for countertraction. A second blunt instrument may be used for countertraction if it is significantly loose and/or decentered. When there is extensive zonular loss or weakness, it may be necessary to begin the tear by cutting the anterior capsule with a sharp-tipped 15-degree blade or a diamond blade while providing counter traction with a second blunt instrument. The capsulotomy should be made large enough to allow for easy nucleus manipulation. A 5.5-mm to 6.0-mm capsulorrhexis should be adequate.

Furthermore, it may be necessary to stabilize the capsular bag with a dull second instrument or with an iris retractor to complete the capsulorrhexis. It is important to note that the capsulorrhexis should be made "off-center" in an eye with significant lens subluxation so that the capsulorrhexis will be centered after placement of a CTR or MCTR.

These PMMA rings can be inserted into the capsular bag at any point after the capsulorrhexis; however the bulk of the nucleus can make visualization and placement of the CTR difficult. If implantation before phacoemulsification is chosen, the device is inserted using dull forceps or a specially designed injector. Before inserting the CTR, create a space between the peripheral capsular bag and any remaining lenticular material with viscoelastic. Doing so will help prevent entrapment of cortex under the CTR, which can be difficult to aspirate. If the CTR is placed before phacoemulsification, loop a "safety-suture" (10.0 Prolene) through the leading eyelet. This suture is left trailing out of the incision and can be used to retrieve the CTR should the capsule break during phacoemulsification. Additionally, if the CTR is difficult to place, this suture can be used to help "coax" the leading haptic around the capsular bag periphery. Once the CTR is in place, one can proceed with the remainder of the procedure with the advantage of having a CTR-stabilized capsular bag.

Once capsulorrhexis has been completed, if the surgeon has chosen to proceed with phacoemulsification prior to capsular tension ring implantation, the surgeon may need to stabilize the capsular bag by hooking the capsulorrhexis edge with 1 to 4 iris retractors placed through limbal stab incisions (Figure 4-3).[14] The silicone stop on the hook is adjusted to pull the capsulorrhexis edge toward the scleral wall, thereby supporting the loose capsular bag for safer phacoemulsification.

Hydrodissection is then performed carefully, yet thoroughly, to maximally free the nucleus and thereby decrease zonular stress during manipulation of the nucleus. If the nucleus is soft, hydrodissection of the nucleus completely into the anterior chamber will greatly simplify its removal and will virtually eliminate zonular stress during phacoemulsification.[15]

Phacoemulsification should be performed using low vacuum and aspiration settings in order to keep the bottle height and flow rate at a minimum.[16] It is important, however, not to lower the bottle so much as to allow chamber collapse because this can lead to vitreous prolapse. Chop techniques are preferred for the dense nuclei to minimize zonular stress during phacoemulsification. The surgeon must be careful to apply equal forces in opposing directions to avoid displacing the nucleus. It is very helpful to "viscodissect" the nuclear halves or quadrants free from the cortex in areas of zonular weakness.[17] Viscoelastic injected between the nuclear quadrants and peripheral capsular bag will lift the nuclear fragments while expanding and stabilizing the

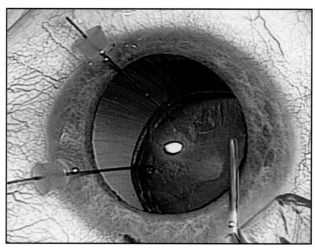

**Figure 4-3.** Disposable nylon iris retractors are used to grasp the capsulorrhexis edge and stabilize the loose lens.

bag. Nucleus manipulation must be performed gently when using iris hooks to support the loose lens in order to prevent the hook from tearing the capsulorrhexis edge.

Cortical viscodissection prior to aspiration will also limit the stress on remaining zonules.[17] Viscoelastic is injected against the residual anterior capsular rim and peripheral capsular bag, separating the cortex from its adhesions to the capsule. It may be helpful to aspirate cortex manually using a 24- to 27-gauge cannula while the anterior segment is filled with viscoelastic material. Whenever cortex is aspirated, strip along a vector tangential to the capsular bag periphery to decrease the risk of further damaging the zonules.

Before inserting the CTR or MCTR, the surgeon should place viscoelastic just under the surface of the residual anterior capsular rim to create a space for the ring and to dissect residual cortex away from the peripheral capsule, making cortical entrapment less likely (Figure 4-4). Insertion of a CTR is performed as described above; however, it is notably easier after removal of the lens material. Insertion of the MCTR begins by preplacing a 9.0 Prolene or Gortex suture, double-armed with CIF-4 needles, through the eyelet of the fixation hook. Alternatively, the suture can be single-armed and the free end of the Prolene tied to the fixation hook eyelet. We no longer recommend 10.0 Prolene suture due to several cases of late suture breakage more than 1 year after surgery. The MCTR is inserted with smooth forceps through the main incision and dialed into the capsular bag (Figure 4-5). The fixation hook will often "capture" anterior to the capsulorrhexis edge. If it does not, the hook is easily manipulated anteriorly with a Y-hook and a second dull instrument to retract the capsulorrhexis edge. The Y-hook is used to "dial" the MCTR until the eyelet is centered at the site of zonular dehiscence or zonular weakness. Next, displace the fixation hook to the scleral wall to be certain that the chosen location will result in bag centration (Figure 4-6). A scleral

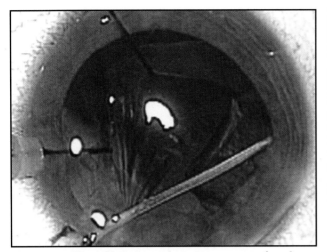

**Figure 4-4.** Viscoelastic is used to create a space for placement of the MCTR and viscodissect any remaining cortex so that it will not become entrapped by the ring.

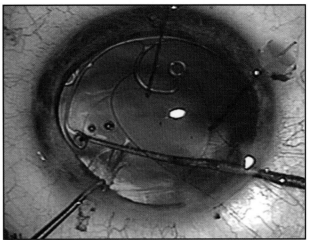

**Figure 4-5.** A Cionni chopper (Duckworth and Kent, St. Louis, Mo) and Osher Y-hook (Duckworth and Kent) are used to place the MCTR, model 1-L into the capsular bag.

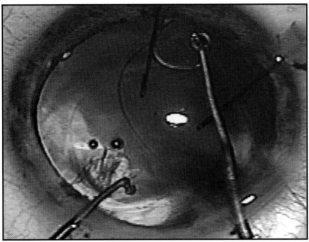

**Figure 4-6.** The fixation hook of the MCTR model 1-L is displaced to the scleral wall with an Osher Y-hook to determine the best axis for suture fixation.

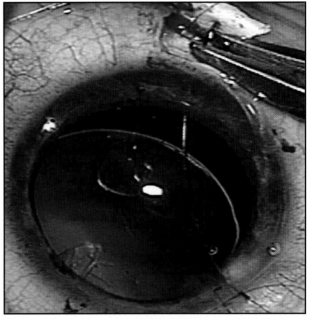

**Figure 4-7.** Each needle of the double-armed 9.0 Prolene suture is passed through the main incision, anterior to the anterior capsule, and out through the ciliary sulcus and scleral wall to exit beneath a partial thickness flap.

flap is fashioned at this site so that once the Prolene suture is tied the suture and knot can be covered. Viscoelastic is then used to create space between the undersurface of the iris and the anterior capsule in preparation for needle passage. The needles are placed through the incision, into the pupil, and behind the iris. The needle and suture should remain anterior to the anterior capsule at all times (Figure 4-7). The 2 needles should exit the scleral wall approximately 1.5 mm apart and 1.5 mm posterior to the corneal-scleral junction. This will position the fixation hook posterior enough to prevent postoperative iris chaffing. The sutures are then cinched to verify centration, and a temporary knot is tied (Figure 4-8). If a single-armed suture is used, the needle is passed through partial-thickness scleral beneath the scleral flap and then tied to itself. After suture fixation of the MCTR, any remaining cortex can be aspirated manually with a 24- to 27-gauge cannula. Alternatively, one can use an automated irrigation/

aspiration device, but vitreous prolapse may be more likely. The capsular bag is then reinflated with viscoelastic prior to PCIOL insertion.

We have found it easiest to insert a foldable-style PCIOL into the capsular bag in these cases. We currently favor the Alcon (Fort Worth, Tex) AcrySof SA 60 and Monarch II (Alcon) delivery system, which can be injected completely into the capsular bag through a 3.0-mm incision. This lens material is especially useful in younger patients because it

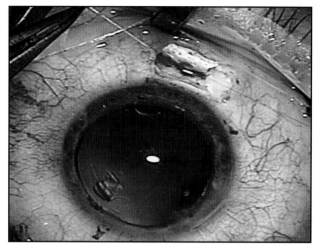

**Figure 4-8.** The 9.0 Prolene suture is tightened and a temporary knot tied, centering and stabilizing the capsular bag.

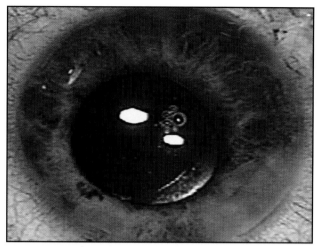

**Figure 4-9.** The single-piece acrylic PCIOL is centered within the capsular bag at the end of the procedure.

does not elicit a significant inflammatory response and because it has a low rate of posterior capsule opacification.[18-21]

Once the PCIOL is in place, the temporary knot is released and a permanent knot is tied with just enough tension to center the IOL. The knot can then be rotated beneath the sclera, or simply buried beneath the scleral flap. If the 2-hook model (2-L) is used, the fixation site for each hook must be ascertained by displacing each hook to the scleral wall prior to suturing. Depending on the size of the capsular bag, the best centration may be obtained with the hooks less than 180 degrees apart. Viscoelastic is removed manually through the side-port incision or with an automated irrigation/aspiration handpiece. Miochol is instilled to ensure that the pupil rounds. Conjunctiva is reapproximated over the scleral flap and the corneal incision is hydrated and checked to be certain that it is watertight (Figure 4-9).

# COMPLICATIONS AND MANAGEMENT

If vitreous presents at any time during the procedure, it should be carefully and completely removed from the anterior chamber. We have developed a technique using Kenalog (Alcon) (triamcinolone suspension) to identify vitreous in the anterior chamber.[22] Kenalog is injected into the anterior chamber where they become imbedded in the vitreous gel. The white suspension provides the surgeon better visualization of the location and the extent of prolapsed vitreous, allowing for a more thorough anterior vitrectomy (Figure 4-10). It also allows for the surgeon to observe the vitreous behavior and avoid maneuvers that increase vitreous traction or prolapse.

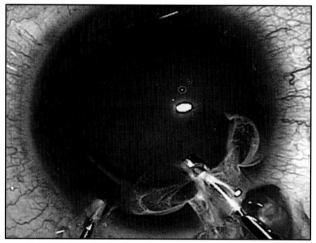

**Figure 4-10.** Demonstrates Kenalog-assisted anterior vitrectomy. Note how the Kenalog particles highlight the location and extent of vitreous prolapse, as well as the movement of the vitreous to the vitrector.

Before injecting Kenalog into the anterior chamber we exchange the preservative-containing vehicle of Kenalog for BSS. To remove the preservative, Kenalog suspension is prepared exactly as follows. Withdraw 0.2 ml of well shaken Kenalog (40mg/ml) into a tuberculin syringe. Replace the needle with a 5-μm syringe filter (Sherwood Medical). The plunger is then depressed forcing the suspension into the 5-μm filter, allowing the vehicle to pass through, yet capturing the Kenalog particles. The filter is then transferred to a 6-ml syringe containing 2 ml of BSS. The plunger is depressed causing the BSS to rinse through the filter and the Kenalog. Without removing the filter from the syringe, a 22-gauge needle is placed on the distal end of the filter, and approximately 5 ml of BSS is drawn up into the syringe, resuspending the Kenalog. The syringe is inverted several times to ensure thorough resuspension and washing of the Kenalog particles. The plunger is then depressed, expressing all of the fluid through the filter and re-capturing the Kenalog particles. Finally, 2 ml of BSS is drawn into the syringe through the filter to resuspend the Kenalog particles. The filter is removed and the washed Kenalog suspension is transferred to a sterile 3-ml syringe. Before injecting the washed Kenalog the syringe must be inverted several times to ensure thorough suspension. The Kenalog is then injected into the anterior chamber through a 27-gauge cannula.

Small amounts of vitreous can be removed by using a "dry" vitrectomy technique with an automated vitrector and an anterior chamber filled with viscoelastic.[23] Significant vitreous prolapse is best handled by Kenalog-assisted bimanual vitrectomy. After injecting Kenalog into the anterior chamber, a side-port incision can be used for irrigation with a 25-gauge cannula. The vitrectomy handpiece can be inserted through the initial incision or through a pars plana sclerotomy.[24]

CTRs and MCTRs of any model should not be used if a complete continuous capsulorrhexis is not attained or if a posterior capsule tear occurs since the expansile forces may cause the capsular bag to rupture. In such a case, the surgeon may choose to suture the IOL to the iris or to the scleral wall. Alternatively, an anterior chamber IOL can be implanted.

# CONCLUSION

The CTR has been FDA approved; however, the MCTR has not yet been approved by the FDA. These devices afford us the possibility of saving the capsular bag, recentering the capsular bag and even placing a PCIOL within the capsular bag. This surgery can be performed through a 3.0-mm incision, giving the patient a rapid visual recovery. This is most important in young children, as prolonged visual deprivation could result in dense amblyopia.

At the time of this writing, the CTR and MCTR are not yet FDA approved for use in the United States despite their widespread availability throughout the rest of the world. While these newer devices have improved the operative management of zonular weakness, the surgeon must be familiar with each of these advanced surgical techniques since these cases represent some of the most difficult procedures that we encounter. Yet skilled and knowledgeable management will usually result in a satisfying outcome for both the patient and his surgeon.

# REFERENCES

1. Jensen AD, Cross HE. Surgical treatment of dislocated lenses in Marfan's syndrome and homocystinuria. *Trans Am Acad Ophthalmol Otolaryngol.* 1972;76:1491-1499.

2. Varga B. The results of my operations improving visual acuity of ectopia lentis. *Ophthalmologica.* 1971;162:98-110.

3. Maumenee IH. The eye in Marfan's syndrome. *Trans Am Acad Ophthalmol Soc.* 1981;79: 684-733.

4. Straatsma BR, Allen RA, Pettit TH, Michael MO. Subluxation of the lens with iris photocoagulation. *Am J Ophthalmol.* 1966;61:1312-1324

5. Cionni RJ, Osher RH. Management of zonular dialysis with the endocapsular ring. *J Cataract Refract Surg.* 1995;21:245-249.

6. Cionni RJ, Osher RH. Management of profound zonular dialysis or weakness with a new endocapsular ring designed for scleral fixation. *J Cataract Refract Surg.* 1998;24:1299-1306.

7. Zetterstrom C, Lundvall A, Weeber Jr H, Jeeves M. Sulcus fixation without capsular support in children. *J Cataract Refract Surg.* 1999;25:776-781.

8. Dick HB, Augustin AJ. Lens implant selection with absence of capsular support. *Curr Opin Ophthalmol.* 2001;12(1):47-57.

9. Menezo JL, Martinez MC, Cisneros AL. Iris-fixated Worst claw versus sulcus-fixated posterior chamber lenses in the absence of capsular support. *J Cataract Refract Surg.* 1996;22(10):1476-84.

10. Hara T, Hara T, Yamada Y. "Equator ring" for maintenance of the completely circular contour of the capsular bag equator after cataract removal. *Ophthalmic Surg.* 1991;22:358-359

11. Legler U, Witschel B, et al. The capsular tension ring, a new device for complicated cataract surgery. Presented at the *Amer Soc Cataract Refract Surg.* Seattle, Wa: May 1993.

12. Osher RH. *Video journal of cataract and refractive surgery.* 1997;8:1.

13. Pfeifer V. Video presentation at the American Society of Cataract and Refractive Surgery. San Diego, Calif: April 1998.

14. Merriam J, Zheng L. Iris hooks for phacoemulsification of the subluxated lens. *J Cataract Refract Surg.* 1997;23:1295.

15. Maloney WF. Supracapsular phaco: achieving greater efficiency with phaco outside of the capsular bag: a 3-year experience. Presented at the American Society of Cataract and Refractive Surgery. Seattle, Wa: April 1999.

16. Osher RH. Slow motion phacoemulsification approach (Letter). *J Cataract Refract Surg.* 1993;19:667.

17. Cionni RJ, Osher RH. Complications of phacoemulsification. In: Weinstock FJ, ed, *Management and care of the cataract patient.* Cambridge, MA: Blackwell Scientific Publications Inc; 1992;209-210.

18. Hollick EJ, Spalton DJ, Ursell PG, Pande MV. Biocompatibility of poly(methylmethacrylate), silicone, and AcrySof intraocular lenses: randomized comparison of the cellular reaction on the anterior lens surface. *J Cataract Refract Surg.* 1998;24:361-366.

19. Ursell PG, Spalton DJ, et al. Relationship between intraocular lens biomaterials and posterior capsule opacification. *J Cataract Refract Surg.* 1998;24:352-360.

20. Linnola RJ, et al. Adhesion of fibronectin, vitronectin, laminin, and collagen type IV to intraocular lens materials in pseudophakic human autopsy eyes: part 1 histological sections. *J Cataract Refract Surg.* 2000;26:1792-1806.

21. Linnola RJ. Adhesion of fibronectin, vitronectin, laminin, and collagen type IV to intraocular lens materials in pseudophakic human autopsy eyes: part 2 explanted intraocular lenses. *J Cataract Refract Surg.* 2000;26:1807-1818.

22. Burk SE, Da Mata AP. Visualizing vitreous using Kenalog suspension. *J Cataract Refract Surg.* In press.

23. Osher RH. Dry vitrectomy. *Video J Cataract Refract Surg.* 1992;8(4).

24. Snyder ME, Cionni RJ, Osher RH. Management of intraoperative complications. In: Gills JP, ed, *Cataract Surgery: The State of the Art.* Thorofare, NJ: SLACK Incorporated; 1998: 149-152.

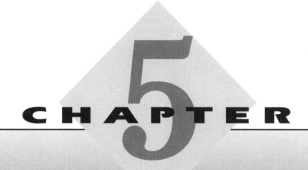

# CHAPTER 5

# CATARACT WITH DISLOCATED AND SUBLUXATED LENSES

*Steve Charles, MD*

Over 2 million cataract surgery procedures are performed in the United States every year and approximately 98% are said to be successful. Although most papers suggest that the incidence of anterior vitrectomy in cataract surgery is 1%, there are approximately 5 anterior vitrectomy packs sold for every 100 phacoemulsification packs. This data suggest that at least 100,000 cases of capsule rupture and anterior vitrectomy in the United States occur every year. It is likely that this number is similar to occurrence rates outside the United States.[1]

Business publications today emphasize the need for focus to achieve better performance. It is the author's contention that many surgeons place as much focus on operating time, incision size, and emmetropia as on prevention of capsular rupture. Even more critically, there appears to be more emphasis on prevention of posterior dislocation of lens material than on iatrogenic retinal detachment. There is no credible evidence that posterior dislocation of lens material causes *any* mechanical damage to the retina. This is even true for dense, "sharp," nuclear fragments. Damage to the retina in these cases is caused by inappropriate approaches used to remove lens material and because of less than ideal vitrectomy methods. Clearly, retinal detachment is a more serious complication than posterior dislocation of lens material.

## PREVENTION OF CAPSULAR RUPTURE

Flow limiting using systems like the Alcon (Fort Worth, Tex) MicroFlare ABS as well as cortical cleaving hydrodissection decrease capsular rupture rates during phaco procedures. The new Alcon silicone-tipped I/A tools appear to significantly reduce capsular incursion during cortical cleanup.

## TIMING OF INTERVENTION

Lens material may cause inflammation and/or phacolytic glaucoma if the material is left in place for an extended period. This is not an argument for instant or emergency surgery to remove dislocated lens material. Timing can be nearly as important as technique with respect to surgical outcomes. Posterior vitrectomy requires excellent visualization to produce optimal outcomes. Striate keratopathy, corneal edema, and pupillary miosis are often present intraoperatively and for 1 to 2 weeks after complicated cataract surgery. Waiting until the cornea is clearer and the pupil is able to be dilated is a better approach than chasing lens material around the vitreous cavity at the time of cataract surgery. Similarly, it is better to wait for a few days or even weeks until the cornea

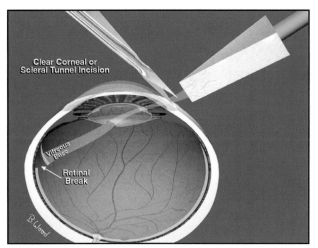

**Figure 5-1.** Cellulose sponges to remove vitreous means substantial pulling on the vitreous, which can cause retinal breaks and subsequent a retinal detachment.

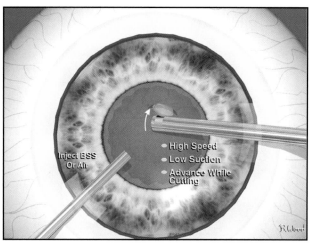

**Figure 5-2.** Vitreous cutters should always be used with the highest cutting rates to reduce vitreoretinal traction. Low suction and advancement of the probe while cutting works best.

clears to remove posteriorly dislocated lens material. If severe inflammation or significant phacolytic glaucoma presents the surgeon should proceed with vitrectomy.

# ANTERIOR VITRECTOMY

Cellulose sponge vitrectomy was a major contribution when introduced over 30 years ago but has been overused for over 2 decades. Cellulose sponges remove vitreous via a wick-like mechanism, which means that substantial pulling on the vitreous occurs even before it is lifted to cut it with the scissors (Figure 5-1). Many surgeons use the term "simple anterior vitrectomy," but the reality is that anterior vitreous fibers are firmly attached to the peripheral retina at the vitreous base. The peripheral retina has 1/100 the tensile strength of the posterior retina. There is nothing simple about a procedure that can cause retinal breaks and subsequent retinal detachment.

It is a common misconception that vitrectomy causes inflammation when, in fact, eyes undergoing total pars plana vitrectomy have virtually no postoperative inflammation. The inflammation associated with anterior vitrectomy is primarily caused by mechanical trauma to the iris from the hydrated sponge as it is withdrawn through the pupil. Cellulose fibers are often seen on the anterior vitreous after sponge vitrectomy raising the question of inflammation from retained material.

The so-called Charles sleeve is an obsolete device for anterior vitrectomy because it causes turbulent flow because of proximity between inflow and outflow. Using a sideport for injection of air during vitrectomy avoids turbulent flow. A soft eye can lead to suprachoroidal hemorrhage; therefore a viscoelastic, BSS, or air must be injected. Air is the best infusate choice because the interface between vitreous and

viscoelastics is invisible and BSS causes hydration of the vitreous. Injecting air through a second incision keeps the anterior vitreous back via surface tension and prevents vitreous strands from being incarcerated in the wound.

Sweeping the wound for vitreous with a spatula causes unacceptable vitreoretinal traction and should be avoided. The focus should be on retinal detachment prevention; not just vitreous in the wound. Mechanized anterior vitrectomy using air infusion through the sideport is very effective at eliminating vitreous from the wound.

Vitreous cutters should always be used with the highest possible cutting rates to reduce vitreoretinal traction. High cutting rates reduce pressure variation per port open-close cycle and prevent uncut vitreous from being pulled through the port (Figure 5-2). Higher cutting rates also limit sudden flow through the port like the Alcon Legacy MicroFlare ABS phaco tip. Flow limiting is crucial when using the vitreous cutter to remove lens material or scar tissue. When dense tissue elastically deforms through the port, it is followed by a flow surge that can cause retinal breaks. Using the lowest vacuum or flow rate that will effectively remove vitreous reduces vitreoretinal traction and the likelihood of retinal breaks and detachment. Moving the port away from vitreous while vacuum is applied also creates traction; it is better to advance the port toward the tissue anytime aspiration is applied.

# REMOVAL OF DISLOCATED LENS MATERIAL

The phacoemulsification probe should *never* be used to remove lens material anywhere in the vitreous body or to

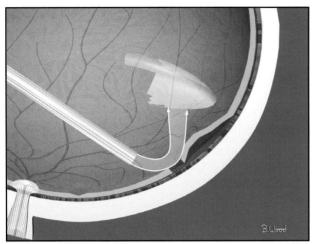

**Figure 5-3.** A jet of BSS can be used to wash the lens fragment into the anterior segment but it may cause a retinal detachment.

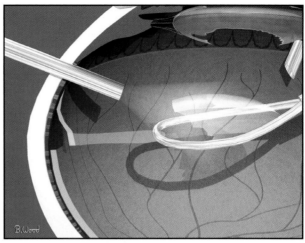

**Figure 5-4.** A lens loop can be used to "fish" the nucleus out of the vitreous but it causes significant vitreoretinal detachment.

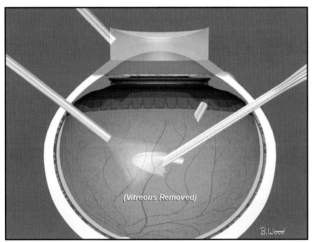

(Vitreous Removed)

**Figure 5-5.** All of the vitreous is removed except for the most peripheral vitreous before removing any lens material. An Accurus fragmenter is used to remove the nuclear material.

perform vitrectomy. Ultrasonic energy breaks up hyaluronic acid, giving the appearance of vitrectomy but it cannot safely cut vitreous collagen fibers.[2]

Some surgeons suggest using a jet of BSS to move the lens or nucleus into the anterior chamber when it becomes dislocated during cataract surgery. A jet of fluid can create experimental retinal detachments. Forceful irrigation of the vitreous cavity causes vitreoretinal traction even if the jet of fluid does not penetrate the retina (Figure 5-3).

Lens loops have been used by some surgeons to "fish" the nucleus or lens out of the vitreous. It can be readily seen that IOL haptics cause significant vitreoretinal traction when an attempt is made to reposition dislocated IOLs making it obvious that a lens loop will do the same (Figure 5-4).

Pars plana vitrectomy is the safest and most efficient method to remove dislocated lens material. It is essential to use the best possible visualization for this procedure. A fundus contact lens (hand-held or sew-on) or a wide angle system is absolutely necessary; an operating microscope can only focus to a point just behind the lens without an additional optical system. An indirect ophthalmoscope leaves only 1 hand free; therefore, modern day 3-port vitrectomy technique cannot be used. In addition, an inverted view is very difficult to learn which may lead to retinal damage. A fiberoptic endoilluminator is essential as it provides illumination without glare from light scattered and reflected light by the cornea and IOL.

It is essential to remove all except the most peripheral vitreous before removing *any* lens material. Trying to use vitreous to "support" lens material is unwise and increases the likelihood of vitreoretinal traction. It is better to allow lens material to fall posteriorly as the vitreous is removed. The Alcon (Fort Worth, Tex) Accurus fragmenter uses the same ultrasonics as the Legacy and is ideal to remove nuclear material after vitreous removal (Figure 5-5). Twenty-gauge fragmenters are best used with continuous aspiration to cool the needle, which is far more thermally efficient than trying to irrigate the needle externally. Continuous sonification coupled with continuous, proportionally controlled ultrasound energy is the most efficient and safe approach for removing lens material. A vacuum-only technique is used to pick up the lens material and then fragmenter power is applied and increased until lens material begins entering the port. If the fragmenter needle penetrates the lens, the endoilluminator can be used to push the lens material off the needle. This technique resembles 2-handed phacoemulsification. Alternatively, the endoilluminator can be used to crush a "speared" lens fragment in order to split the fragment or push it in the fragmenter port. Some surgeons have advocat-

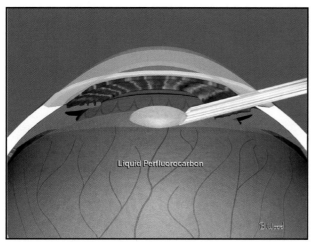

**Figure 5-6.** Perfluorocarbon liquid is used to float the lens material away from the retina so that the lens can be removed through the cataract wound.

ed using a phacoemulsification probe in the vitreous cavity but this requires a larger wound, causes greater turbulence, and has no advantages over the fragmenter.[3]

Perfluorocarbon liquids can be used to float lens material away from the retina but this step is unnecessary in most cases. A very dense nucleus can be floated up to the anterior chamber and removed through a cataract wound with a lens loop, cohesive viscoelastic, or vectis (Figure 5-6).

## SUBLUXATED LENSES

In most instances it is safer to remove all vitreous except that in close proximity to the vitreous base before removing a subluxated lens. Often the remaining zonules will create a hinge, causing the lens to swing down against the peripheral retina when the patient is supine and the vitreous has been removed. Extreme care must be taken to avoid creating vitreous base traction when the lens is near peripheral retina. Careful removal of vitreous around the lens can facilitate severing the remaining zonules in a controlled fashion. It is desirable to create posterior dislocation of the lens so it can be removed with the fragmenter without causing a peripheral retinal traction and retinal breaks.

## CONCLUSION

The goal of this chapter is to emphasize safe vitrectomy techniques and methods to remove lens material that becomes dislocated posteriorly during cataract surgery. Retinal detachment prevention should be the focus of these efforts rather than rapid removal of lens material. The time is now to eliminate unsafe, cellulose sponge vitrectomy in this world of high-tech, sophisticated small incision cataract surgery.

## REFERENCES

1. Al-Khaier A, Wong D. Determinants of visual outcome after pars plana vitrectomy for posteriorly dislocated lens fragments in phacoemulsification. *J Cataract Refract Surg.* 2001;27(8):1199-206.

2. Hutton WL, Snyder WB. Management of surgically dislocated intravitreal lens fragments by pars plana vitrectomy. *Ophthalmology.* 1978;85(2):176-89.

3. Mittra RA, Connor TB. Removal of dislocated intraocular lenses using pars plana vitrectomy with placement of an open-loop, flexible anterior chamber lens. *Ophthalmology.* 1998;105(6):1011-4.

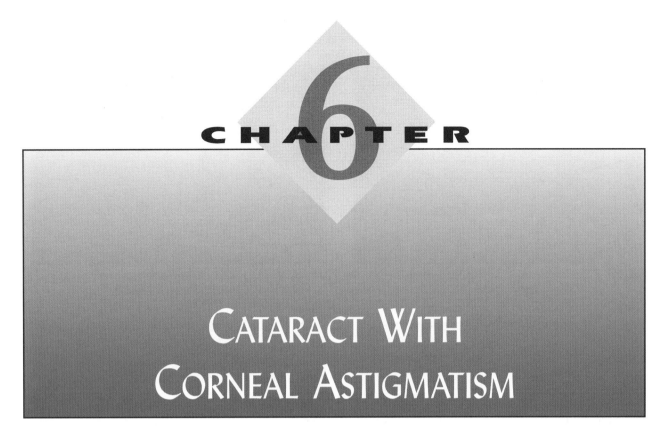

# CHAPTER 6

# CATARACT WITH CORNEAL ASTIGMATISM

*Harry B. Grabow, MD*

## INTRODUCTION

As anterior segment ophthalmic surgeons, we have come to realize—as we exit the 20th century and enter the 21st century (and a new millennium)—that any surgery we perform on the anterior segment will now be judged by doctor and patient alike according to the refractive outcome. Be it corneal, lenticular, or glaucoma surgery, we now include in our surgical planning the refractive consequences of our procedures and the refractive options available to us. Thus, a glaucoma surgeon who performs combined phacotrabeculectomy through a superior incision and consistently induces against-the-rule cylinder change may now consider the options of LRIs, astigmatic keratotomy, or toric IOL with these procedures. Increasingly, cataract and refractive surgeons are having to remove lenses in eyes that have had previous keratorefractive surgery. Not only is implant power calculation technology evolving for these eyes, but correction of residual or induced astigmatism must now be considered, as well as surgical planning so as not to induce new astigmatism in an eye that was previously made emmetropic by a keratorefractive procedure. The only area of concern that may require secondary (or tertiary) surgical intervention is that of induced irregular astigmatism. Jorge Alio reported an incidence of up to 5% of induced irregular astigmatism following LASIK[1]; other studies have reported up to 13% inci-

dence. These eyes may come to wavefront-guided custom corneal ablation following a phaco-IOL procedure. In this chapter, I will address methods and techniques for achieving astigmatism reduction as it relates to lens replacement surgery, either cataract or refractive clear lens exchange.

## ASTIGMATISM

Astigmatism may be classified as either corneal or lenticular. Posterior (scleral-choroidal-retinal) astigmatism has never been classified, but may be a consideration in the future. An eye with a spherical cornea that demonstrates refractive cylinder has been believed to have "lenticular astigmatism," but is never known for certain until the lens is removed and replaced with a spherical IOL. Eyes with posterior staphylomata or retinal elevation from some pathologic process may have posterior astigmatism, which may or may not be refractively correctable by an anterior technique. This form of astigmatism still remains elusive to diagnosis; however, it may be suspected in eyes with spherical corners and spherical IOLs if demonstrated by wavefront technology. Custom laser keratorefractive surgery may be able to neutralize these astigmatic aberrations.

Lenticular astigmatism may, therefore, be defined as refractive astigmatism with a spherical cornea and without

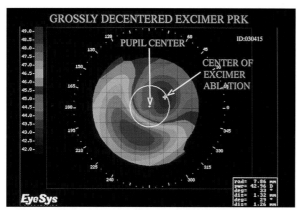

**Figure 6-1.** A topographic example of irregular corneal astigmatism. (Courtesy of EyeSys Vision, Inc.)

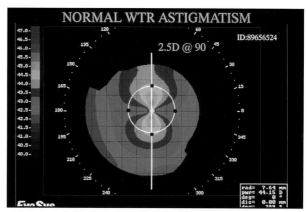

**Figure 6-2.** A topographic example of symmetric corneal astigmatism. (Courtesy of EyeSys Vision, Inc.)

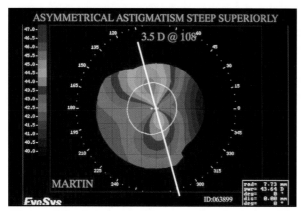

**Figure 6-3.** A topographic example of asymmetric corneal astigmatism. (Courtesy of EyeSys Vision, Inc.)

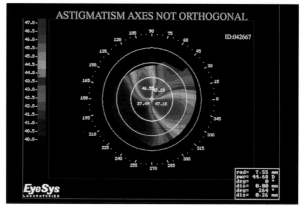

**Figure 6-4.** A topographic example of non-orthogonal corneal astigmatism. (Courtesy of EyeSys Vision, Inc.)

posterior pathology. In this situation, simple lens removal and replacement with a spherical IOL, assuming an astigmatically neutral incision, will correct the pre-existing astigmatism. Corneal astigmatism is further classified as regular versus irregular (Figure 6-1); and regular astigmatism is further subclassified as symmetric (Figure 6-2) versus asymmetric (Figure 6-3) and orthogonal versus nonorthogonal (Figure 6-4). These classifications may only become apparent following corneal topography. Keratometry alone, usually measuring the central 3 mm of the corneal apex, cannot detect or demonstrate asymmetric or nonorthogonal astigmatism, and this can affect the refractive outcome of anterior segment surgery. Therefore, if corneal modulation is to be included in anterior segment surgical planning, corneal topography must be available to the surgeon. Newer technology, such as Orbscan (Bausch & Lomb, Rochester, NY) evaluation of corneal thickness and the posterior corneal surface can provide even more valuable information. The value of wavefront aberrometry, in addition, may provide even more detailed information, which, regarding lenticular surgery, is just beginning to be studied.

# INCISIONAL CORRECTION OF ASTIGMATISM

Astigmatic keratotomy (AK) was first successfully performed in Moscow by Svyatoslav Fyodorov[2] (Figure 6-5) in the 1970s, originally combined with radial keratotomy for the correction of myopia (Figure 6-6). AK was further developed in the United States in the 1980s as straight tangential incisions, *T cuts*, by Spencer Thornton (Figure 6-7) and as arcuate incisions by Thornton,[3] Lindstrom,[4,5] and others[6,7] (Figure 6-8). The CRIs were then moved to the limbus[8] in the 1990's, and nomograms were developed for these by Gills (Figure 6-9) and Nichamin[9] (Figure 6-10). An elaborate system of AK was developed by Oliveira of Brazil[10] to reduce the incidence of a phenomenon he called *keratopyramis* (Figure 6-11) and attempt to produce a more spherical cornea.

When planning incisional correction of astigmatism, the surgeon must determine how many incisions are necessary, at what axis (or axes), at what optical zone(s) (distance from

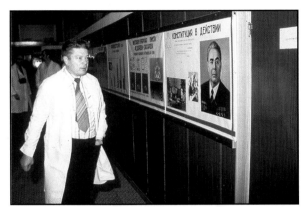

**Figure 6-5.** Svyatoslav Fyodorov, Moscow 1981. (Courtesy of Richard J. Knox.)

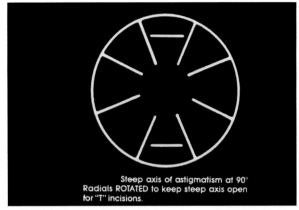

Steep axis of astigmatism at 90°
Radials ROTATED to keep steep axis open
for "T" incisions.

**Figure 6-6.** Diagram of typical 8-incision RK combined with straight tangential ("T cuts") AK for incisional correction of myopia with with-the-rule astigmatism.

the corneal apex), what shape, what length, and what depth. These decisions are based on how much cylinder is present, as determined by keratometry; at what axis, as determined by topography; at what depth, as determined by pachymetry (or empirically); and according to the patient's age. The older the patient, the greater is the effect of incisional keratotomy.

In addition, what effect will the phacoemulsification incision have on the corneal curvature? Can the phacoemulsification incision be used to reduce preexisting astigmatism?[11] A scleral-pocket incision (SPI), being farther from the cornea, has less effect on altering corneal curvature than do limbal and clear corneal incisions (CCI). In addition, the shape of the scleral incision also determines its effect on corneal curvature (Figure 6-12). A curved limbus-parallel SPI will cause more flattening at that meridian than a straight incision; and the *frown*[12] or *suspension-bridge*[13] curved SPI has even less effect and may be *astigmatically neutral*. However, either a straight or a limbus-parallel SPI, because each flattens the cornea at the meridian of placement, can be used to reduce up to approximately 2.00 D of astigmatism, depending on the patient's age. An even greater effect can be obtained with a clear-corneal incision. Using CCIs *on-axis* to reduce astigmatism was popularized by Gills.[14]

The clear-corneal phaco incision can be constructed in two ways, and each can have a slightly different effect on corneal curvature.[12] If the CCI is made as a 3.2-mm, 1-step single-plane stab incision (Figure 6-13), it will flatten the cornea usually no more than 0.37 D, and only in that hemimeridian. If a 2-step, biplane, grooved CCI is made (Figure 6-14), the vertical groove can act as an LRI and cause more flattening, up to about 1.25 D, depending on the patient's age. Additionally, the length of the limbal arc groove and the depth are variables. The length may be up to 12 mm, according to some LRI nomograms. The depth may vary from 300 μm to 600 μm, as suggested by Langerman.[16] The deeper the groove, the more flattening of the adjacent cornea (Figure 6-15).

Both the phacoemulsification incision and an AK or LRI can be used in combination to reduce higher degrees of corneal astigmatism. For example, a moderate degree of against-the-rule (ATR) astigmatism may be corrected with a temporal grooved CCI combined with a nasal AK or LRI. Performing lens surgery with this combination of incisions, a grooved CCI and an opposing AK or LRI, has been called *keratolenticuloplasty* by Kershner.[17,18]

Instrumentation for incisional keratotomy progressed through the years as the technology advanced. In the beginning, straight incisions were made with razor blade fragments held in special in instruments called *blade holders*. The amount of blade exposure was measured on a metal ruler (Figure 6-16). Metal blades are manufactured today with blade exposures preset at the factory determined by a metal footplate or guard (Oasis Medical, Glendora, Calif). They can be used for on-corneal AK or for the limbal groove of a CCI. Terry designed a metal-blade astigmatome (Oasis) (Figure 6-17), which has 1 or 2 metal blades set at fixed exposures designed to make reproducible accurate AKs by manual rotation of the trephine-like astigmatome (Figure 6-18). For those with an unlimited surgical equipment budget, Rhein manufactures an automated suction trephine designed by Jorg Krumeich in Germany[16] called the guided trephine system (GTS) (Figures 6-19 and 6-20). This vacuum trephine was originally designed for penetrating keratoplasty for front-cutting of both the donor and host corneal buttons. The instrument works like a LASIK microkeratome, obtaining purchase by vacuum-suction and using a rotating blade system. Another precise instrument for arcuate keratotomy is the Hanna arcitome (Moria, France)[19,20] (Figure 6-21), which has diamond blades and the ability for the blades to translate forward and backward for incision redeepening.

Many surgeons performing CCI phacoemulsification today use diamond blades for their incisions and diamond blades for their AKs or LRIs. It has become the preference of this surgeon to perform on-corneal straight-T 3-mm AKs using the Feaster diamond blade (Rhein, Tampa, Fla)

## THORNTON NOMOGRAM FOR ASTIGMATIC KERATOTOMY -
### (Must be corrected for actual age, intraocular pressure and other modifiers)

### CYLINDER CORRECTED BY PAIRED STRAIGHT TRANSVERSE INCISIONS

| Target | Length of One Pair Transverse Incisions at 7 mm OZ |
|--------|------------------------|
| 0.50 D | 1.3 mm |
| 0.75 D | 1.5 mm |
| 1.00 D | 1.7 mm |
| 1.25 D | 1.8 mm |
| 1.50 D | 2.1 mm |
| 1.75 D | 2.3 mm |
| 2.00 D | 2.5 mm |
| 2.25 D | 2.7 mm |

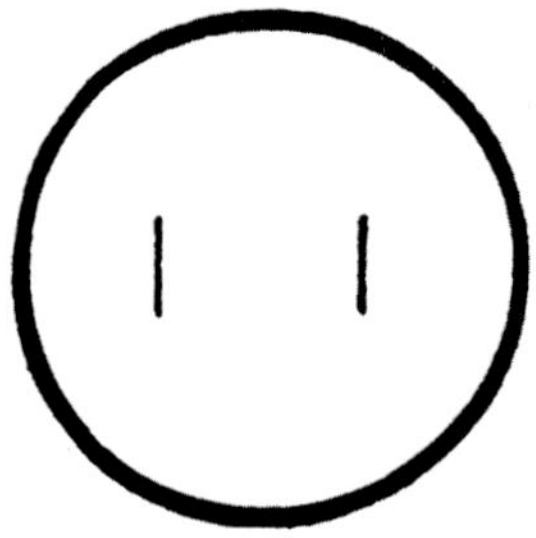

| Target | Length of Two Pair Transverse Incisions | |
|--------|---------|---------|
|        | 6 mm OZ | 8 mm OZ |
| 2.00 D | 1.3 mm | 1.7 mm |
| 2.25 D | 1.5 mm | 2.0 mm |
| 2.50 D | 1.7 mm | 2.3 mm |
| 2.75 D | 1.9 mm | 2.6 mm |
| 3.00 D | 2.1 mm | 2.9 mm |
| 3.25 D | 2.3 mm | 3.2 mm |
| 3.50 D | 2.5 mm | 3.4 mm |
| 3.75 D | 2.7 mm | 3.6 mm |

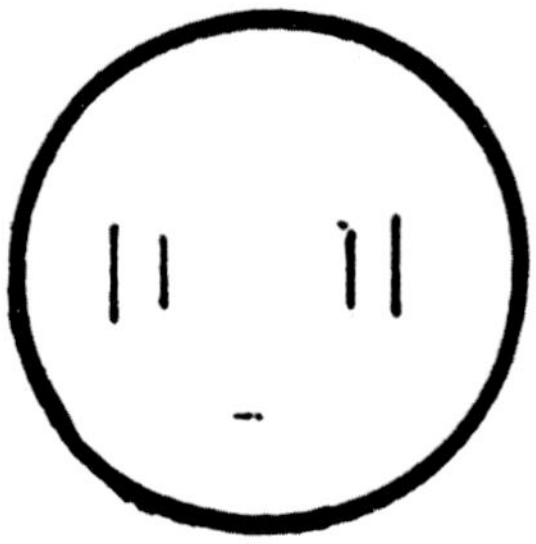

| Target | Length of Three Pair Transverse Incisions | | |
|--------|---------|---------|---------|
|        | 6 mm OZ | 7 mm OZ | 8 mm OZ |
| 3.25 D | 1.3 mm | 1.5 mm | 1.7 mm |
| 3.50 D | 1.5 mm | 1.8 mm | 2.0 mm |
| 3.75 D | 1.8 mm | 2.1 mm | 2.3 mm |
| 4.00 D | 2.0 mm | 2.3 mm | 2.6 mm |
| 4.25 D | 2.3 mm | 2.6 mm | 2.9 mm |
| 4.50 D | 2.5 mm | 2.9 mm | 3.2 mm |
| 4.75 D | 2.7 mm | 3.1 mm | 3.5 mm |
| 5.00 D | 2.9 mm | 3.3 mm | 3.7 mm |

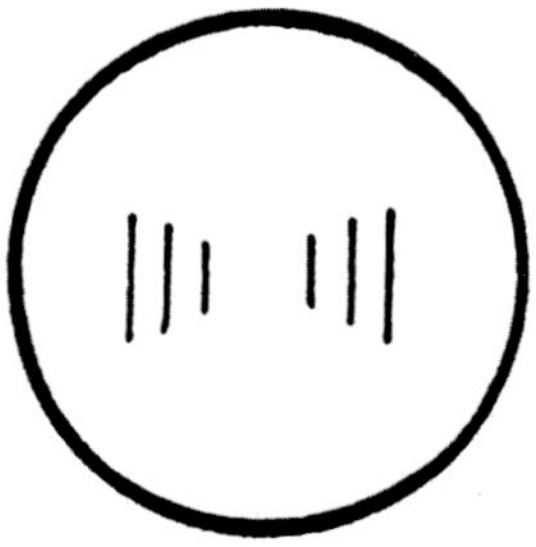

**Smaller OZ (5.5 mm to 7.5 mm) → 0.5 D to 1.0 D more**

**Figure 6-7.** Nomograms for correcting symmetric corneal astigmatism using straight ("T cuts") AK incisions. (Reprinted with permission from Thornton SP. Theory behind corneal relaxing incisions/Thornton nomogram. In: Gills JP, Martin RG, Sanders DR, eds. *Sutureless Cataract Surgery*. Thorofare, NJ: SLACK Incorporated. 1992;123-143.)

## CYLINDER CORRECTED BY PAIRED ARCUATE TRANSVERSE INCISIONS

### Chord Length of One Pair Arcuate Transverse Incisions

| Target | Degrees Arc | 7 mm OZ |
|--------|-------------|---------|
| 0.50 D | 20° | 1.2 mm |
| 0.75 D | 23° | 1.3 mm |
| 1.00 D | 25° | 1.5 mm |
| 1.25 D | 28° | 1.7 mm |
| 1.50 D | 32° | 1.9 mm |
| 1.75 D | 35° | 2.1 mm |
| 2.00 D | 38° | 2.3 mm |
| 2.25 D | 42° | 2.5 mm |
| 2.50 D | 45° | 2.7 mm |

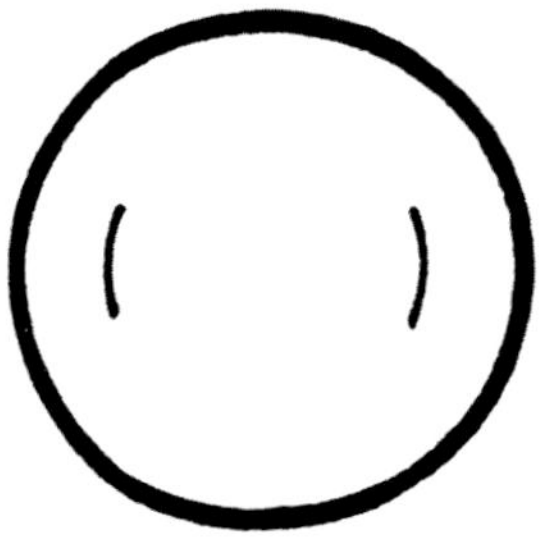

### Chord Length of Two Pair Arcuate Transverse Incisions

| Target | Degrees Arc | 6 mm OZ | 8 mm OZ |
|--------|-------------|---------|---------|
| 2.00 D | 23° | 1.2 mm | 1.5 mm |
| 2.25 D | 27° | 1.4 mm | 1.8 mm |
| 2.50 D | 31° | 1.6 mm | 2.0 mm |
| 2.75 D | 35° | 1.8 mm | 2.3 mm |
| 3.00 D | 39° | 2.0 mm | 2.6 mm |
| 3.25 D | 43° | 2.2 mm | 2.9 mm |
| 3.50 D | 47° | 2.4 mm | 3.1 mm |
| 3.75 D | 48° | 2.6 mm | 3.3 mm |

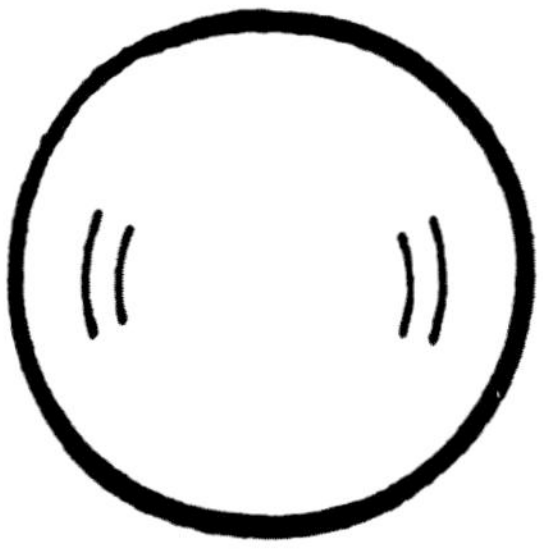

### Chord Length of Three Pair Arcuate Transverse Incisions

| Target | Degrees Arc | 6 mm OZ | 7 mm OZ | 8 mm OZ |
|--------|-------------|---------|---------|---------|
| 3.25 D | 22° | 1.1 mm | 1.3 mm | 1.5 mm |
| 3.50 D | 26° | 1.3 mm | 1.5 mm | 1.8 mm |
| 3.75 D | 30° | 1.5 mm | 1.8 mm | 2.1 mm |
| 4.00 D | 35° | 1.8 mm | 2.1 mm | 2.4 mm |
| 4.25 D | 40° | 2.0 mm | 2.4 mm | 2.7 mm |
| 4.50 D | 45° | 2.3 mm | 2.7 mm | 3.1 mm |
| 4.75 D | 50° | 2.5 mm | 3.0 mm | 3.4 mm |
| 5.00 D | 54° | 2.7 mm | 3.2 mm | 3.6 mm |

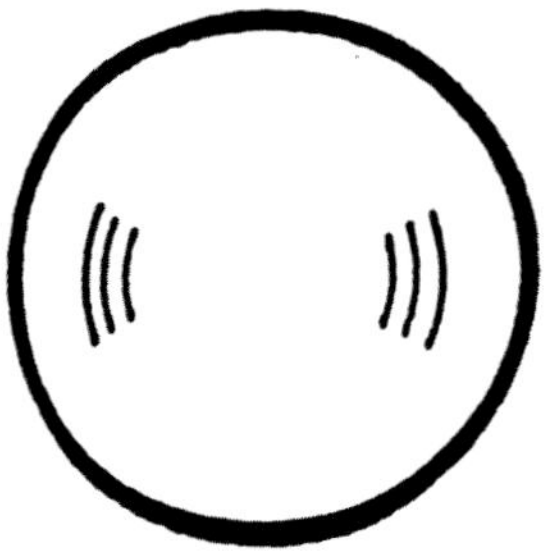

Smaller OZ (5.5 mm to 7.5 mm) → 0.50 D to 1.00 D more

**Figure 6-8.** Nomograms for correcting symmetric corneal astigmatism using arcuate AK incisions. (Reprinted with permission from Thornton SP. Theory behind corneal relaxing incisions/Thornton nomogram. In: Gills JP, Martin RG, Sanders DR, eds. *Sutureless Cataract Surgery*. Thorofare, NJ: SLACK Incorporated. 1992;123-143.)

# Correction of Astigmatism with Cataract Surgery

The following nomogram was developed for limbal relaxing incisions to correct astigmatism at the time of surgery. This nomogram applies to patients older than 73 years of age. Patients younger than 73 require longer incisions to achieve the same effect.

## LRI Nomogram (Modified Gills)

| CYL | LRI (mm) | # INC |
|------|----------|-------|
| 1.00 | 6 | 1 |
| 2.00 | 6 | 2 |
| 3.00 | 8 | 2 |
| 4.00 | 10 | 2 |
| 5.00 | 12 | 2 |

Blade setting: 600 microns for most patients.
(Exception: Blade setting of 500 microns for patients over 80 and for those with corneo-scleral thinning.)

**Figure 6-9.** Nomogram for correcting symmetric corneal astigmatism using LRI's. (Courtesy of Dr. James Gills.)

## ASTIGMATISM STRATEGY
## FOR
## CLEAR CORNEAL PHACO SURGERY

**NEUTRAL:** +0.75 X 90 ◄———————► +0.50 X 180

*"Neutral" temporal clear corneal incision*

**ATR (Steep Axis 0-30° / 150-180°):** Intraoperative keratoscopy determines exact incision location

Neutral temporal clear corneal plus:

| PRE-OP CYLINDER | | 30-50 yo | 51-70 yo | 71-85 yo | >85 yo |
|-----------------|--|----------|----------|----------|--------|
| +0.75 → +1.50 | nasal limbal arc = | 50° | 45° | 30° | – |
| +1.75 → +2.50 | *paired arcuate incisions = | 60° | 50° | 45° | 30° |
| +2.75 → +3.50 | *paired arcuate incisions = | 90° | 75° | 50° | 45° |
| +3.75 → +4.50 | *paired arcuate incisions = | reduce o.z. (i.e., 7.0 mm) | 90° | 75° | 60° |
| | | | degrees of arc to be incised | | |

*\*Temporal clear corneal incision followed by temporal and nasal peripheral arcuate incisions*

**WTR (Steep Axis 45°- 145°):** Intraoperative keratoscopy determines exact incision location

Neutral temporal clear corneal plus:

| PRE-OP CYLINDER | | 30-50 yo | 51-70 yo | 71-85 yo | >85 yo |
|-----------------|--|----------|----------|----------|--------|
| +1.00 → +1.75 | Paired limbal arcs on steep axis = | 40° | 35° | 30° | – |
| +2.00 → +2.75 | Paired limbal arcs on steep axis = | 60° | 50° | 45° | 30° |
| +3.00 → +3.75 | Paired limbal arcs on steep axis = | 75° | 60° | 50° | 40° |
| | | | degrees of arc to be incised | | |

**Figure 6-10.** Nomograms for correcting symmetric against-the-rule (ATR) and with-the-rule (WTR) corneal astigmatism. (Courtesy of Dr. Nichamin.)

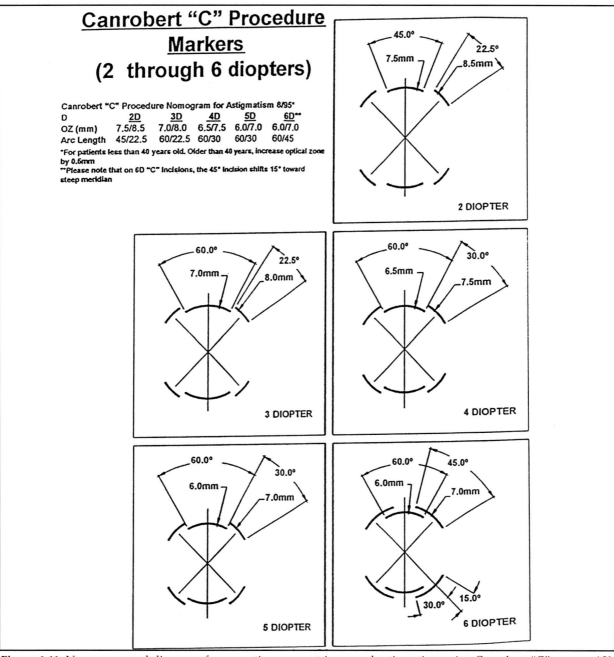

**Figure 6-11.** Nomogram and diagrams for correcting symmetric corneal astigmatism using Canrobert "C" arcuate AK. (Courtesy of Mastel.)

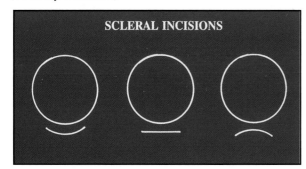

**Figure 6-12.** Limbus-parallel (left), straight (center), "frown" (right) scleral incisions.

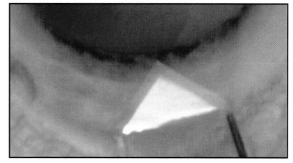

**Figure 6-13.** Single-plane 1-step clear-corneal incision with diamond blade. (Courtesy of Grabow.)

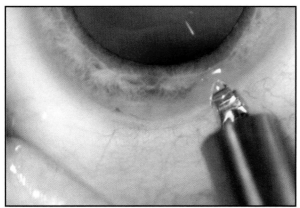

**Figure 6-14.** Groove LRI with guarded diamond blade as first step of 2-step biplane CCI. (Courtesy of Grabow.)

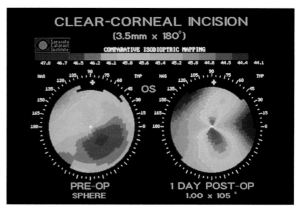

**Figure 6-15.** Flattening effect of temporal CCI as observed as the dark blue zone in the 1-day postoperative topography.

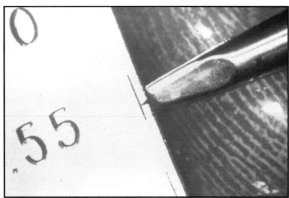

**Figure 6-16.** Setting metal blade exposure on metal gauge for incisional keratotomy as performed in the 1970's and 1980's.

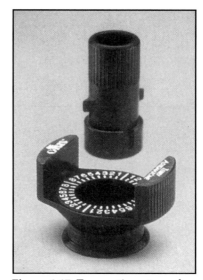

**Figure 6-17.** Terry astigmatome for metal-blade arcuate astigmatic keratotomy. (Courtesy of Oasis.)

## Terry Astigmatome - Nomogram

### WTR - 8mm OZ

| CYL | LRI | # INC |
| --- | --- | --- |
| 1.00 | 60° | 2 |
| 2.00 | 80° | 2 |
| 3.00 | 100° | 2 |

### ATR - 10mm OZ

| CYL | LRI | # INC |
| --- | --- | --- |
| 1.00 | 90° | 1 |
| 2.00 | 60° | 2 |
| 3.00 | 80° | 2 |
| 4.00 | 100° | 2 |

**Figure 6-18.** Nomograms for correcting for WTR and ATR corneal astigmatism using the Terry astigmatome.

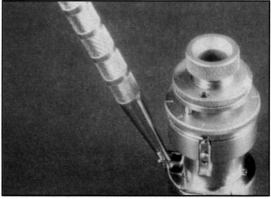

**Figure 6-19.** Krumeich Guided Trephine System (GTS) for vacuum astigmatic keratotomy and lamellar keratectomy. (Courtesy of Rhein.)

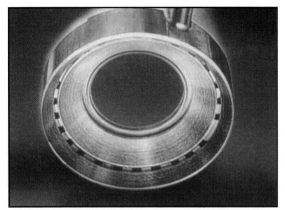

**Figure 6-20.** View of suctioning ports of Krumeich Guided Trephine System. (Courtesy of Rhein.)

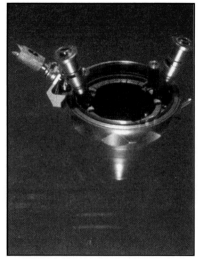

**Figure 6-21.** Hannah Arcitome for diamond-blade astigmatic keratotomy.

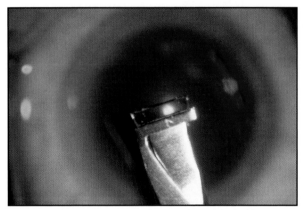

**Figure 6-22.** Feaster 3 mm diamond AK blade (Courtesy of Rhein) for straight T-cut astigmatic keratotomy.

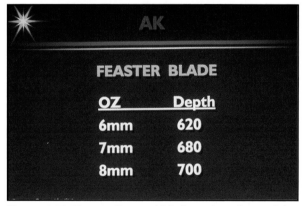

**Figure 6-23.** Feaster diamond blade settings for straight 3-mm astigmatic keratotomy. (Courtesy of Grabow.)

(Figure 6-22). This blade was designed by Fred Feaster and is 3 mm long and designed to be used by indentation rather than translation. It is not infrequently observed with translating keratotomy that an epithelial flap or abrasion may occur due to the toxic effects of topical medication, weak epithelial-basement membrane attachment, and/or the age of the typical cataract patient. The accuracy of free-hand arcuate keratotomy may also not be as consistent and reproducible as with the fixed-length indentation system. With every AK being 3 mm long, the length of the AK is no longer a factor in the surgical plan to reduce astigmatism. The optical zone, the axis, the number of AK incisions, and the blade exposure remain as factors to be determined. From personal experience, this surgeon has established a table of Feaster blade exposure settings related to optical zone sizes (Figure 6-23). Because indentation keratotomy pushes stroma ahead of the blade, incisions may be shallower than expected for the same exposure of a translating blade. Therefore, the empiric blade exposures for each optical zone are greater than would be used for translational keratotomy.

The Feaster system includes a Mendez axis gauge and optical zone markers (Figure 6-24). In addition, a Thornton

ring is available to stabilize the globe and create a more firm cornea during indentation keratotomy. The Feaster blade is then placed on the epithelial mark and rocked back-and-forth, heel-to-toe, allowing the blade to cut through Bowman's and stroma full-depth to the footplate (Figure 6-25). The blade is then simply withdrawn and the perfectly straight linear 3-mm AK can be observed without disturbance of the overlying epithelium. These AKs are usually performed at the beginning of surgery, before any incisions into the anterior chamber. In this way, the eye is more firm and there is no chance of the indentation pressure causing a wound leak or flat chamber. However, some surgeons prefer to perform AK at the end of the phacoemulsification procedure, either with viscoelastic still in the eye, or with the eye temporarily inflated to a firm IOP.

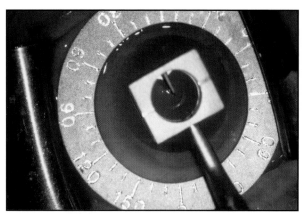

**Figure 6-24.** Mendez gauge and optical zone marker for Feaster diamond blade astigmatic keratotomy. (Courtesy of Rhein.)

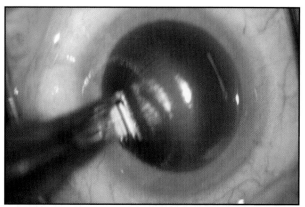

**Figure 6-25.** Feaster diamond blade indentation astigmatic keratotomy. (Courtesy of Grabow.)

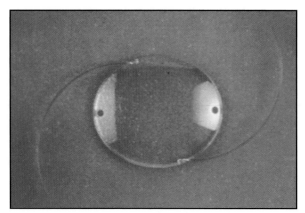

**Figure 6-26.** Three-piece PMMA toric IOL with 5.5- x 6.5-mm optic and 13.0-mm polypropylene haptics implanted by Shimizu (Nidek, Japan).

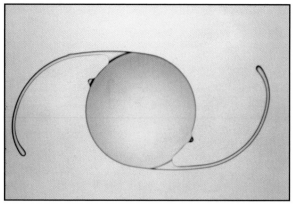

**Figure 6-27.** One-piece PMMA toric IOL with 5.25-mm optic and 12.5-mm haptics implanted by Shimizu (Nidek, Japan).

# Intraocular Correction of Astigmatism

The use of an intraocular lens (IOL) to correct a refractive error was first conceived and performed, as we know, for aphakia by Harold Ridley in England in 1949.[22] These first rigid PMMA lenses, and their subsequent foldable successors, were spherical models able to correct only the spherical component of refractive errors. In 1986, spherical phakic IOLs made their re-entry into the surgical arena,[23,24] after initial failure in the 1950's.[25-30] In the early 1990's toric aphakic IOL implantation began on 2 continents. In Japan, Kimiya Shimizu[31] began implantation with a 3-piece PMMA loop-haptic toric aphakic IOL manufactured by Nidek (Figure 6-26). This 3-piece loop-haptic design was shown to have rotated off axis 20 degrees or more in 30% of eyes. Shimizu later implanted a series of 1-piece loop-haptic all PMMA toric IOLs (Figure 6-27). Now, in the first decade of the new millennium, toric phakic IOL implantation has

begun, both with the Artisan iris-fixated lens (Ophtec, the Netherlands) and with the ICL (implantable contact lens [STAAR, Monrovia, Calif]) in the posterior chamber, first performed in Europe by Tobias Neuhann of Munich and in North America by Howard Gimbel[32] of Calgary.

In the same time period, the first foldable silicone toric IOLs were implanted in a STAAR Surgical FDA clinical trial. The first prototype lens to be studied, the STAAR AA4203T,[33] was a 1-piece plate-haptic TIOL with small 0.3 mm haptic fenestrations (Figure 6-28). This model was 10.8 mm in diagonal length and had a 2.25-D toric correction on 1 optic surface. The side of the optic with the toric correction was marked at the optic haptic junction with alignment marks and was designed to be placed anteriorly. The alignment marks were also used at surgery to aid the surgeon in aligning the long axis of the IOL with the steep axis of corneal curvature. They were also useful in allowing the surgeon to evaluate the IOL axis postoperatively. The 2.25 D of front-surface toric correction were shown to correct approximately 1.25 D of refractive cylinder at the spectacle plane. This length plate-haptic toric showed a rate of 8% off-axis

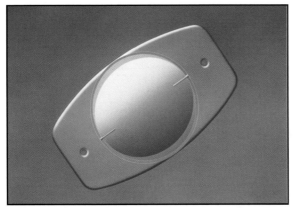

**Figure 6-28.** First-generation 1-piece silicone plate-haptic toric IOL with 0.03-mm haptic fenestrations (STAAR AA4203T).

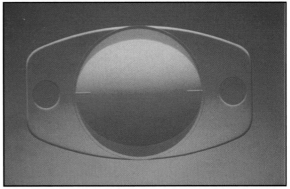

**Figure 6-29.** Second-generation 1-piece silicone plate-haptic toric IOL with 1.15-mm haptic fenestrations (STAAR AA4203TF).

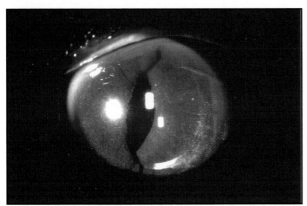

**Figure 6-30.** Anterior dislocation of one haptic of plate-haptic IOL. (Courtesy of Grabow.)

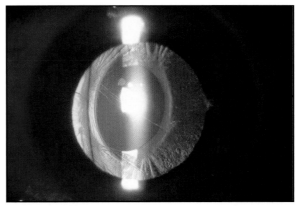

**Figure 6-31.** Short-axis decentration of a plate-haptic IOL. (Courtesy of Grabow.)

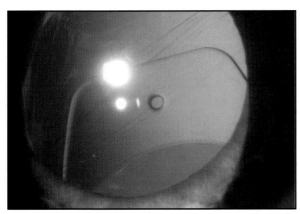

**Figure 6-32.** Subluxation of a plate-haptic IOL through unstable opening in posterior capsule. (Courtesy of Grabow.)

rotation of 30 degrees or greater. A subsequent model is now manufactured that is 11.2 mm long (STAAR AA4203TL) that is also available with 3.50 D of toric correction that corrects 2.25 to 3.00 of refractive cylinder. The longer length is designed to reduce the rate of off-axis rotation. In addition, the newer models have larger 1.15-mm haptic fenestrations

(Figure 6-29), designed to allow fibrotic fusion of the anterior and posterior lens capsules to prevent late post-YAG-capsulotomy IOL dislocation.

The technique of aphakic toric IOL implantation involves removing the lens nucleus and cortex through a small incision, usually 3.2 mm or less, and through an anterior continuous curvilinear capsulorrhexis (CCC) of 5.5 mm or less. It is not recommended to implant a plate haptic silicone IOL through an anterior CCC that is not continuous because late capsular fibrosis can cause anterior dislocation of one haptic (Figure 6-30) with subsequent optic decentration along the long axis of the IOL. Anterior CCC openings that are greater than the optic 6.0-mm diameter can allow anterior-posterior capsular fusion lateral to one side of the optic, which can result in optic decentration along the short axis of the IOL (Figure 6-31). It is also not recommended to implant a plate-haptic IOL in an eye with an unstable opening in the posterior capsule as subluxation (Figure 6-32) or posterior dislocation (Figure 6-33) may occur; a stable posterior CCC may be implanted.

The steep corneal axis may be marked prior to surgery in several ways. Some surgeons use a sterile gentian violet marking pen to mark the limbus, either using a reticle in a slit

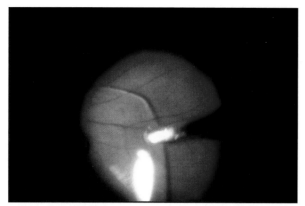

**Figure 6-33.** Total posterior dislocation of a plate-haptic IOL through unstable opening in posterior capsule.

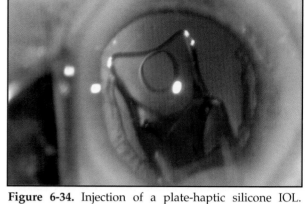

**Figure 6-34.** Injection of a plate-haptic silicone IOL. (Courtesy of Grabow.)

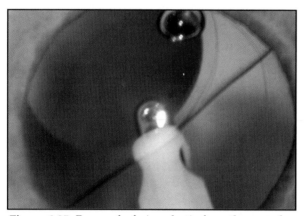

**Figure 6-35.** Removal of viscoelastic from the capsular bag with the irrigation-aspiration tip behind the plate-haptic IOL. (Courtesy of Grabow.)

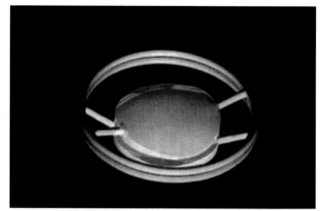

**Figure 6-36.** Piggyback bitoric PMMA IOL system for postoperative cylinder power and axis adjustment. (Courtesy of H-R Koch, Germany.)

lamp or using a Mendez gauge. Some surgeons prefer to mark the vertical meridian and the steep meridian, or just the vertical meridian and then use a Mendez gauge at the time of implantation to align the IOL with the steep axis. Some surgeons prefer to mark the peripheral cornea with a cautery after topical anesthesia as the gentian violet marks may wash away with copious corneal irrigation.

The STAAR toric IOL is injected into the capsular bag in one step (Figure 6-34). The IOL is then rotated so that the long axis is approximately 90 degrees to the phacoemulsification incision to allow removal of viscoelastic from the capsular bag, behind the IOL (Figure 6-35). The IOL is then rotated to the steep corneal axis with the I/A tip.

High degrees of astigmatism may require combinations of procedures. An eye may require both corneal modulation, with AKs or LRIs and toric IOL implantation. Gills[34] has recently demonstrated the use of 2 STAAR toric IOLs sutured together for piggyback toric IOL implantation. Hans-Reinhardt Koch in Germany designed a primary bitoric piggyback IOL system (Figure 6-36) in which the apposing optic surfaces are planar and the non-apposed optic

surfaces are toric. The haptics are complete 360-degree circles allowing for the postoperative adjustment of cylinder and axis by the rotation of the anterior IOL. The initial prototypes of these IOLs were 1-piece PMMA requiring 6.5-mm incisions. Another company in Germany, Dr. Schmidt Intraocularlinsen, manufactures a PMMA toric IOL in sphere powers of -3 to +30 and toric powers of +1 to +12 for very high degrees of astigmatism.

Recently, Alex Hatsis in New York performed a combination of procedures he called trioptics. He placed a STAAR toric IOL in the bag (monoptic); an AMO (Santa Ana, Calif) Array multifocal IOL in the sulcus (bioptics); and then, as a second procedure, LASIK (trioptics) to fine-tune the refractive result.

# TORIC IOL OFF-AXIS ROTATION

The plate-haptic toric IOLs are fixed-length IOLs without the expansile properties of longer loop-haptic IOLs. Therefore, if one is shorter than the diameter of the newly evacuated capsular bag, the IOL may rotate off-axis. Those that rotate usually do so within the first 24 hours after surgery before capsular contraction has begun. For this reason, it is recommended that all toric cases be evaluated 1 day postoperatively by dilatation to determine the IOL axis. It has been shown by Donald Sanders[33] that a 2.25 toric IOL that rotates up to 20 degrees off axis will still reduce the astigmatism, but not fully as though the IOL were right on-axis. A toric IOL that rotates between 20 degrees and 30 degrees off-axis will theoretically not reduce any astigmatism and will act like a spherical IOL. A toric IOL that rotates 40 degrees or more off-axis can add to the existing astigmatism.

The decision to surgically rotate a toric IOL back on-axis depends on the patient's and the surgeon's refractive desires. It is recommended that IOL rotation be performed between 7 to 14 days postoperatively. Some IOLs that were rotated within the first week rerotated off-axis. Waiting at least 7 days allows for initial capsular contraction. Waiting longer than 3 weeks may result in fibrosis through the haptic fenestrations and peripheral fibrotic contraction around the square corners of the plate haptics, both of which can make IOL rotation difficult or impossible without placing the zonule at risk.

If IOL rotation is desired, it can be performed in the operating room at the same time the second eye is to have surgery, 1 to 2 weeks following the first eye procedure, using separate sterile set-ups. The IOL may be rotated with a sterile 30-gauge cannula on a BSS or lidocaine syringe, through the initial sideport incision, through the dilated pupil, under topical anesthesia. In rare cases, particularly in the second eye of a very cooperative patient, the IOL can be rotated at the slit-lamp. This requires dilatation and topical anesthesia also, possibly a lid speculum, and a sterile 30-gauge cannula also. Topical antibiotics are also recommended, just as would be used if performed in the operating room.

# SIX STEPS TO SPHERICITY

## *A Personal Astigmatism Management System*

This approach to the surgical correction of astigmatism involves 6 combinations of 4 variables: (1) ungrooved uniplanar CCIs; (2) grooved biplanar clear-corneal incisions; (3) astigmatic keratotomy; and (4) toric IOLs. The system is designed to be used with temporal CCIs only. For the purposes of this system and its application to astigmatism reduction, "temporal" is defined as within 30 degrees of the horizontal axis. I do not choose to perform unsutured clear-corneal phaco-and-foldable incisions obliquely or superiorly, as I believe incisions at these axes have demonstrated higher degrees of corneal endothelial cell loss and an increased risk of early postoperative infectious endophthalmitis. Albeit, many American and European surgical colleagues have safe-

ly and successfully mastered "on-axis" oblique and superior incisions, even with unsutured 5-mm incisions for PMMA lenses. All of my CCIs are now temporal, not only for the aforementioned reasons, but also for efficiency and ergonomics. It has simply become easier now to be temporal. There is better limbal exposure without working over the bony brow and better red reflex.

Six different "steps" or choices of astigmatism-reducing procedures have been designed for approaching eyes that are to have lens replacement surgery combined with astigmatism reduction (Figure 6-37).

### STEP 1

The first step to sphericity is applied to eyes with virtually *spherical corneas*. In these cases, the goal is to have the postoperative corneal curvature equal to the preoperative curvature. The incision, therefore, must be astigmatically neutral, resulting in either no change in astigmatism or no more than a 0.37-D induction WTR. Therefore, a simple single-plane, 1-step ungrooved peripheral temporal stab incision is used (see Figure 6-13).

### STEP 2

For *mild astigmatism ATR of 0.50 D to 1.25 D*, a 2-step peripheral temporal clear-corneal grooved incision is used (see Figure 6-14). The groove depth used in this system is 550 μm. However, depths of 400 μm (Williamson)[35] or 600 μm (Langerman)[16] can be used. The deeper the groove, the greater the effect. In addition, as with all pure incisional keratorefractive procedures (RK and AK), age is a factor. The 60-year-old clear lensectomy patient might result in only a 0.50 D change in cylinder, whereas the 80-year old cataract patient may get a 1.25-D shift from the same incision.

### STEP 3

For *moderate ATR astigmatism of 1.50 D to 3.00 D*, a 2-step grooved incision is used; however, the groove is not made at the limbus but is moved 0.5 to 1.0 mm centrally on the corneal surface. Moving the vertical groove (or LRI) centrally effectively reduces the optical zone of the "arcuate AK" portion of the 2-step phaco-foldable incision, thereby increasing its effect. Again, the effect is age-related.

### STEP 4

For *higher degrees of ATR astigmatism, 3.00 D to 6.00 D*, the centrally placed 2-step incision is used, as in Step 3; however, an AK incision is added across the cornea 180 degrees away, for more effect. For 4.00 D, the full-thickness phaco incision would be placed at an OZ of 8.0 mm and an AK incision would be added at the 8.0 mm OZ 180 degrees away, as well as 2 additional AK incisions (a pair) more centrally at the 7.0 mm OZ. For 6.00 D of astigmatism, a triple set of incisions may be desired, especially in a younger patient, at optical zones of 6.0, 7.0 and 8.0. *Beware: the full-thickness grooved phacoemulsification incision moved in on the cornea can be very powerful in the elderly, over 80 years of age.* Also, remember that WTR astigmatism is visually preferable to ATR astigmatism. Therefore, overcorrection of ATR and undercorrection of WTR is recommended.

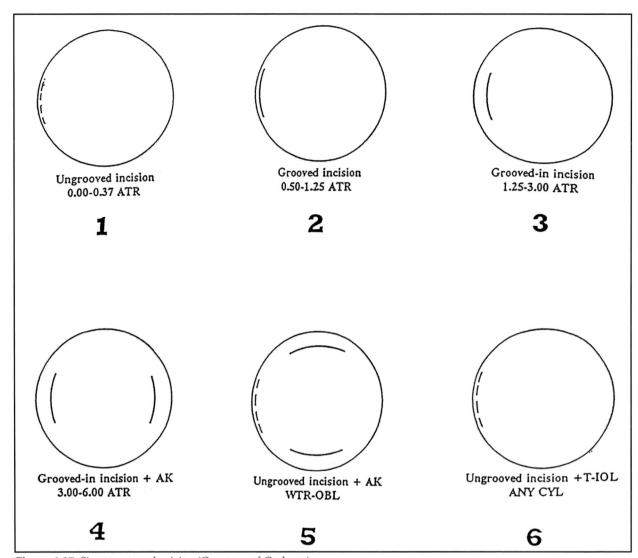

**Figure 6-37.** Six steps to sphericity. (Courtesy of Grabow.)

STEP 5

For *oblique-axis or WTR astigmatism*, the astigmatically neutral, single-plane, ungrooved T-CCI is used and the appropriate AK incisions are placed at the oblique or vertical axis. The AK incisions are made first, before entering the eye with the phaco-foldable incision, as the eye is more firm and the incision depths are more consistent.

STEP 6

This is the ultimate step which can add to or replace many of the previous steps in this system of astigmatism management: *the toric IOL*. The STAAR aphakic toric IOL is the only toric IOL currently available in the United States. At present, 2 toric powers are available: 2.00 D toric for up to 1.25 D of astigmatism and 3.50 D for 2.25 D to 3.00 D of astigmatism. The toric IOL may be used alone through a simple single-plane CCI for cylinder up to 3.25, or in combination with LRI or AK for cylinder 3.50 and more. These toric IOLs are presently available in 2 lengths: 10.8 mm

(AA4203TF) and 11.2 mm (AA4203TL). The longer length is recommended for axis stability whenever available. High degrees of astigmatism may also be corrected with 2 toric IOLs (piggyback) sutured together at both ends, as described by James P. Gills.

# REFERENCES

1. Alio JL, Belda JI, Shalaby AMM. Correction of irregular astigmatism with excimer laser assisted by sodium hyaluronate. *Ophthalmol*. 2001;108:1246-1260.

2. Fyodorov SN, Durnev VV. Surgical correction of complicated myopic astigmatism by means of dissection of circular ligament of cornea. *Ann Ophth*. 1981;115-118.

3. Thornton SP. Astigmatic keratotomy: a review of basic concepts with case reports. *J Cataract Refract Surg*. 1990;16:430-435.

4. Lindstrom RL. Pre/post cataract astigmatism: to treat or not to treat. Presented at AAO Annual Meeting; 1987.

5. Lindstrom RL, Lavery GW. Correction of post-keratoplasty astigmatism. In Sanders DR, Hofman FR, Salz JJ, eds. *Refractive Corneal Surgery.* Thorofare, NJ: SLACK Incorporated; 1986:215-240.

6. Lavery GW, Lindstrom RL. Clinical results of the Ruiz astigmatic keratotomy. *J Refract Surg.* 1985;1(2):70-74.

7. Price FW. Astigmatism reduction clinical trial: a multicenter prospective evaluation of the predictability of arcuate keratotomy. *Arch Ophthal.* 1995;113:277-282.

8. Muller-Jensen K, Fischer P, Siepe U. Limbal relaxing incisions to correct astigmatism in clear corneal cataract surgery. *J Refract Surg.* 1999;15:586-589.

9. Nichamin LD. Astigmatism management during phaco surgery. *Rev Refract Surg.* Apr 2001;41-45.

10. Oliveira C. The "keratopyramis phenomenon" and the Canrobert "C" procedure. Presented at the Pre-AAO meeting of ISRK. Chicago; Nov 1993.

11. Rao NR, Konoroal A, Murchison AE, Epstein RJ. Enlargement of the temporal clear corneal cataract incision to treat pre-existing astigmatism. *J Refract Surg.* 2002;18,463-467.

12. Singer JA. Frown incision for minimizing induced astigmatism after small incision cataract surgery. *J Cataract Refract Surg.* 1991;17:677-688.

13. Fukasaku H. The no-stitch suspension bridge incision. *Ocular Surg News.* Sept 1, 1991;76-77.

14. Gills JP, Gayton JL. Reducing pre-existing astigmatism. In: Gills JP, ed. *Cataract Surgery: State of the Art.* Thorofare, NJ: SLACK Incorporated; 1998;53-66.

15. Grabow HB. The clear-corneal incision. In Fine IH, Fichman RA, Grabow HB, eds. *Clear-Corneal Cataract Surgery and Topical Anesthesia.* Thorofare, NJ: SLACK Incorporated; 1993:29-62.

16. Langerman, DW. Architectural design of a self-sealing corneal tunnel single-hinge incision. *J Cataract Refract Surg.* 1994;20:84-88.

17. Kershner RM. Keratolenticuloplasty. In Kershner RM, ed. *Refractive Keratotomy for Cataract Surgery and the Correction of Astigmatism.* Thorofare, NJ: SLACK Incorporated; 1994:25-41.

18. Kershner RM. Clear corneal cataract surgery and the correction of myopia, hyperopia, and astigmatism. *Ophthalmology.* 1997;104:381-389.

19. Krumeich JH, Knulle A, Daniel J. Improved technique of circular keratotomy for the correction of corneal astigmatism. *J Refract Surg.* 1997;13:255-262.

20. Hannah KD, Hayward M, Hagen KB, et al. Keratotomy for astigmatism using an arcuate keratome. *Arch Ophthal.* 1993;111;998-1004.

21. Hannush SB. Arcuate keratotomy: how to get the mechanical edge. *Rev Ophthal.* Mar 1995;93-96.

22. Ridley H. Intraocular acrylic lenses. *Trans Ophthalmol Soc UK.* 1951;71:617-621.

23. Fechner PU, VanDerHeijde GL, Worst JGF. The correction of myopia by lens implantation into phakic eyes. *Am J Ophthalmol.* 1989;107:659-663.

24. Fyodorov SN, Zuyev VK, Tumanyan EB, Larionov YV. Analysis of long-term clinical and functional results of intraocular correction of high myopia. *Ophthalmosurgery.* 1990;2:3-6.

25. Strampelli B. Soppontabilita di lent acriliche in camera anterione nella afachia o nei vizi di refrazione. *Ann Oftalmol Clin Oculist Parma.* 1954;80:75.

26. Barraquer JM. Lentes plasticoes de camera anterior. *Estudios C Informaciones Oftalmologicas.* 1954;6:15.

27. Strampelli B. Complication de l'operation de Strampelli. *Anne Therapeutique et Clinique En Ophtalmologique.* 1958;9:349-370.

28. Barraquer J. Anterior chamber plastic lenses—results and conclusions from five years' experience. *Trans Ophtalmol Soc UK.* 1959;79:393.

29. Barraquer JM. Complications de la inclusion segun los diversos tipos de lentes. *Annules de Instituto Barraquer.* 1962; 3:588-592.

30. Choyce P. *Intraocular Lenses and Implants.* London: HK Lewis; 1964:153-155.

31. Shimizu K, Misawa A, Suzuki Y. Toric intraocular lenses: correcting astigmatism while controlling axis shift. *J Cataract Refract Surg.* 1994;20:523-526.

32. Gimbel HV, Ziemba SL. Management of myopic astigmatism with phakic intraocular lens implantation. *J Cataract Refract Surg.* 2002;28:883-886.

33. Sanders DR, Grabow HB, Shepherd J, Raanan MG. STAAR AA4203T Toric Silicone IOL. In Martin RG, Gills JP, Sanders DR, eds. *Foldable Intraocular Lenses.* Thorofare, NJ: SLACK Incorporated; 1993;237-250.

34. Gills JP. Piggyback toric lenses. In: Gills JP, ed. *A Complete Surgical Guide for Correcting Astigmatism.* Thorofare, NJ: SLACK Incorporated; 2003;161-164.

35. Williamson CH. Williamson surgical technique. In: Martin RG, Gills JP, Sanders DR, eds. *Foldable Intraocular Lenses.* Thorofare, NJ: SLACK Incorporated; 1993;136-147.

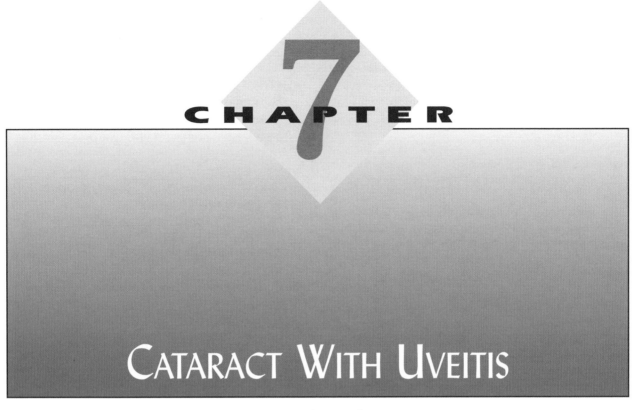

# CHAPTER 7

# CATARACT WITH UVEITIS

*Gustavo Barbosa Abreu, MD*

## INTRODUCTION

Perhaps one of the most intriguing and complex chapters in the surgical treatment of cataract is its association with uveitis.

Whereas patients with a history of uveitis and cataract represent a small contingent among indications for cataract surgery, cataract is a frequent complication among patients with intraocular inflammation.

The ophthalmologist will be required to do his or her utmost when faced with such a difficult and challenging situation. He or she must have a thorough knowledge of general medicine, ophthalmic examination, and therapeutics. In addition, he or she must be experienced in treating these conditions and also be surgically skilled. These attributes are indispensable for achieving satisfying results in the management of this severe disease.

Uveitis represents a wide range of conditions with different presentations and complications requiring various treatment strategies. Despite the excellent therapies established, structural eye injuries repaired by surgery alone are common. Among these, cataract formed by inflammation or use of topical and systemic corticosteroids appears as one of the leading causes of low visual acuity.

In the past, due to a large number of complications such as postoperative inflammatory exacerbations, ocular hypotony, and phthisis, there was a strong tendency toward a conservative approach in patients with uveitis. Although now it is still not regarded as a conventional cataract surgery, given the various factors involved, better control of inflammation and indisputable advances in ocular microsurgery have contributed to a safer surgery, thus improving visual results.[1]

It must be taken into account that each eye with uveitis is unique in its anatomic changes. Surgical intervention should be planned at an appropriate time. During the perioperative period, patients must be offered special care and each case should be evaluated individually.

## WHEN TO INDICATE SURGERY

Once the diagnosis of cataract is made in a patient with uveitis, doubts may arise whether or not to indicate surgery and the optimal time for its performance.

Among reasons for indicating surgery in these cases is improvement of visual function, which is one common to patients with cataract. Nevertheless, because of a higher risk of complications, surgery is not justified when there is only a mild reduction in visual acuity. Another reason would be the need for a transparent media to allow better assessment, follow-up and treatment of diseases involving the posterior segment of the globe. These 2 reasons, added to phacogenic uveitis with its prompt surgical indication and cataract associated with uveitis in children whose battle against amblyopia must be won are the cardinal reasons for indicating surgery.

Although it is not in our interest to rashly indicate surgery, we should not forget that delaying it may also lead to a permanent loss of vision, preventing adequate visualization and treatment of inflammatory disease and its complications.

In conclusion, we would like to emphasize that corneal and vitreous opacities, epiretinal membranes, and CME, among other conditions, may also be concurrent with cataract, accounting for part or all of the low visual acuity found. Therefore, only a sound clinical judgement will actually determine the indication and best time for surgery.

# PREOPERATIVE EVALUATION

Once cataract surgery is indicated in a patient with uveitis, the ophthalmologist must use all the clinical methods available to gather as much information as possible about the case, specifically the eye to be operated, because uveitis is essentially multifaceted. This includes, when necessary, the use of special testing methods. Only in this manner may preoperative management, indication of the surgical technique, and postoperative care be suitably defined and planned in order to achieve the best results. It is very important to determine the cause of ocular inflammation whenever possible because of its relevant prognostic role. Preoperative laboratory tests for etiological investigation should be ordered in a directed manner, according to ophthalmic findings, thus avoiding the very expensive nondirected standardized tests.

After the diagnosis is made, cases of Fuchs' heterochromic cyclitis, granulomatous, and nongranulomatous anterior uveitis, chorioretinitis, pars planitis, juvenile rheumatoid arthritis, Vogt-Koyanagi-Harada syndrome, sarcoidosis,[2] herpetic keratouveitis, and numerous other forms of uveitis will be treated on an individual basis, according to the natural history of the specific disease. We should keep in mind that many cases of ocular inflammation remain without an etiological diagnosis, but still receive medical or surgical treatment when necessary.[2]

## *Diagnostic Evaluation*

Ophthalmic examination should properly define whether we are dealing with a case of anterior, posterior or diffuse, granulomatous or nongranulomatous, acute or chronic uveitis, as well as the degree of disease activity. During slit-lamp examination and funduscopy we should pay special attention to the following findings:

1. *Cornea:* presence of melting, herpetic keratitis, and keratopathy in strips, among others.

2. *Anterior chamber:* presence of keratic precipitates, goniosynechiae, iris bombé, posterior synechiae, synchysis, pupillary membrane, rubeosis, among others.

3. *Posterior chamber:* type of cataract (predominantly anterior subcapsular, or posterior, nuclear, cortical, nigra, or hypermature) and phacodonesis (when present, it indicates extreme zonular laxity).

4. *Intraocular pressure:* presence of glaucoma or acute or chronic hypotony.

5. *Posterior segment:* direct examination when possible should be able to clarify the presence of cyclitic membrane; vitreous membranes; hemorrhage; inflammatory cells; fibrovascular membranes; retinal vascular occlusions; choroidoretinitis; macular pathology (notably, CME), macular pucker, and epiretinal membranes; inflammatory, ischemic, or granulomatous optic neuropathy; and retinal detachment.

## *Special Testing Methods*

### ULTRASOUND BIOMICROSCOPY

When it is not possible to directly evaluate the anterior segment of the globe up to the area corresponding to the anterior vitreous and ciliary body, we can use this method.[3]

In our opinion, in cases of uveitis it is mainly indicated for diagnosis and evaluation of cyclitic membrane and its correlation with the ciliary body, which may or not lead to ocular hypotony.

### ULTRASONOGRAPHY

Ultrasonography is used in opaque media for evaluation of the posterior segment of the globe, in order to detect vitreous inflammation and/or hemorrhages, vitreous membranes, fibrovascular membranes, and retinal detachment. In extreme cases, it is also used to examine the macular and papillary area.[3]

### FLUORESCEIN ANGIOGRAPHY

In media where it is permitted, even partially, fluorescein angiography is mandatory mainly to investigate CME and poorly perfused capillary areas.

### POTENTIAL ACUITY METER

When possible, this method will indicate the functional status of the macula, which is indispensable for final good visual acuity.[4] In cases where potential acuity meter (PAM) is unsatisfactory, we should caution the patient, although there are cases in which definite macular injury has not occurred yet and adequate treatment may reverse it.

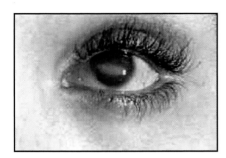

**Figure 7-1.** Band keratopathy.

# PREOPERATIVE MANAGEMENT

## Control of Inflammation

In cases in which surgery must be performed despite the presence of acute inflammation, as occurs in phacoantigenic uveitis, and in those in which no sign of inflammatory activity is found, we believe prophylactic therapy is not indicated. Anti-inflammatory treatment should be initiated after surgery. In other conditions in which we find some degree of inflammatory activity, preoperative therapy is mandatory.

There is no doubt even today that corticosteroids are the mainstay of anti-inflammatory treatment. These drugs act in reactions mediated by leukocytes and macrophages, as well as in those mediated by lymphocytes. Nevertheless, it is clear that we should use all the necessary and available methods to control inflammation and guide the various treatments instituted, including noncorticosteroidal anti-inflammatory and immunosuppressive drugs, which are prescribed on an individual basis.

In general, the disease must be under control for a period of 2 to 3 months before surgery is performed. However, this does not necessarily mean a total lack of cells. In fact, there are cases in which no matter how much medication is given, we still find a certain degree of activity, possibly due to a permanent breakdown of the blood-aqueous barrier. It should be considered that in predominantly posterior uveitis with dense cataracts, adequate evaluation of inflammatory activity may be impossible.

For reasons mentioned above, we must maximally suppress preoperative ocular inflammation in uveitis patients avoid further delay in surgery. Otherwise, these patients may become debilitated and we may be unable to adequately follow-up the posterior segment. In these cases, we routinely use topical (dexamethasone, 4 to 8 times/day) and subtenon corticosteroids (0.5 ml of triancinolone, 40 mg/ml, for 5 to 15 days) and nonsteroidal anti-inflammatory drugs (indomethacin). In the presence of CME or if there is a high risk of its occurrence, we use topical nonsteroidal anti-inflammatory drugs (ketorolac tromethamine, 4 times/day).

If inflammation persists, despite the medication given, we initiate treatment with anti-inflammatory doses of prednisone (1 mg/kg/day).

We must remember that the continuous administration of systemic corticosteroids also produces adverse effects. The use of these drugs in children and diabetics is a matter of concern.

And finally, in our clinical judgement, if this medical treatment does not adequately suppress ocular inflammation, we administer immunosuppressive drugs, especially cyclosporine in consultation with an immunologist.

## Control of Pain and Photophobia

The symptoms and signs of uveitis that compromise primarily or secondarily the anterior segment of the globe are mainly due to iritis. In these cases, mydriatics and cycloplegics are essential not only to relieve patient discomfort, but also to reduce stimuli to inflammation and pupil movements, lysing the existing synechiae and preventing the occurrence of newly formed ones.

## Special Situations

### BAND KERATOPATHY

The presence of band keratopathy is a sign of chronic ocular inflammatory disease, especially juvenile rheumatoid arthritis, sarcoidosis and some forms of pars planitis. The latter must be removed days before cataract surgery. Treatment includes chelation therapy with 1% or 2% sodium EDTA, superficial keratectomy, and excimer laser phototherapeutic keratectomy (PTK).

We prefer superficial keratectomy under local or general anesthesia (in children) because of the ease of the surgical procedure and our especially satisfying results.[5] PTK, although an elegant indication, only removes calcium from the central region of the cornea and we know that band keratopathy usually occurs from limbal white to limbal white in the interpalpebral fissure. Another inconvenience is the occurrence of a hyperopic shift. In our opinion, this further limits its use (Figure 7-1).

### HERPETIC KERATOUVEITIS

In cases of viral keratouveitis, either caused by *herpes simplex* or *varicella zoster*, postoperative inflammation is exacerbated, requiring intensive corticotherapy, which in turn may lead to the recurrence of inflammation.

We believe the prophylactic use of topical antiviral agents (acyclovir) is recommended in both cases. Systemic antiviral agents are recommended for patients with *v. zoster* 2 days before surgery.

### TOXOPLASMOSIS

Reactivation of inactive retinochoroiditis manifests itself by satellite lesions quite often after surgical trauma.[5]

In cases with areas of old retinochoroiditis adjacent to areas crucial to visual function, such as the macular papillary bundle and the juxtafoveal region, specific prophylactic medication is indicated. We use a combination of sulfamethoxazole and trimethoprim, starting 2 days before surgery and extending from 3 to 6 months depending on the severity of the case.

### GLAUCOMA

There is a common association between cataract and glaucoma in more severe cases of uveitis. Glaucoma may be described as chronic with an open-angle, chronic with a closed-angle, and acute with a closed-angle.

Regardless of the type of glaucoma found, it is imperative to begin its clinical or surgical treatment before cataract surgery. In our experience, results are not good when these surgeries are combined. If we are fortuitously required to perform the combined surgeries, we think that a 2-incision technique would be suitable.

In cases of chronic angle-closure glaucoma, if there is still an important block component and the eye is quiet, we use argon laser associated with Nd-YAG laser to try to achieve a wide and patent iridotomy. Iridotomies performed only with Nd-YAG laser in patients affected by uveitis, even with active disease, have a strong tendency to close.

In cases of acute glaucoma caused by pupillary block in patients with uveitis, a patent iridectomy is unlikely. However, we should use anti-inflammatory drugs, cycloplegics, mydriatics, intravenous osmotic agents (mannitol), oral acetazolamide, and eye drops of hypotensive agents in an attempt to reverse the situation. If successful, we must perform iridotomy using argon laser associated with Nd-YAG laser. If this fails, not rare in these cases, we should attempt to perform a surgical peripheral iridectomy, giving special preference to the superior nasal quadrant. We try to leave normal conjunctiva at the 12-o'clock position and in the superior temporal quadrant for a possible filtering procedure.

### OCULAR HYPOTONY

There are 3 causes of ocular hypotony in uveitis that must be carefully analyzed:

1. Hypotony secondary to acute and severe inflammatory disease such as observed in some cases of herpetic keratouveitis and Vogt-Koyanagi-Harada syndrome. In these conditions, treatment of the underlying disease is sufficient to reverse the process.

2. Hypotony caused by traction of the ciliary body by a cyclitic membrane. In this case, only confirmed by ultrasound biomicroscopy (UBM), surgery is mandatory.

3. Failure of the ciliary body, in which case only the ophthalmologist can judge whether the performance of surgery is still possible or if there is a strong chance that phthisis will ensue.

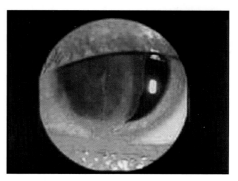

**Figure 7-2.** Luxated lens in anterior chamber.

# CHOICE OF SURGICAL TECHNIQUE

The truth about cataract surgery in patients with uveitis is that it may produce absolutely unexpected results. Clinical experience, therefore, should always be finely tuned to choose the best surgical plan.

Cataract surgery has been divided into 5 types for didactic purposes:

1. Intracapsular
2. Extracapsular by irrigation/aspiration or phacoemulsification without IOL
3. Extracapsular by irrigation/aspiration or phacoemulsification with IOL
4. Extracapsular by irrigation/aspiration or phacoemulsification with IOL associated with posterior vitrectomy
5. Lensectomy combined with vitrectomy

## Intracapsular Surgery

Intracapsular cataract surgery, which until only recently was considered one of the best techniques for cataract extraction in phacoantigenic uveitis, has currently been relegated to those few cases, nearly always senile patients, who present long-term uveitis, or those who present signs of a luxated or extensively subluxated crystalline lens.

In cases of uveitis and hypermature cataract, cataract extraction using the extracapsular technique, either by irrigation/aspiration or phacoemulsification, and a meticulous removal of cortical material, in conjunction with anti-inflammatory therapy have been sufficient to eradicate the process (Figure 7-2).

## Extracapsular Surgery by Irrigation/Aspiration or by Phacoemulsification Without Intraocular Lens

This technique may be indicated when we intend to leave the posterior capsule intact to act as a barrier and limit

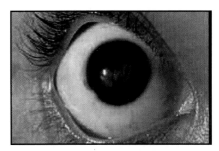

**Figure 7-3.** Synechiae in 270 degrees with pupillary membrane in a white and soft cataract.

uveitis to the anterior segment. This technique is also useful if an IOL is implanted at a later date.

In our opinion, with the current advances in ocular therapeutics and surgical techniques, this indication has practically ceased to exist. It is possible to maintain the posterior capsule without the risk of forming posterior synechiae, pupillary and cyclitic membranes, and many other inconveniences. In addition, an IOL, now highly biocompatible, may be implanted. On the other hand, there are cases in which we believe IOL placement may put patients at greater risk for inflammation. In these cases, removal of substrate at the pupillary and ciliary body sites involved in posterior capsule preservation, produces a unicameral ocular globe.

In conclusion, special attention must be given to those cases in which frequently formed iridocapsular synechiae, pupillary symphysis, iris bombé, pupillary membranes, and posterior capsular opacity requiring capsulotomy make IOL implant in a secondary procedure more difficult or even impossible.

## Extracapsular Surgery by Irrigation/Aspiration or by Phacoemulsification With Intraocular Lens Implant

Extracapsular cataract surgery associated with IOL implant is now considered the surgery of choice for the majority of uveitis cases. The main reason for this is the undeniable fact that pseudophakic patients enjoy a better quality of life than aphakic patients. Unquestionably, the latter have limitations in their daily activities. In addition, improvement in anti-inflammatory treatments and in surgical techniques, as well as better IOL designs, have made it possible to operate a greater number of eyes with ocular inflammation.

The advantage of this technique is that it preserves the posterior capsule intact, which in conjunction with the IOL, acts as a barrier to the diffusion of mediators originating in the anterior segment. This reduces the incidence of CME among other complications.[6]

Its disadvantage is greater difficulty in dealing with posterior synechiae and pupillary membranes in the periopera-

tive period. There is a higher incidence of synechiae formation and complications in the postoperative period than a combined lensectomy and vitrectomy technique. However, we must remember that synechiae are formed between the iris and capsular remnants, and never between the iris and the IOL (Figure 7-3).

This technique is indicated in cases without CME; vitritis or with mild vitritis controlled for a minimum of 3 months (occurring in some more benign cases of pars planitis and sarcoidosis); Fuch's heterochromic cyclitis; anterior uveitis HLA B27 positive and inactive uveitis lasting over a year; adults with a previous history of juvenile rheumatoid arthritis and uveitis who had mild to moderate inflammation, but now present quiet, apparently healthy eyes; and phacogenic uveitis.

Indication for inserting an IOL during the surgical procedure involves complex considerations, mainly because these lenses are capable of inciting inflammatory and foreign-body response, as well as the activation of the complement pathway and coagulation cascade.[7] However, suitable biocompatible lenses with better designs, and accurately placed in the bag, seem to be very well tolerated in selected cases in which uveitis has been quiescent for a prolonged period before surgery. Rigid PMMA lenses, which are less biocompatible and cannot fold, are less commonly used today. We can even affirm that their days are numbered because they are not suitable in small incisions. Likewise, 3-piece lenses (because of their loops, made of polyimide, PMMA, or polypropylene) are avoided in favor of 1-piece lenses.

We should also remember that anterior chamber IOLs are contraindicated in cases of uveitis, because they propagate inflammation, produce fibrosis of the angle with a resultant increase in IOP, and produce deleterious effects on the corneal epithelium.

Extracapsular extraction using the I/A technique is restricted to a few conditions in which phacoemulsification is contraindicated, mainly in the presence of cataract nigra (owing to its large volume and very hard nucleus). This is due to an inflammatory response produced by a large scleral or corneoscleral incision, ocular globe decompression, increased contact with the uvea, and a greater likelihood of perioperative prolapse and postoperative hernia of the iris. However, when this technique is indicated we use a 7.0-mm optical zone IOL without holes because it is less likely to decenter. This IOL is coated with heparin, rendering it hydrophilic and preventing surface cell deposits.

In all other conditions in which extracapsular extraction is recommended, the preferred technique is a small-incision phacoemulsification in a clear cornea, using a one-piece, foldable acrylic, hydrophilic lens. Its margins preferably have sharp edges, which are highly biocompatible, and therefore cause less inflammatory response. They also have a prolonged barrier function to the proliferation of lens epithelial cells, retarding the posterior capsule opacification process, especially undesirable for eyes with uveitis. Phacoemulsification is the best option and we can safely indicate it in most cases because the procedure is currently secure even in small pupils and hard nuclei. In addition, there is a perceptible reduction in the inflammatory response due to less aggressive surgery.

Major advances in cataract surgery using the emulsification technique are the continuous anterior circular capsulotomy and the valvular and self-sealing corneal incision. Advances in viscoelastic surgery—consisting of the concurrent use of cohesive and dispersive viscoelastic materials and finally in the development of foldable IOLs and phacoemulsification devices—have occurred.

Continuous capsulorrhexis has permitted surgery within the capsular bag, ensuring placement of the IOL in this situation. This reduces inflammatory stimulus because the IOL does not touch the uvea, resulting in less optic decentration and pupillary capture. In addition, it permits earlier use of mydriatics and cycloplegics. Capsule contraction syndrome has appeared as an adverse effect both in capsulotomies smaller than 5.0 mm in diameter and incomplete removal of lens epithelial cells, which are not rare in cases of uveitis with small pupils. This complication may lead to complete luxation of the capsular bag with IOL toward the vitreous chamber, if it is concurrent with extreme zonular laxity (Figure 7-4).

A small incision of about 3.0 mm dispenses with peritomy and suture—in a "vertical seesaw" movement, since it is unlikely to be in the same plane as the iris and crystalline lens—facilitates surgery. In addition, it causes less trauma, iris prolapse, bleeding, and other perioperative complications. That is why this technique can be used without restrictions in the presence of goniosynechiae. It offers better exposure to all types of orbits, primarily if it is performed through the temporal route. It permits working in a closed system with virtually constant intraocular pressure, a constantly reformed anterior chamber, and a more stable mydriasis. It also leads to less surgical trauma, shorter surgical duration, less induced astigmatism, and prompt refraction stability. In addition, it benefits earlier follow-up and treatment of the posterior segment when necessary.

Concurrently used cohesive and dispersive viscoelastic materials offer great protection to the corneal epithelium and provide more anterior chamber stability and a wider mydriasis. Also, these materials facilitate lysis of synechiae. At the end of surgery, they should be completely removed to prevent IOP elevation and postoperative inflammation.

Foldable IOLs are now more biocompatible, meaning that they are more capable of remaining inert, especially 1-piece acrylic lenses, followed in order by hydrogel and silicone lenses.

A decrease in diameter and change in design of the currently used phacoemulsification tip have produced greater

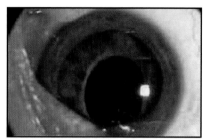

**Figure 7-4.** Beginning of capsular contraction.

cavitation, as well as permitted work with higher vacuum and shorter ultrasound time, without the undesirable occurrence of the "surge effect" or anterior chamber collapse.

## Extracapsular Surgery by Phacoemulsification With Intraocular Lens Associated With Posterior Vitrectomy

Although at first this technique may seem to be less frequently indicated, in fact it is increasingly being used, especially in cases associated with cataract in which there are old vitreous opacities preventing visualization of the fundus, in cases of epiretinal membranes in the posterior pole that must be removed, or in cases of macular pucker or hole.

This surgery is also well employed in cases of mild and moderate vitritis.

## Lensectomy and Posterior Vitrectomy

The majority of cataracts associated with uveitis occur in young patients who undergo earlier surgery. Cataracts are softer and often can simply be removed through the anterior route using I/A or increased vacuum and minimum ultrasound. When surgery is performed through the pars plana, cataracts may be removed by a phacofragmentation device (phacoemulsifier) or vitrophage.

Thus, in cases that for various reasons it does not seem important to leave any type of substrate, support, or framework at the pupillary and ciliary body plane, we believe removal of the crystalline lens associated with a wide posterior vitrectomy should be performed. If the cataract is soft enough, its removal can be indicated using the posterior route with a vitrophage. However, if it is hard, especially in patients over 40 years of age, we perform a phacoemulsification surgery with a 2.75-mm self-sealing incision in a clear cornea. Proceeding through the posterior route, we remove anterior capsule remnants, posterior capsule and zonular remnants. Only then do we perform the actual posterior vitrectomy.

The main drawback of this technique is removal of the barrier, a function of the capsule, as well as the potential risk of increased hemorrhage, rupture, and retinal detachment. In contrast, it decreases cell accumulation and clouding during the inflammatory process.[8] In addition, it prevents the formation of posterior synechiae, cyclitic membranes, and phthisis. It also permits the performance of iridoplasties, which in some cases is fundamental for follow-up of the posterior segment.

The technique is indicated for cases with chronic and/or recurrent inflammation—which will probably persist in the postoperative period—such as cases of juvenile rheumatoid arthritis in children, Vogt-Koyangi-Harada syndrome, sympathetic ophthalmia, and recurrent granulomatous uveitis with extensive synechiae formation, as occurs in sarcoidosis. Ocular hypotony associated with cataract is another condition for which lensectomy associated with vitrectomy is indicated, especially one in which the presence of cyclitic membrane exerting traction on the ciliary body is observed by direct examination or UBM.

Finally, we would like to emphasize that we would rather see our patients aphakic than submit them to unnecessary risks that might lead to permanent loss of vision.[9]

# Performance of Surgery

Whatever the technique indicated for surgery, we must be sure whether or not we need to administer perioperative corticosteroids. If we do, dosage must be tailored in each specific case. Thus, subconjunctival dexamethasone, 0.5 ml, subtenon triancinolone, 40 mg/ml, intraocular triancinolone 4mg/0.1 ml, and intravenous methylprednisolone 50 to 100 mg may and should be used.

Mydriatics, cycloplegics, and NSAIDs should be instilled every 15 minutes, 1 to 2 hours before surgery, in order to obtain pupil dilation that is as wide and long lasting as possible. An exception is made for intracapsular surgery in which preoperative dilation is contraindicated. When performing surgery using an intracapsular technique or an IOL capsular bag implant or a combined lensectomy and vitrectomy, mydriatics and cycloplegics should be instilled at the end of surgery, thus minimizing the inflammatory response. In cases in which we implanted an IOL in the sulcus or we are not sure it was implanted in the bag, we must delay use of these eye drops.

Intraocular tissue plasminogen activator (tPA) for perioperative therapy has been gaining ground and is being used for rapid reabsorption of fibrin, inflammation, and clots.

Regarding surgical technique, a well-indicated intracapsular surgery offers no greater difficulty and requires no comments.

Extracapsular cataract surgery either using irrigation/aspiration or phacoemulsification is rendered more difficult in the presence of findings such as stromal iris pathology, represented by iris atrophy and pupillary sphincter sclerosis, vascular iris anomalies accounting for perioperative hemorrhage, anterior synechiae, symphysis, iris bombé, and zonu-

lar laxity. In cases in which extracapsular extraction is performed by irrigation/aspiration and the nucleus is removed by expression, special care must be taken during the scleral or corneoscleral incision in order to prevent bleeding; during lysis of the synechiae, which must be done under a closed system and anterior chamber filled with viscoelastic material; and during capsulotomy, preferably continuous and circular, large enough to facilitate nucleus expression and prevent the capsular retraction syndrome. When it is not possible to perform a sufficiently large capsulorrhexis, we must use the can-opener technique and place the lens in the sulcus. We must remember that in this technique, there is a significant increase in synechiae formation, possibly due to capsular flaps.

Because the eye has been sectioned with a large enough incision to permit performance of iridectomy, this portion of the procedure should be done. We can perform sector iridectomy immediately at the beginning of surgery to facilitate capsulotomy and nucleus expression or we can do a peripheral iridectomy only at the end of surgery.

In phacoemulsification surgery, we must make both the main and accessory incisions in a clear cornea. After this, we inject viscoelastic material into the anterior chamber and with the cannula itself we proceed to lyse the synechiae (if any exist) injecting viscous into the retroiris space. If this maneuver is not sufficient, we use 2 iris hooks or a bimanual technique to perform microsphincterectomies and subsequent pupil dilatation. When none of these alternatives meet with success, especially in the presence of pupillary membrane, it may be possible to remove the cataract before this procedure. Sometimes we can extract it using the capsulorrhexis forceps. If the cataract is too dense it can only be removed after being sectioned. For this purpose, we use the vitrectomy scissors because it allows adequate work through a small corneal incision. It may seem amazing, but using these procedures we have never needed to use either the De Juan iris retractors or serial sphincterectomies, although these also appear to be excellent indications. Once sufficient pupil dilation is obtained, we must reinject viscoelastic material for an even wider and stable pupil dilation. Only then do we proceed with the capsulotomy.

As we have previously mentioned, this incision should be circular, continuous, sufficiently centered, and wide. If possible, it should be even wider than the diameter of the optical portion of the IOL, which is foldable and no larger than 6 mm in diameter. We must remember that in cases of small pupils it is not always easy to achieve this goal.

There are cases of white cataracts with loss of the red reflex in which the use of vital dyes, especially trypan blue is mandatory. The best way to stain the anterior capsule is to initially inject air into the anterior chamber, followed by injection of the dye. We wait 2 to 3 minutes and then inject the viscoelastic material, filling all the anterior chamber and removing the excess dye.

After performing capsulotomy, hydrodissection, and hydrodelineation, we begin phacoemulsification. We must pay close attention to anterior chamber depth because when too deep, it indicates zonular laxity. In this situation, we must maximally lower the height of the infusion bottle.

After nucleus removal, we aspirate as much cortical remnants as possible, in order to avoid proliferation of lens epithelial cells, which ultimately leads to capsule opacification.

If surgery has gone well thus far, a 1-piece acrylic lens, preferably with sharp-edged margins may be inserted with the aid of an injector. There is no need to enlarge the incision. When for any reason there is a small rupture of the posterior capsule, we may try to implant the same IOL in the bag; however, if this lens is suspected to be unsuitable for the sulcus, we can replace it with a 3-piece foldable acrylic lens and place it in the sulcus over the anterior capsule.

In cases of phacoemulsification and in-the-bag IOL implant, peripheral iridectomy is not frequently performed; however, if we believe this technique is necessary, a corneal tunnel incision may be hazardous. A limbal incision would be the optimal access, if possible, at the superior nasal quadrant.

When proceeding with the surgery and IOL implant combined with posterior vitrectomy, we must take a few precautions. The first and perhaps most important is insertion of the infusion cannula through the pars plana, which must be entered before the anterior segment surgery is performed. We must proceed with phacoemulsification, place the IOL and fill all the anterior chamber with viscoelastic material. This material, added to the self-sealing incision, is a great aid in stabilizing the anterior chamber for the performance of vitrectomy. Following this, we check whether the cannula is really in the vitreous chamber and not behind the uvea or retina, and only then do we start the posterior infusion, perform the other pars plana and vitrectomy incisions. At the end of the posterior vitrectomy, we return to the anterior chamber and remove the viscoelastic material.

There are other reasons for indicating the lensectomy and vitrectomy technique, in addition to cataract extraction, such as removal of all substrate in the pupillary and ciliary body plane, thus preventing any support that facilitates the formation of pupillary and cyclitic membranes. In this situation, we must also place the infusion cannula into the pars plana, but maintain it disconnected. We perform the 2 accessory incisions and another one in a cornea clear enough to introduce a Butterfly number 27, through which we proceed with the infusion. Following these incisions, we perform needling of the crystalline lens, taking care to introduce the needle through the pars plana route, parallel to the iris plane, avoiding premature rupture of the posterior capsule. After this is done, we introduce the infusion through the anterior route and the vitrophage through the posterior route. Then we remove the anterior capsule and as much lens material as possible. Using the scleral depression technique, we remove anterior capsule remnants, more peripherally located cortical remnants, the zonule, and finally the posterior capsule. Once lensectomy is performed—we interrupt the anterior infusion—check if the cannula fixated in the pars plana route is appropriately placed in the vitreous chamber. If it is, we inject air into the anterior chamber, start the infusion and proceed with the posterior vitrectomy, removing vitreous, epiretinal and internal limiting membranes, ultimately all that is necessary. We can even perform endolaser in selected cases of fibrovascular membranes.

# POSTOPERATIVE PERIOD

In general uveitis patients who have been suitably submitted to cataract surgery present improved visual acuity.[10] When the final visual results are not good, either in procedures performed through the anterior or posterior route, these are due to preexisting structural injuries. Therefore, better control of inflammation and its ocular sequelae before surgery is imperative.

As occurs in eyes without uveitis, postoperative results may be complicated by corneal decompensation, glaucoma, posterior synechiae, iris capture, IOL dislocation, posterior capsule opacity, capsule rupture, pupillary and cyclitic membranes, capsular retraction syndrome, vitreous loss, retinal detachment, infectious endopthalmitis and others. Control of postoperative inflammation is obviously mandatory in cases of uveitis. Daily control in the first week after surgery is essential. Due to preoperative and postoperative medication, the eye may appear quiet during the first few days but as time goes by, inflammation may intensify. It may be necessary to increase the initial corticosteroid therapy. We basically use drops of antibiotic and steroids, 4 to 6 times a day, and maintain the oral prednisone given in the preoperative period, increasing or decreasing its dosage according to the course of each case.

In the presence of CME, we use drops of NSAIDs for a minimum period of 2 months. Oral acetazolamide, which is known to have beneficial effects on the Irvine-Gass syndrome, may also be used in these cases in an attempt to reduce macular compromise.

Subconjunctival, tPA, subtenon, and intravitreal corticosteroids may also be used both perioperatively and postoperatively to try to minimize the inflammatory response.

Treatment with mydriatics and cycloplegics must be promptly begun in patients receiving in-the-bag IOLs or aphakic patients and vitrectomized, unlike patients receiving sulcus-fixated IOLs or when there is doubt about accurate IOL placement in the bag because there is a high incidence of iris capture in the latter patients.

Among the leading causes of postoperative complications are posterior synechiae formation, iris bombé, and closed-

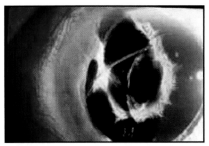

**Figure 7-5.** Iridocorneal synechiae with disengagement of IOL. Notice that the optical portion of IOL is almost entirely covered by the anterior capsule.

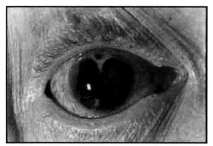

**Figure 7-6.** Iris bombé in a patient operated by the extracapsular technique, without IOL. Observe the iridocapsular synechiae.

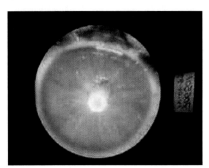

**Figure 7-7.** Small pupil of the Vogt-Koyanagi-Harada syndrome, where a peripheral iridotomy was done with the association of YAG-laser and Argon-laser. Notice the wide iridotomy consequent.

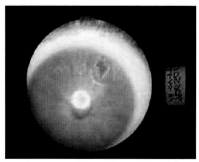

**Figure 7-8.** Peripheral iridotomy done with YAG-laser and Argon-laser.

angle glaucoma, hypotony, cyclitic membrane formation, iris capture, posterior capsule opacification, capsular retraction syndrome, and necessary IOL explant.

## Posterior Synechiae

Synechiae lead to IOL dislocation, pupil seclusion with glaucoma, and may prevent adequate examination of the posterior segment of the globe. These are formed between the iris and the capsule. The incidence of synechia formation is higher in can-opener capsulotomies than in capsulorrhexis. They are rarely formed between the iris and the inflammatory membrane that coats the IOL but never between the iris and the IOL (Figure 7-5).

## Iris Bombé (Figure 7-6)

Although it is known that Nd-YAG laser has been widely used for the performance of iridotomies, membranotomies and even pupillotomies for prompt relief of a hypertensive crisis, in fact only rarely do we achieve a patent iridotomy in an acute glaucoma case with an underlying ocular inflammatory disease. Because it is a noninvasive method, we must use all the medical treatment available to try to reverse the hypertensive disorder and maintain the lowest intraocular pressure possible. We perform iridotomy associating argon laser with Nd-YAG laser, in an attempt to obtain a wide and patent iridotomy. If this does not occur in the primary procedure, we prefer to perform a surgical iridectomy (Figures 7-7 and 7-8).

## Iris Capture

This complication does not occur if the IOL is in the bag and only manifests itself when the IOL has at least 1 haptic in the sulcus, especially in cases in which a can-opener capsulotomy was performed. If the capture has recently occurred, the simple use of mydriatics and miotics may solve the problem. If this is not successful, we use an insulin needle connected to a syringe with the miotic agent and enter the anterior chamber by the limbal route, replace the IOL, and inject the miotic agent.

In more severe cases, we mobilize the pupil with mydriatics and cycloplegics, use topical corticosteroids, and perform a combined capsulotomy and pupilloplasty with Nd-YAG laser or vitrophage through the pars plana (Figures 7-9 and 7-10).

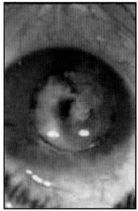

**Figure 7-9.** Pupillary membrane capturing IOL preoperative period when the membrane was excised via pars plana.

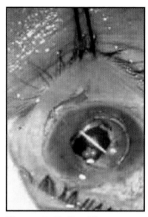

**Figure 7-10.** Pupillary membrane capturing IOL postoperative period when the membrane was excised via pars plana.

## Posterior Capsule Opacity

It occurs in a quarter of healthy eyes submitted to cataract surgery in 5 years and is considered the legal cause of low visual acuity in successful surgeries.

Posterior capsule opacity is observed more frequently in uveitis. This may be due to the underlying pathology, surgical difficulty that limits the removal of lens epithelial cells, or the patient's young age. The type of lens and its position also have an influence on the higher incidence of this complication. The 1-piece acrylic lens appear to work as a true barrier to the migration of lens epithelial cells.

When opacities occur, we must perform a small capsulotomy with Nd-YAG laser, especially when dealing with a silicone lens to avoid its luxation toward the vitreous.

It is important to be aware that capsulotomy with Nd-YAG laser is not a totally innocuous procedure. It may lead to CME, retinal detachment, increased IOP, and IOL luxation among other complications; therefore, it must be delayed as much as possible.

## Capsule Retraction Syndrome

It is due to a combination of various factors such as small anterior capsulotomy (usually less than 5 mm in diameter), incomplete clean-up of lens epithelial cells and finally, increased zonular laxity, which at times may be so intense that it leads to luxation of the IOL and capsular bag toward the vitreous chamber.[12] In these cases, we must make relaxing radial incisions on the anterior capsule with the Nd-YAG laser.

## IOL Removal

Even in apparently well-indicated cases of IOL placement, this procedure seems to propagate ocular inflamma-tion.[13] Thus, in eyes with medically uncontrolled, chronic, or subclinical uveitis that predisposes to pupillary, perilenticular, or cyclitic membrane formation, there is no other alternative but to remove the IOL along with the whole framework represented by the membranes and posterior capsule. The devastating effects of ocular hypotony and end-stage phthisis produced by these membranes are thus prevented.

## REFERENCES

1. Nussenblatt RB, Whitcup SM, Palestine AG. *Uveitis: Fundamentals and Clinical Practice.* 2nd ed. St. Louis, Mo: Mosby; 1996;135-142.

2. Beniz J. Catarata e Uveítes. In: Rezende F, ed. *Cirurgia da catarata.* Rio de Janeiro: Cultura Médica; 2000;Cap44:415-25.

3. Mitre J, Allemann N, Andrade M. In: Abreu G, ed. *Ultra-sonografia ocular: Atlas e Text.* Rio de Janeiro: Cultura Médica; 2000;Cap44:415-25.

4. Foglar R, Biswas J, Ganesh SK, Ravishankar K. Evaluation of cataract surgery in intermediate uveitis. *Ophthalmic Surg Lasers.* 1999;30(3):191-8.

5. Bosch-Driessen LH, Plaisier MB, Stilma JS, Lelij AV, Rothova A. Reactivations of ocular toxoplasmosis after cataract extraction. *Ophthalmology.* 2002;109(1):41-5.

6. Holland GN, Horn SDV, Margolis TP. Cataract surgery with ciliary sulcus fixation of intraocular lenses in patients with uveitis. *Am J Ophthalmol.* 1999;128(1):21-30.

7. Rauz S, Starou P, Murray PI. Evaluation of foldable intraocular lenses in patients with uveitis. *Ophthalmology.* 2000;107(5):909-18.

8. Akova YA, Foster CS. Cataract surgery in patients with sarcoidosis associated uveitis. *Ophthalmology.* 1994;101(3):473-9.

9. Probst LE, Holland EJ. Intraocular lens implantation in patients with juvenile rheumatoid arthritis. *Am J Ophthalmol.* 1996;122(2):161-70.

10. Okhravi N, Lightman SL, Towler HMA. Assessment af visual outcome after cataract surgery in patients with uveitis. *Ophthalmology.* 1999;106(4):710-22.

11. Dana MR, Chatzistefanou K, Schaumberg DA, Foster CS. Posterior capsule opacification after cataract surgery in patients with uveitis. *Ophthalmology.* 1997;104(9):1387-94.

12. Trindade FC. Facectomia e uveíte. In: Orefice F, ed. *Uveíte: Clínica e Cirúrgica: Atlas e Text.* Rio de Janeiro: Cultura Médica; 2000;2:Cap60:1099-104.

13. Foster CS, Stavrou P, Zafirakis P, Rojas B, Tesavibul N, Baltatzis S. Intraocular lens removal patients with uveitis. *Am J Ophthalmol.* 1999;128(1):31-7.

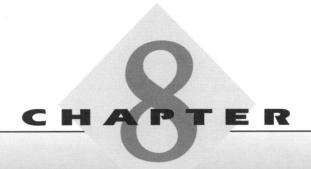

# CHAPTER 8

# DISLOCATION AND DECENTRATION OF INTRAOCULAR LENSES

*Lisa Brothers Arbisser, MD*

## INTRODUCTION

Since Harold Ridley's era, rehabilitation after cataract surgery has been revolutionized by the implantation of an IOL. The IOL restored, and often even improved the focus of light rays upon the retina. Unfortunately, Ridley's own lens design may have been abandoned due to the nearly 10% dislocation rate. Improvements in surgical technique and lens material and design have markedly reduced malpositions. Although incorrect lens power has become the leading reason for explantation in recent years, the incidence of malposition remains significant.[1]

Malpositions can be divided into 3 categories:
1. *Dislocation* (luxation), complete loss of the lens into the vitreous cavity, occurs with an incidence of 0.8% to 1.2%.
2. *Clinically significant decentration* (subluxation), some part of the lens still in the posterior chamber, is noted in about 3% of cases.
3. *Clinically insignificant decentration*, defined as non-coincident optic and pupillary centers without symptoms or signs of inflammation, is estimated to occur in 25% of implantations.[2]

Another characteristic that separates cases of malposition and gives clues as to its etiology is the timing of the onset after surgery. Initial presentation may range from the time of implantation to a decade or more postoperative. The majority of malpositioned PCIOLs are discovered within 3 months of surgery.[3]

## SYMPTOMS

Implant malposition may cause significant visual disability. Optical aberrations include decreased contrast sensitivity, glare, monocular diplopia, chromatic visual distortion, and uncorrected aphakic acuity. Symptoms associated with a decentered IOL's image contrast are inversely proportional to the size of the aphakic portion of the pupil. Light passing through this aphakic crescent forms a blurred secondary image on the retina. For example, when 50% of the pupil is exposed, it causes a 50% decrease in contrast.[4] Although most optics today are 5.5 to 6.0 mm in diameter the effective zone of best acuity may be smaller according to the lens design and material. Multifocal implants employ an even more limited central zone for best distance acuity.

When a luxated lens lies adjacent to the macula, patients have been reported to see the color and position of the lens haptic and are even able to draw its shape and details. One accurately counted the pits from Nd:YAG laser capsulotomy on the lens optic.[5,6]

# ETIOLOGY

Although postoperative trauma can certainly be associated with IOL malposition, its etiology most commonly begins with the initial surgery. Over time, the types of malpositions have evolved with changes in implant styles and surgical technique. Subluxation was most commonly seen with the iris-fixated lenses of the 1970's and 1980's. Subsequently, pupillary capture of the optic was most common in sulcus-fixated lenses without haptic angulation. Haptic malposition from the posterior chamber into the anterior chamber, often through the peripheral iridectomy, which was still in vogue at the time, was common. Elaborate discussion of sunrise, sunset, and windshield wiper syndromes gave clues to the possible etiology of the conditions. This led to better lens design as well as improvements in surgical technique.[7] Today most cases are associated with discontinuity of the capsular bag or the zonular apparatus occurring as complications of cataract surgery. Preexisting conditions that predispose to a weakness of these structures or conditions that restrict the surgeon's view during implantation may lead to a greater likelihood of malposition.

Pseudoexfoliation syndrome, prior trauma, prior surgery such as pars plana vitrectomy, systemic connective tissue disease like Marfan's syndrome, extreme advanced age, and prior miotic therapy may all increase risk. These patients should be preoperatively counseled. In these cases meticulous surgical technique, efforts at inspection prior to implantation and the choice of lens style and material can influence long-term outcome. It is now well recognized that acrylic IOL material causes the least fibrosis and contraction of capsule in the postoperative period, and this should influence lens choice in these patients. Increasing zonular support with CTRs, sutured and unsutured as circumstances require, clearly makes a difference in stabilizing the iris-lens diaphragm intraoperatively and possibly in the postoperative period.[8]

Large pupils may convert a clinically insignificant minor decentration into a symptomatic one. Optic diameter choice and careful centration are all the more critical for these patients. Large anterior segments may also be outsized for the average optic and haptic diameters affecting centration, particularly if sulcus placement is required. Hinting at sulcus size, but not defining it, a white-to-white limbal measurement greater than 13 mm should alert the surgeon that an other-than-standard lens might be appropriate. Plate haptic lenses are a poor choice for these eyes as are 5.5-mm optics or 12- to 12.5-mm diameter haptic 3-piece lenses. The 1-piece foldable acrylic lens, which does not auto-center—but can be positioned at the surgeon's will and expected to adhere in place to the capsule—would be a good choice. Alternatively, if only a standard 3-piece IOL was available and sulcus placement required, the haptics should be sulcus implanted and the optic captured in the posterior chamber through a well-centered and sized capsulorrhexis. A lens with elastimide haptics, which is 14 mm from haptic to haptic, is the best choice for these eyes. A 7-mm optic, 13.5- or 13.75-mm haptic lens would require a larger incision negating the advantage of the clear corneal incision as would an iris-imbricating anterior chamber lens, though these can result in reliable centration in these uncommon circumstances.

Dislocation associated with Nd:YAG laser posterior capsulotomy has been described, almost exclusively with plate haptic silicone lenses. This tendency is also noted to a lesser degree with the newer large hole models.[9-11] A spiral rather than cruciate capsulotomy strategy along with anterior capsule rim relaxing incisions can reduce this risk.

# PREVENTION

Perhaps the single most important improvement in operative technique that reduced lens decentration rates over the last decade has been the continuous circular capsulorrhexis (CCC).[12] Prior techniques all entailed linear tears in the anterior capsule allowing radial propagation of the tears intraoperatively or postoperatively. This prevented reliable endocapsular placement of haptics. Strategies were devised to reduce decentration by placing the haptics away from the area of tears to avoid unfolding of small anterior capsule flap remnants leading to decentration.[13] These noncontinuous edges, however, still allow asymmetric forces to develop with unpredictable anterior-posterior capsule flap adhesions. Moderate decentration, especially late onset, can result.[14] Late-onset decentrations can also be due to initial asymmetric fixation of the haptics with or without an intact CCC. For example, with bag inferior and sulcus superior haptic placement, inferior capsule contraction forces the implant to rise. This error is seen far less commonly with CCC except in small pupil cases. Direct visualization should be performed by retracting the pupil margin to confirm symmetric bag placement. In the era of the can-opener capsulorrhexis, 1 post-mortem study revealed that 48.7% of posterior chamber lenses had a bag-sulcus haptic fixation pattern and that this group had a far higher incidence of decentration. Approximately 60% of all asymmetrically fixated IOLs showed a decentration value of 0.8 mm or more. This can correspond to a loss of at least 17% of the effective optical zone. Interestingly, 16% of sulcus-sulcus implanted lenses compared with only 2% of bag-bag implanted lenses were decentered more than 1 mm. This implies that the sulcus, even without discontinuity of the capsular bag, is not a very reliable place to implant.[15]

The current gold standard is a centered, continuous capsulorrhexis that ideally covers the optic for 360 degrees in a symmetric fashion. The aim is to have the CCC 0.5 to 1 mm smaller in diameter than the optic so all edges are overlapped. This will almost assure good long-term IOL centration. If the rhexis is too large, it may stray into the zone of zonular attachment. If it is too small it may promote capsular phimosis.[16] This can promote zonular weakness requiring intervention with Nd:YAG laser relaxing incisions. Once the IOL is placed, it is not difficult to secondarily enlarge the CCC to the appropriate size, and this maneuver should not be overlooked. If the CCC strays asymmetrically off of the IOL optic it will spoil the sandwich effect, which reduces posterior capsule opacity by limiting lens epithelial cell growth outside the visual axis. Asymmetry of the CCC may also allow the anterior and posterior leaves of the capsule to seal, squeezing the optic off center. Again the risk increases with plate-haptic lens styles. The pursuit of the perfect CCC is a lofty goal contributing to ideal centration in the anterior-posterior direction as well as laterally. This is critical in promoting predictable and stable refractive outcomes. The ideal size CCC has the added advantage of allowing reliable centration of the IOL in the event of a posterior capsule rupture by permitting the sulcus fixation of haptics with the optic captured in the posterior chamber by the CCC. This is undoubtedly the second best place to full bag fixation for securing IOLs. This author knows of no reports of decentration or dislocation of a lens when placed in this fashion.

A newly recognized phenomenon of late spontaneous dislocation of the entire IOL and bag with complete zonular dehiscence has been described.[17] One case posttrauma and several spontaneous luxations with pseudoexfoliation syndrome have been reported.[18] There seems to be a common theme of CCC centripetal fibrosis. We may recognize the patients most at risk by their very shallow preoperative anterior chamber depth measurements of less than 2.5 mm.[19] This phenomenon is another inducement to strive for adequate sizing of the CCC, choice of capsule-compatible lens material and zonular friendly surgical techniques. It remains to be seen whether the placement of CTRs will reduce the risk of this phenomenon by stabilizing the equator of the lens.

An intact CCC is a prerequisite for implantation of a CTR. These devices are definitely helpful in achieving in the bag placement in the case of zonular weakness or zonulolysis. Even a severely subluxated bag can be centered with the Cionni modified ring, as the added islet permits suturing the bag to the sclera without breaching the integrity of the capsule itself.

At each step of the cataract procedure there is an opportunity to lessen the chance of IOL malposition. Wound construction should be tight and tailored to the phacoemulsification tip allowing minimal leak. This reduces the chance that a post-occlusion surge will lead to posterior capsule rupture. Attention should be paid to keeping the paracentesis at 0.5 mm to promote a formed chamber.

Upon IOL insertion, the incision size must be adequate to manage the haptics through the tunnel without damage if forceps implanting, or to prevent stretching and tearing the incision during cartridge insertion. Adequate in-service for scrub personnel loading the IOL into the cartridge for insertion is essential. If a haptic is crimped or torn it will not resume its normal configuration with time. PMMA haptics are quite unforgiving. A haptic can potentially be externalized and coaxed back to an acceptable contour with forceps but immediate explantation and lens exchange should be considered if it doesn't center ideally after this maneuver. If a lens looks asymmetric on the table it won't improve postoperatively. If the incision fails to seal water-tight, along with the risk of endophthalmitis comes the potential for chamber shallowing that can promote optic-pupillary capture in the presence of a large CCC.

Meticulous hydrodissection and delineation will promote gentle rotation of the nucleus averting zonular stress and facilitating cortical clean-up. Capsule and zonule sparing techniques like vertical phacoemulsification chop are optimal. Although supracapsular and flip techniques are zonule friendly, they require the CCC to be tailored to the size of the nucleus rather than the optic of the IOL. Maintaining a stable anterior chamber in the presence of elastic tissues in high myopes and pediatric eyes reduces movement of the vitreous body and accompanying zonular stretch. Using the nondominant hand instrument to lift the iris away from the anterior capsule flap will relieve reverse pupillary block and restore normal chamber depth in these cases.

The anterior leaf of cortex should be aspirated rather than the posterior leaf to avoid residual wisps of cortex. These become the nidus for lens epithelial cell (LEC) growth causing asymmetric forces on the bag and leading to late subtle decentration. Subincisional cortex can be effectively removed with curved I/A tips or bimanual approaches. Sommering's ring, which can cause progressive IOL decentration, emanates from missed clumps of residual cortex that can be avoided by sequential removal of cortex, leaving no skip areas. If complete removal is questioned, the automated I/A setting can be put on a vacuum mode and the capsular fornix safely probed for remaining cortical capsular adhesions. In the case of a small pupil, the iris can be retracted for inspection. Vacuum mode should be used routinely to polish the anterior capsule flaps free of LECs for as close to 360 degrees as possible. These cells can undergo fibrous metaplasia and increase the risk of capsule contraction, especially with silicone IOL materials. There is controversy as to whether these cells may be helpful in creating the sandwich effect and therefore should be left for their role in reducing posterior capsule opacity. The posterior capsule should be polished to minimize the need for Nd:YAG capsulotomy. Attention to all of these details will significantly reduce the incidence of malposition.

## DAMAGE CONTROL

In a routine case with normal anatomy the chances of IOL malposition are small. When a complication occurs, take measures that will significantly influence the likelihood of immediate or delayed subluxation or luxation. Once a complication is recognized, the next step is to control the damage by compartmentalization with a dispersive viscoelastic or viscoadaptive.

A central or paracentral posterior capsule tear requires conversion to a circular capsulorrhexis if at all possible. Even when the posterior tear appears round it still lacks resistance to extension unless it is converted. Insinuate a small amount of viscoelastic through the tear to retroplace the intact vitreous face. Zoom the microscope to high magnification and grasp the edge of the tear with forceps. A proper centripetal vector (directed centrally) minimizes the size of the opening. If there is no edge, one must initiate a tiny cut made with a micro-scissor or intraretinal scissor. This challenging maneuver results in a stable tear and facilitates safe in-the-bag implantation after vitreous and lens material clean up.

It is imperative to make the best effort to maintain the integrity of the CCC for an adequate platform for IOL implantation. If the CCC restricts a large fragment of nucleus from forward movement, it can be enlarged. Under viscoelastic control, a tangential cut is made and forceps used to enlarge the continuous tear to the minimum effective size. Alternatively, radial relaxing incisions are the default maneuver to prevent a tear, which can extend around the equator to the posterior capsule. Before choosing a lens style and position, stop and inspect. Verify a clean bag and the absence of residual vitreous prolapse. Evaluate the intactness of the CCC and the extent of the posterior capsule tear. Note any defects in the zonular apparatus and assess residual sulcus support.

An IOL should be placed in a bag with a posterior tear only if the tear has been converted to a true posterior CCC. A possible exception to this rule may be that the 1-piece acrylic lens, which does not release any pent-up energy on unfolding, does not need to be dialed, and does not create asymmetric forces on the bag with haptic expansion once in place. If these conditions are not present then, if the anterior CCC is intact, a 3-piece lens should be used for sulcus haptic placement with the optic captured through the CCC into the posterior chamber (Figure 8-1).

The 1-piece acrylic is also the lens of choice for bag placement in the presence of an anterior capsulorrhexis edge tear. After inspection to insure that an anterior tear does not extend into the peripheral region of zonular attachment, a 3-piece IOL can also be considered. This must be placed with a 2-handed technique that avoids dialing and therefore pressure on the torn edge. It has been suggested that once in position a radial cut, just through the CCC edge, be made 180 degrees away from the unintended tear to distribute postoperative contractile forces and minimize the risk of late subluxation.

In the absence of both an intact posterior and anterior CCC, a sulcus-style IOL may be placed entirely in the sul-

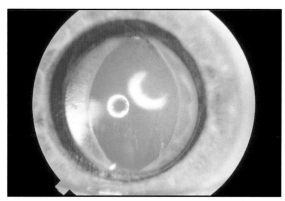

**Figure 8-1.** Haptics in sulcus and optic captured through CCC. Note ovaling of capsulorrhexis at optic haptic junction. (Courtesy of Eye Surgeons Associates, PC.)

cus if there is adequate posterior capsule support 180 degrees apart. Plate-haptic and 1-piece acrylic lenses are not intended for the sulcus. A plate lens can only appropriately be implanted into an intact capsular bag with a perfect CCC.

In cases of zonular weakness or zonulolysis with an intact capsule and CCC, placement of a CTR is optimal. If the bag is not centered or if there is more than 4 clock hours of lysis, the Cionni model that allows scleral fixation should be chosen. This then permits in-the-bag implantation of an IOL. With less than 2 clock hours of lysis an IOL can be considered for the bag without the CTR. When employing a 3-piece style, the haptic should be oriented to support the equator of the bag over the area of missing zonules.

In the absence of scleral support, one could employ a sutured posterior chamber lens or an anterior chamber open loop lens according to surgeon preference. Consider reducing operative time and trauma after a difficult case by the choice of the anterior chamber lens. When appropriately sized for an eye, the modern style lenses have not been associated with an increased risk of corneal decompensation or glaucoma.[20]

If the surgeon has been unable to clean the posterior chamber, there is significant edema and reduced view, and if posterior loss of lens material is confirmed or suspected, temporary aphakia may be the wisest option. A poorly placed or an unstable lens may increase inflammation and hamper a subsequent vitreoretinal surgery.

Once a lens has been placed, certain maneuvers can promote centration and security. A 3-piece posterior chamber lens in an uncomplicated case can be rotated in the bag to assure that no part of the capsule is snagged or tucked. This is most important with a multifocal lens where minimal decentration may distort the vision due to the blend zones around the central distance optical zone becoming axial. If a 3-piece lens does not appear centered despite rotation, suspect that 1 haptic is in the sulcus and the other in the bag. Manual inspection with a lens manipulator can reveal and

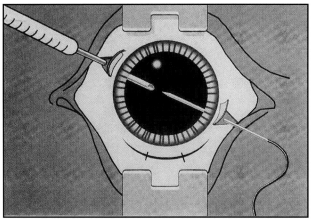

**Figure 8-2.** On a straight needle, a 10-10 polypropylene suture enters a 28-gauge barrel insulin syringe. (Reprinted from *Ophthalmology*, 100[9], Lewis JS, Sulcus fixation without flaps, 1346-1350, Copyright [1993], with permission from Elsevier Science.)

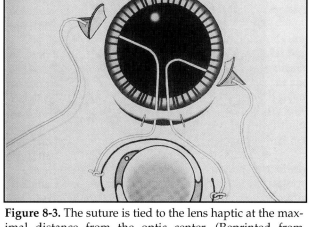

**Figure 8-3.** The suture is tied to the lens haptic at the maximal distance from the optic center. (Reprinted from *Ophthalmology*, 100[9], Lewis JS, Sulcus fixation without flaps, 1346-1350, Copyright [1993], with permission from Elsevier Science.)

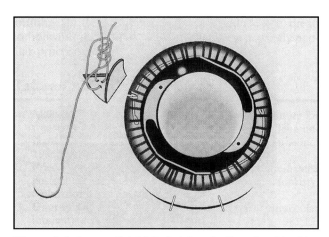

**Figure 8-4.** A superficial bite is taken in the scleral bed to secure the externalized supporting suture. (Reprinted from *Ophthalmology*, 100[9], Lewis JS, Sulcus fixation without flaps, 1346-1350, Copyright [1993], with permission from Elsevier Science.)

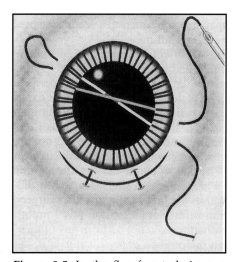

**Figure 8-5.** In the flap free technique, a second transscleral pass is made with the original 10-0 polypropylene suture. (Reprinted from *Ophthalmology*, 100[9], Lewis JS, Sulcus fixation without flaps, 1346-1350, Copyright [1993], with permission from Elsevier Science.)

correct the error. If, after identifying the anterior capsule edge, appropriate placement is confirmed, the decentered lens has a distorted or bent haptic and steps must be taken to reshape it or replace it.

After placing a sulcus lens be sure that the optic remains centered and the haptics are well supported. A tap test may reveal an unstable lens. The effects of gravity in the recumbent position may otherwise be deceiving. If in doubt as to sulcus support, a temporary rescue suture may be placed around a haptic and temporarily tied to avoid loss of a lens posteriorly during implantation. The suture can then be untied intracamerally and removed once the tap test proves the lens position secure. When intentionally suturing a lens into the sulcus the ideal position, ab externo, for the suture is 0.8 mm behind the limbus. Many techniques involve accurate measurement and placement of hollow bore needles to allow the internal suture-swedged needle to be guided out through the ideal position. This can avoid rotational and tilt-induced aberrations in these lenses (Figures 8-2 through 8-8). There is evidence that 10-0 prolene may not be sufficient and 9-0 may be more stable over time when an eyelet haptic implant is employed. A posterior chamber lens may be secured by suturing the haptics with 10-0 prolene to mid-peripheral iris.

When placing anterior chamber lenses, sizing is critical. There are those that say there are 2 sizes—too big and too small. Modern Kelman-style 4-point fixation lenses are more flexible than previous closed loop lens models and have dis-

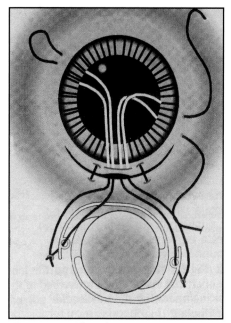

**Figure 8-6.** After the sutures are rescued through the limbal incision, they are cut and threaded through the lens islets. The suture pairs are tied. (Reprinted from *Ophthalmology,* 100[9], Lewis JS, Sulcus fixation without flaps, 1346-1350, Copyright [1993], with permission from Elsevier Science.)

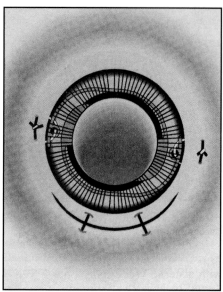

**Figure 8-7.** After lens insertion, the externalized supporting sutures are tied with a standards 3-1-1 square knot. (Reprinted from *Ophthalmology,* 100[9], Lewis JS, Sulcus fixation without flaps, 1346-1350, Copyright [1993], with permission from Elsevier Science.)

crete points of fixation rather than broad contact with the trabecula. This is why the traditional "white-to-white plus one" measurement usually results in a well-fit lens. If the lens is small there will be decentration in the plane of the haptics; if too large, pupil distortion may result. In the extreme, a cyclodialysis cleft may form. Either scenario can be associated with chronic inflammation, pressure problems, or microhyphema (UGH syndrome). To avoid malposition of a correctly sized anterior chamber IOL there are 3 preventable pitfalls. The position of the lens must prevent subluxation of the haptic through the peripheral iridectomy. The trailing haptic must clear the internal Descemet's shelf or the limbal wound edge. Finally, the haptic feet must not tuck the iris peripherally. To position the lens on implantation, the haptics are alternately compressed centrally with a positioning hook to "walk" the lens into an optimal position and release any entrapped peripheral iris.

# TREATMENT

The type of IOL, the location and extent of the malposition, and the patient's symptoms and associated ocular sequelae contribute to the treatment decision process. The course of action may comprise observation, medical symptom abatement, surgical repositioning, or implant removal

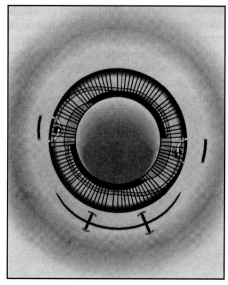

**Figure 8-8.** The polypropylene knot is rotated, buried, and covered with conjunctiva. (Reprinted from *Ophthalmology,* 100[9], Lewis JS, Sulcus fixation without flaps, 1346-1350, Copyright [1993], with permission from Elsevier Science.)

or exchange. Timing of onset is another factor to be considered. If malposition is noted at the time of primary cataract surgery, obviously immediate intervention is indicated. In late-onset subluxation the timing will be based on individual assessment of risks and benefits.

In cases of mild posterior chamber lens decentration, medically inducing miosis in mesopic and scotopic conditions may be sufficient to allow a stable symptom-free outcome. First line choice would be brimontadine hydrochloride for its minimal side-effect profile. This creates a subtle miosis in most eyes and may be sufficient to allow glare-free night driving when this is the predominant complaint. A somewhat more powerful and inexpensive choice would be pilocarpine 0.5% to achieve the same goal. The patient must be warned of the symptoms of retinal tears and the peripheral retina examined for any need for prophylaxis prior to beginning therapy. As long as the patient can tolerate residual imperfection and there is no iritis, pigment dispersion, or CME this may be the treatment of choice.

Surgical intervention is indicated when visual symptoms from a decentered posterior chamber lens cannot be tolerated with medical therapy or the lens is unstable. Dynamic slit lamp examination can reveal pseudophakodonesis, which makes intervention more pressing. IOL rotation is recommended provided there is an intact capsule, acceptable lens power and nondeformed haptics. Paracentesis tracts provide access for 2 Sinskey hooks placed in the optic haptic junction of the decentered lens with viscoelastic to stabilize the anterior chamber. The hooks are used to inspect the edge of the capsulorrhexis. If the lens is seen to be partially in the bag and partially in the sulcus, viscodissection can free the lens for rotation and allow the sulcus haptic to be rotated into the bag. A 2-handed technique using a "y" hook through the paracentesis is most effective. The lens should then reliably center. If the capsulorrhexis is not intact, the optic is rotated into the pupillary space and the haptics into the ciliary sulcus. Once centered, the optic is tapped to assure stability and the iris retracted to inspect the peripheral capsular and zonular ring. If the lens cannot be easily rotated, then viscodissection may avert further compromise of the scarred bag and avoid vitreous presentation. If this maneuver fails to free up the lens, then the haptics should be amputated and the IOL exchanged.

If the lens cannot be centered reliably, or is unstable to the tap test, the reason may be a deformed haptic, or capsular or zonular ruptures. A decision must be made to fixate the current lens by suturing to the iris or the sclera or to explant the lens. The antiquated idea of rotating the entire IOL into the anterior chamber was abandoned because of complications.[21]

Meticulous vitreous cleanup is always critical. The goal is to avoid traction with its higher likelihood of CME and retinal tears. A pars plana incision should be considered for the bimanual vitrector hand piece. Irrigation through an anterior paracentesis avoids hydration of vitreous and further vitreous prolapse. A modified McCannel suture[22] or sliding knot suture, which spares traction on the iris, can be used for fixation.[23-25] One or both haptics are sutured to iris or scle-

ra as needed. Maintenance of potentially self-sealing incisions results in excellent control of the anterior chamber and consistent pressurization, leading to quiet postoperative eyes.

To iris fixate the lens, the optic is elevated with the 2 Sinskey hooks to induce pupillary capture. Miocol E is instilled. This will peak the pupil along the axis of the optic-haptic junction and make the silhouette of the haptics evident against the posterior surface of the iris guiding suture placement. A CTC-6 or CIF-4 needle with 10-0 Prolene suture (Ethicon Inc, Sommerville, NJ) is ideal. The bites should be mid-peripheral (to allow pupillary dilation postoperatively), small, and not overly tight to avoid peaking the pupil. The suture ends should be cut short to avoid rabbit ears irritating the corneal endothelium. The optic is then repositioned behind the iris and viscoelastic exchanged for BSS.[26]

Long-term data in postmortem eyes show that iris-fixated lenses are well tolerated.[27]

When scleral fixation is preferred there are many techniques that have been described over time in the literature. They all have certain goals in common. Strategies to avoid both vitreous entrapment, and to prevent suture erosion are required. Reliable placement of the haptics anatomically in the sulcus and precisely 180 degrees apart avoids torsion and tilt.

There is consensus that when the lens is completely luxated into the posterior segment, a 3-port pars plana vitrectomy, often with perfluorocarbon liquid to float the lens off the macula is indicated.[28-30] These liquids have a specific gravity greater than water and a high-surface tension. Of the 4 types in clinical use, the perfluorophenanthrene is the only one that can be retained in the eye without toxicity for up to 30 days in the event of concurrent retinal detachment. The technique of viscolevitation through the pars plana described by Chang can salvage an IOL dislocated into the anterior vitreous without involvement of a posterior segment surgeon depending on the surgeon's comfort with this maneuver.[31] Once the lens is restored to the pupillary plane it can be treated like a subluxated lens without exchange if it is a 3-piece posterior chamber style, is undamaged, and provides the appropriate refractive power.

There are many ways to secure a haptic. Because vitreoretinal surgeons are usually involved in luxation cases, their techniques and instrumentation have become part of the armamentarium for these patients. Sutures must be placed symmetrically at the bend of the haptic, or at the point of greatest distance between them. To accomplish this, the surgeon may pursue a choice of strategies. Temporary externalization of the haptic reduces intraocular gymnastics. It has been advocated through the limbus, through the pars plana, but it is probably best done through horizontal sclerotomies at the ciliary sulcus where final 2- or 4-point fixation can occur. The suture may be attached with a triple throw knot. Slip knots have also been advocated to reduce the time and complexity of the manipulations involved. Cautery can be applied to bead up the end of the haptic and prevent the suture from sliding off.[32-34]

Intracameral suture attachment to haptics has been accomplished by many techniques. The simple use of double-armed sutures placed above and below the bend of the haptic affecting a loop around it does not require visualization of the tip of the haptic.[35] This is a quick and simple technique and may be adequate when only 1 haptic needs to be secured because of some residual capsule support. Similarly, the "luggage-tag" suture fixation is applicable in this situation and may provide better stability to avoid torque. This technique involves "passing an untied loop of double-armed suture under the haptic so that it emerges upward between the haptic and the optic. The loop of suture is regrasped from above the haptic and externalized. The free ends are passed through the loop in a manner analogous to a luggage tag, and the knot is secured."[36] When the haptic end is visible, techniques to secure the haptic with a suture snare,[37] or a special threaded needle[38] have been ingeniously devised. A special 25-gauge forceps has been designed to facilitate many of these maneuvers as well.[39] These challenges seem to bring out the cowboy in the ophthalmologist as there are many variations such as the lens lasso and the cow-hitch knot.[40-42]

Anatomic considerations require accurate suture placement transclerally no more than 0.5 to 1 mm from the surgical limbus. Sutures must be perpendicular to the sclera in order to have a hope of true sulcus placement and to avoid hemorrhage from the ciliary body or the major arterial circle.[43] The actual location is 0.83 mm in the vertical meridian and only 0.46 mm posterior to the limbus in the horizontal meridian. Many techniques utilize 26- or 27-gauge hypodermic needles for accurate ab externo positioning as a guide. The internal suture-swedged needle is threaded into the bore and externalized at the precise location.[44-45] Interestingly, an UBM study of unsutured posterior chamber IOL implantation after capsular tear showed that half the patients had optic tilt. More than half the IOLs were not actually located in the intended location of the sulcus even in experienced surgeons.[46] In an evaluation of sutured posterior chamber IOLs in pseudophakic postmortem eyes, some showed sutures through iris stroma as well as the pars plicata.[47] Endoscopy is not widely available and has a steep learning curve; however, it could be useful as the only way to visualize what is actually taking place behind the iris. Suture placement, haptic alignment, and vitreous incarceration would be directly observed.[31] Another common technical error is possible asymmetric placement of the suture on the haptics. This can result in tilt or torsion and thus adversely affect the quality of postoperative vision. This is why eyelets were developed on the haptics of lenses used strictly for the purpose of secondary sulcus fixation. This of course requires

explanation of the previous lens and as the lens is currently manufactured only of nonfoldable PMMA, a larger incision is required.

The issue of suture erosion is significant as there are reports of endophthalmitis associated with exposed sutures.[48] To avoid erosion, which occurs in 24% of suture knots covered with conjunctiva, surgeons have used partial thickness scleral flaps which still have an erosion rate of 15%.[49] In cases of knot erosion, trimming, cautery, and occasionally adjunctive surgery with scleral patch grafting is necessary. Methods for internalizing knots by rotation or using the islet of a fixation IOL to house the knot internally, have been developed.[44]

If the suture is ever cut or breaks the chances of redislocation are significant as there is no evidence on histopathology of any fibrous encapsulation of the lens haptics.[50] The patient should be counseled about this danger and the medical records travel with him in the event of a change of ophthalmic care.[51]

If explanation of a foldable IOL is required or preferred, one may avoid the need for a large incision by refolding or cutting the lens intracamerally. To refold, after extricating the lens from the bag or sulcus, a viscoelastic sandwich is formed in the anterior chamber. Through a paracentesis 180 degrees away from the main incision, a sweep is introduced under the optic and folding forceps are brought down over the optic to affect the fold and extract the lens. This can sometimes damage the proximal iris and care must be taken not to entrap it between the edges of the fold thereby causing a dialysis on removal of the lens. Alternatively, with the viscoelastic barrier in place, intraocular scissors are used with counter pressure from an instrument though the standard paracentesis to allow the jaws of the scissor to progress over the full diameter of the optic. It can be completely transected or cut three-fourths of the way through the optic and extracted in one piece. As it opens like a ladybug's wings, half its diameter is presented to the incision with the first haptic. The hinge between the cut sections presents next and then the trailing haptic is withdrawn attached to the second half. Almost any scissor easily sections silicone material. For slightly tougher Acrysof acrylic (Alcon, Fort Worth, Tex), one can use any lens cutting instrument such as a snare or any IOL scissor. However, the Sensar acrylic (Allergan, Irvine, Calif) tends to be tougher and requires a heavier scissor like the MacKool help kit to be efficiently transected. Obviously, if the lens is to be exchanged with a nonfoldable implant these maneuvers are not needed.

Once the offending lens is removed, the choice of lens for exchange must be made. Consider using a lens with eyelets for sulcus fixation whereas a 3-piece foldable lens is ideal for iris fixation. Another viable choice is a modern Kelman style, 4-point fixation anterior chamber lens. Appropriate sizing as described above is needed as well as a peripheral iridectomy. This can be neatly made with the guillotine vitrector and does not require further incision or traction on the iris. Iris-imbricating anterior chamber lens styles are also popular where available. These anterior chamber choices require less time, may involve less tissue trauma and operating microscope light exposure, and require skills that are in the armamentarium of the average anterior segment surgeon. The outcomes for the open-loop trabecular fixated anterior chamber IOLs seem to be compatible and even competitive with other methods.[52-54] Remembering to adjust IOL power for the more anterior position is important.

Although today optimal refractive outcomes are a large part of patient and surgeon satisfaction, the possibility of IOL explantation without exchange should be entertained in extreme cases. Visual rehabilitation through contact lens wear can be a functional option and may give an edematous macula its best chance of recovery.

Some surgeons have advocated retaining a luxated lens in the posterior segment and correcting aphakia or placing a second lens, either fixated or anterior chamber. There are anecdotal reports of lenses, especially plate-haptic silicone styles, which have the highest incidence of luxation, being compatible with long- term good function.[55] These tend not to become sessile, however, and often remain free floating in the vitreous cavity. The consensus regarding "bi-pseudophakia" is that the potential for retinal damage or visual disability outweighs the risk of explantation in most cases. It is not recommended to place a secondary lens with 1 luxated lens present.[56]

## OUTCOMES

By now, it should be obvious that an ounce of prevention is worth a pound of cure. Outcomes for repair of IOL malposition are difficult to assess. The trauma of the original surgical complication or the effect of injury to tissues that led to the dislocation cannot be easily distinguished from results of the subsequent treatment. Another confounding factor is the wide range of etiologies of malposition, of techniques used for fixation, and the variable extent of vitrectomy required. Snellen acuity measurements often do not accurately reflect the extent of visual disability with glare and distortion being frequent preoperative complaints. These issues are not quantitatively assessed preoperatively or postoperatively in studies and this further confounds the information that can be gleaned from the literature. In general, there is a mean of 2 lines of improvement in vision with extreme ranges of outcomes from light perception to 20/20. Outcomes of 20/40 or better vision occur in a range from 57% to 94% of patients in several studies.[57-58] The pathology treated and techniques used in these disparate studies are, however, not comparable.

The most common reason for poor outcome was corneal decompensation and glaucoma in the 1980s and CME in the last decade. An angiographic study after scleral fixation revealed 2 other macular problems. Epiretinal membrane

development may be associated with incomplete vitrectomy and the relationship of the vitreous to the IOL unseen behind the iris. Physical injury compatible with operating microscope light toxicity was also seen in up to 33% of cases, though often asymptomatic.[57] In a recent study of 110 dislocations managed by 2 surgeons with many techniques and a mean followup of 13 months, there was an incidence of retinal detachment of 6.3%, vision limiting CME was seen in 3% and 1 patient suffered phthisis bulbi after suprachoroidal hemorrhage associated with transcleral suturing.[59] In another study of sulcus fixation lenses with a median follow up of 15 months, there was a similar rate of retinal detachment, 26% incidence of CME, a 9% rate of epiretinal membrane and a 14% rate of pupillary capture or redislocation.[60] Although scleral fixation has become popular, the outcomes appear rather dismal.

In a comparison of visual results in eyes treated with pars plana vitrectomy and lens repositioning versus lens exchange, the complications and the results were similar. In this retrospective study with a mean follow up of 3 years, eyes that received a lens exchange with a posterior chamber PCIOL had visual results similar to those receiving an ACIOL though the mean increase in visual acuity was greatest in the anterior chamber group.[61]

A prospective randomized trial of IOL fixation techniques with penetrating keratoplasty for pseudophakic corneal edema compared ACIOL placement, transcleral fixation of PCIOLs and iris fixation cases. The cumulative risk of macular edema was significantly less for the iris-fixated cohort than for either the ACIOL or the scleral fixation group. A significantly lower risk of complication was found for the iris compared to the scleral fixation group of PCIOLs. With the techniques used in this study there was a high rate of tilt causing visual disability in the sulcus cohort. Of great interest was the finding of almost twice the rate of peripheral anterior synechia formation in the scleral fixation group compared to the ACIOL group in this multicenter study, which flies in the face of conventional wisdom.[52] In a major retrospective study of over 4000 explanted ACIOLs encompassing more than 14 years, there was convincing evidence that the open-loop ACIOLs are capable of providing a vastly superior tolerance over a long-term period as opposed to their closed-loop counterparts. The deservedly bad reputation of the discontinued closed-loop rigid ACIOLs should not prevent consideration of their modern successors.[53]

## CONCLUSION

It is very difficult to come to a definitive conclusion as to the best course of action and the best technique for this multifaceted problem. The individuality of the malpositions and anatomic status of each eye make it almost impossible to have a like group of patients for which to create a prospective study. With a wide array of treatment options, and a varied level of ability and experience among surgeons, there are too many variables to compare what amount to anecdotal reports of techniques. Because treatment really needs to be tailored to the findings at the time of surgery, it is hard to randomize patients. I was surprised to find, on review of the literature, no distinct advantage and perhaps a trend to a higher complication rate associated with scleral fixation than either iris fixation or anterior chamber lens implantation. Implant repositioning surgery should not be taken lightly and risk benefit ratios should be carefully discussed with patients. There remains no clear indication of our best course of action to date. We must not aim to please ourselves with a pretty slit-lamp view but plan to serve the patients' needs. The iris can hide many sins that the macula or optics of the eye fail to forgive.

If surgery is indicated, it makes sense to try to reposition a viable existing implant in order to maintain a pressurized eye with minimal invasiveness. Depending upon the surgeon's preference and experience, scleral or iris fixation is optional though the latter seems to have an edge in reduced complications postoperatively. If lens exchange is required, some surgeons with experience in sulcus-sutured lenses will choose this option. As retro as it seems, modern open-loop anterior chamber lenses pose an excellent option in the absence of sulcus support.

# REFERENCES

1. Panton R, Sulewski M, Parker J, Panton P, Stark W. Surgical management of subluxed posterior-chamber intraocular lenses. *Arch Ophthalmol.* 1993;111(7):919-926.

2. Smiddy W, Ibanez G, Alfonso E, Flynn Jr H. Surgical management of dislocated intraocular lenses. *J Cataract Refract Surg.* 1995;21(1):64-69.

3. Shakin E, Carty J Jr. Clinical management of posterior chamber intraocular lens implants dislocated in the vitreous cavity. *Ophthalmic Surg Lasers.* 1995;26(6):529-534.

4. Kumar S, Miller D. Effect of intraocular decentration on retinal image contrast. *J Cataract Refract Surg.* 1990;16(6):712-714.

5. Miedziak A, Carty J Jr. Chromatic visual phenomenon caused by a subluxed intraocular lens. *J Cataract Refract Surg.* 1996;22(5):637-638.

6. Yong V, Lee H, AuEong K, Yong V. Subjective visual perception of a dislocated intraocular lens. *J Cataract Refract Surg.* 2002;28(8):1494-1495.

7. Smith S, Lindstrom R. Malpositioned posterior chamber lenses: etiology, prevention, and management. *Journal of American Intraocular Implant Society.* 1985;11:584-591.

8. Cionni R, Osher R. Management of profound zonular dialysis or weakness with a new endocapsular ring designed for scleral fixation. *J Cataract Refract Surg.* 1998;24(10):1299-1306.

9. Petersen A, Bluth L, Campion M. Delayed posterior dislocation of silicone plate-haptic lenses after neodymium: YAG capsulotomy. *J Cataract Refract Surg.* 2000;26(12):1827-1829.

10. Agustin A, Miller K. Posterior dislocation of a plate-haptic silicone intraocular lens with large fixation holes. *J Cataract Refract Surg.* 2000;26(9):1428-1429.

11. Schneiderman T, Johnson M, Smiddy W, Flynn H Jr, Bennet S, Cantrill H. Surgical management of posteriorly dislocated silicone plate haptic intraocular lenses. *Am J Ophthalmol.* 1997;123(5):629-635.

12. Gimbel H, Neuhann T. Development, advantages, and methods of the continuous circular capsulorrhexis technique. *J Cataract Refract Surg.* 1990;16(1):31-37.

13. Davison J. Analysis of capsular bag defects and intraocular lens positions for consistent centration. *J Cataract Refract Surg.* 1986;12(2):124-129.

14. Assia E, Apple D, Barden A, Tsai J, Castaneda V, Hoggatt J. An experimental study comparing various capsulectomy techniques. *Arch Ophthalmol.* 1991;109(5):642-647.

15. Hansen S, Tetz M, Solomon K, et al. Decentration of flexible loop posterior chamber intraocular lenses in a series of 222 postmortem eyes. *Ophthalmology.* 1988;95(3):344-349.

16. Davison J. Capsule contraction syndrome. *J Cataract Refract Surg.* 1993;19(5):582-589.

17. Jehan F, Mamalis N, Crandall A. Spontaneous late dislocation of intraocular lens within the capsular bag in pseudoexfoliation patients. *Ophthalmology.* 2001;108(10):1727-1731.

18. Zech J, Tanniere P, Denis P, Trepsat C. Posterior chamber intraocular lens dislocation with the bag. *J Cataract Refract Surg.* 1999;25(8):1168-1169.

19. Masket S, Osher R. Late complications with intraocular lens dislocation after capsulorrhexis in pseudoexfoliation syndrome. *J Refract Surg.* 2002;28(8):1481-1484.

20. Apple D, Hansen S, Richards S, et al. Anterior chamber lenses. Part II: a laboratory study. *J Cataract Refract Surg.* 1987;13(2):175-189.

21. Liu J, Koch D, Emery J. Complications of implanting three-piece C-loop posterior chamber lenses in the anterior chamber. *Ophthalmic Surg.* 1988;19(11):802-807.

22. McCannel M. A retrievable suture idea for anterior uveal problems. *Ophthalmic Surg.* 1976;7:98-103.

23. Siepser S. The closed chamber slipping suture technique for iris repair. *Ann Ophthalmol.* 1994;26(3):71-72.

24. Snyder M. Repairing the iris. *Review of Ophthalmology.* 2000;7(10):139-148.

25. Ogawa G, O'Gawa G. Single wound, in situ tying technique for iris repair. *Ophthalmic Surg Lasers.* 1998;29(11):943-948.

26. Panton R, Sulewski M, Parker J, Panton P, Stark W. Surgical management of subluxed posterior-chamber intraocular lenses. *Arch Ophthalmol.* 1993;111(7):919-926.

27. Apple D, Price F, Gwin T, et al. Sutured retropupillary posterior chamber intraocular lenses for exchange or secondary implantation—the 12th annual Binkhorst lecture, 1988. *Ophthalmology.* 1989;96(8):1241-1247.

28. Yoshida K, Kiryu J, Kita M, Ogura Y. Phacoemulsification of dislocated lens and suture fixation of intraocular lens using a perfluorocarbon liquid. *Jpn J Ophthalmol*. 1998;42(6):471-475.

29. Fanous M, Friedman S. Ciliary sulcus fixation of a dislocated posterior chamber intraocular lens using liquid perfluorophenanthrene. *Ophthalmic Surg*. 1992;23:551-552.

30. Greve M, Peyman G, Mehta N, Millsap C. Use of perfluoroperhydrophenanthrene in the management of posteriorly dislocated crystalline and intraocular lenses. *Ophthalmic Surg*. 1993;24(9):593-597.

31. Chang DF. Viscoelastic levitation of posteriorly dislocated intraocular lenses from the anterior vitreous. *J Cataract Refract Surg*. 2002;28(9):1515-19.

32. Kokame G, Atebara N, Bennett M. Modified technique of haptic externalization for scleral fixation of dislocated posterior chamber lens implants. *Am J Ophthalmol*. 2001; 131(1):129-131.

33. Lee S, Tseng S, Cheng H, Chen F. Slipknot for scleral fixation of intraocular lenses. *J Cataract Refract Surg*. 2001;27(5):662-664.

34. Chan C. An improved technique for management of dislocated posterior chamber implants. *Ophthalmology*. 1992; 99(1):51-57.

35. Kwok A, Cheng A, Lam D. Surgical technique for transscleral-fixation of a dislocated posterior chamber intraocular lens. *Am J Ophthalmol*. 2001;132(3):406-408.

36. Virata S, Holekamp N, Meredith T. Luggage tag suture fixation of partially dislocated intraocular lenses. *Ophthalmic Surg Lasers*. 2001;32(4):346-348.

37. Poon A, Clark J, Grey R, Markham R. A simple snare for transscleral fixation of dislocated intraocular lenses. *Aus N Z J Ophthalmol*. 1996;24(4):385-388.

38. Smiddy W, Flynn Jr H. Needle-assisted scleral fixation suture technique for relocating posteriorly dislocated IOLs. *Arch Ophthalmol*. 1993;111(2):161-162.

39. Chang S, Coll G. Surgical techniques for repositioning a dislocated intraocular lens, repair of iridodialysis, and secondary intraocular lens implantation using innovative 25-gauge forceps. *Am J Ophthalmol*. 1995;119(2):165-174.

40. Sangha S, Sangha K, Sangha H. Dislocated intraocular lens fixation using intraocular cowhitch knot. *Am J Ophthalmol*. 2001;132(6):949.

41. Lawrence F, Hubbard W. Lens lasso repositioning of dislocated posterior chamber intraocular lenses. Retina. *The Journal of Retina and Vitreous Diseases*. 1994;4(1):47-50.

42. Navia-Aray E. A technique for knotting a suture around the loops of a dislocated intraocular lens, within the eye, for fixation in the ciliary sulcus. *Ophthalmic Surg*. 1993;24(10):702-707.

43. Duffey R, Holland E, Lindstrom R, Agapitos P. Anatomic study of transsclerally sutured intraocular lens implantation. *Am J Ophthalmol*. 1989;108(3):300-309.

44. Lewis J. Sulcus fixation without flaps. *Ophthalmology*. 1993;100(9):1346-1350.

45. Koh H, Kim C, Lim S, Kwon O. Scleral fixation technique using 2 corneal tunnels for a dislocated intraocular lens. *J Cataract Refract Surg*. 2000;26(10):1439-1441.

46. Loya N, Lichter H, Barash D, Goldenberg-Cohen N, Strassmann E, Weinberger D. Posterior chamber intraocular lens implantation after capsular tear: ultrasound biomicroscopy evaluation. *J Cataract Refract Surg*. 2001; 27(9):1423-1427.

47. *Evaluation of Sutured Posterior Chamber Intraocular Lenses in Pseudophakic Postmortem Human Eyes*. Poster presented at American Society of Cataract and Refractive Surgery Meeting. Boston, Massachusetts; 2000.

48. Schechter R. Suture-wick endophthalmitis with sutured posterior chamber intraocular lenses. *J Cataract Refract Surg*. 1990;16(6):755-756.

49. Holland E, Daya S, Eyangelista A, et al. Penetrating keratoplasty and transscleral fixation of posterior chamber lens. *Am J Ophthalmol*. 1992;114(2):182-187.

50. Lubniewski A, Holland E, VanMeter W, Gussler D, Parelman J, Smith M. Histologic study of eyes with transsclerally sutured posterior chamber intraocular lenses. *Am J Ophthalmol*. 1990;110(3):237-243.

51. Cahane M, Chen V, Avni I. Dislocation of a scleral-fixated, posterior chamber intraocular lens after fixation suture removal. *J Cataract Refract Surg*. 1994;20(2):186-187.

52. Schein O, Kenyon K, Steinert R, et al. A randomized trial of intraocular lens fixation techniques with penetrating keratoplasty. *Ophthalmology*. 1993;100(10):1437-1443.

53. Auffarth G, Wesendahl T, Brown S, Apple D. Are there acceptable anterior chamber intraocular lenses for clinical use in the 1990s? *Ophthalmology*. 1994;101(12):1913-1922.

54. Mittra R, Connor T, Han D, Koenig S, Mieler W, Pulido J. Removal of dislocated intraocular lenses using pars plana vitrectomy with placement of an open-loop, flexible anterior chamber lens. *Ophthalmology*. 1998;105(6):1011-1014.

55. Wong K, Grabow H. Simplified technique to remove posteriorly dislocated lens implants. *Arch Ophthalmol*. 2001;119(2):273-274.

56. Izak A, Apple D, Werner L, et al. Bipseudophakia: clinicopathological correlation of a dropped lens. *J Cataract Refract Surg*. 2002;28(5):874-882.

57. Lanzetta P, Menchini U, Virgili G, Crovato S, Rapizzi E. Scleral fixated intraocular lenses: an angiographic study. Retina. *The Journal of Retinal and Vitreous Diseases*. 1998;18(6):515-520.

58. Mamalis N, Crandall A, Pulsipher M, Follett S, Monson M. Intraocular lens explantation and exchange: a review of lens styles, clinical indications, clinical results, and visual outcome. *J Cataract Refract Surg*. 1991;17(6):811-818.

59. Mello M Jr, Scott I, Smiddy W, Flynn Jr H, Feuer W. Surgical management and outcomes of dislocated intraocular lenses. *Ophthalmology*. 2000;107(1):62-67.

60. Thac A, Dugel P, Sipperley J, et al. Outcome of sulcus fixation of dislocated posterior chamber intraocular lenses using temporary externalization of the haptics. *Ophthalmology*. 2000;107(3):480-484.

61. Sarrafizadeh R, Ruby A, Hassan T, et al. A comparison of visual results and complications in eyes with posterior chamber intraocular lens dislocation treated with pars plana vitrectomy and lens repositioning or lens exchange. *Ophthalmology*. 2001;108(1):82-89.

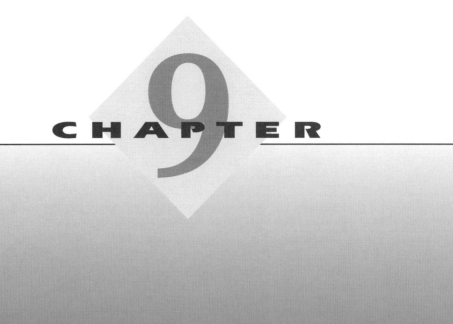

# CHAPTER 9

# INTRAOCULAR LENS EXCHANGE

*Francisco Contreras, MD and Cecilia Contreras, MD*

IOL implantation in cataract surgery began in 1949. If a lens is placed into a previously aphakic eye, we have a secondary implantation of an IOL. If a lens is removed for some unfavorable condition and is replaced by another, we have performed a lens exchange procedure.[1] *Intraocular lens explantation* is removing the IOL without a replacement.[2,3] The incorrect position of an IOL and incorrect power of the lens are presently the most frequent causes of lens exchange.[4,5] Conditions that presently indicate a lens exchange and possible complications of secondary IOLs will be discussed.[6,7]

We will first refer to corneal problems. Reduction or alteration of the endothelial cells due to surgical trauma, inadequate positioning of the IOL or chronic inflammation, may produce edema, bullae, or corneal opacification. It is important to consider the corneal status such as guttata or Fuch's syndrome before cataract surgery.

With regard to the IOL, if we implant an anterior chamber lens (ACL), it is recommended to use those with flexible haptics with the minimal surface of contact with the anterior chamber angle, as the Kelman open-looped lens. Closed-loop lenses are not used today due to uveitis, glaucoma, and possible hyphema.[2,8] If the lens is too small it will be unstable and move, causing inflammation. If the lens is too big it will usually produce pain and the haptic will infiltrate into the uveal stroma, causing chronic inflammation and peripheral anterior synechiae. The iris-supported IOL may move if the iris suture stitches are not placed appropriately, producing pigment dispersion and inflammation.

One of the most frequent causes of the PCIOL being in poor position is that the continuous circular capsulotomy is very big, is eccentric, or has been torn making it possible for 1 or both haptic to exit from the capsular bag, decentralizing and producing optic problems. If the capsulotomy is very small it may present fibrous retraction of the remaining anterior capsular surface and cause capsular phimosis.[9]

The chronic ocular inflammation, besides the mentioned alterations in the corneal endothelium, produces inflammatory infiltration with dispersion of the pigment, central pupillary synechiae, and peripheral anterior synechiae[3] that may also involve the trabecular meshwork and even the main arterial circle of the iris. CME is a disorder that is frequently present after cataract surgeries, more so when there are complications. The topical medical treatment with steroids or non-steroid anti-inflammatory drops should be helpful.[10] When there is a subluxation of the IOL, lens exchange surgery may be useful. We prefer an ACL implant, both for a secondary IOL or a lens exchange.

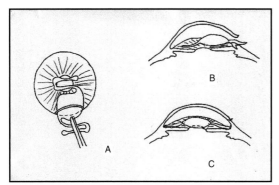

**Figure 9-1A, B, & C.** Introduction of open-looped lens into the anterior chamber is shown in (A) and (B); be careful with the position of the haptics in the anterior chamber angle (C).

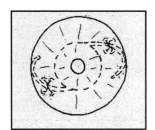

**Figure 9-3.** Lens fixated to the iris. Frontal view of the IOL in final position.

# LENS IN ANTERIOR CHAMBER

This is the easiest technique. This is usually used in older people, with good corneal endothelium, deep anterior chamber, and normal ocular pressure. As in any surgical procedure, the careful previous ocular examination is very important, considering: corrected visual acuity, presence of vitreous in the anterior chamber, gonioscopic examination to detect peripheral or pupillary synechiae, or vitreous bands to a previous corneal or limbal surgical scar. For the ACIOL, it is necessary to measure the horizontal corneal diameter white-to-white and to use an IOL 1 mm longer than the corneal diameter, the lens should be open looped lens with blunt borders. The eye should be hypotonic, and the pupil made small with any miotic. After local anesthesia, we perform a limbal incision parallel to the iris equal in size to the diameter of the optical zone of the lens. An anterior vitrectomy is performed if there is vitreous in the anterior chamber. The IOL is slid over the iris assuring that the iris is not incarcerated. The limbal wound is sutured with 10-0 nylon sutures (Figures 9-1A, B, and C).

# LENS FIXATION TO THE IRIS

To avoid problems that may be present with scleral fixated IOLs, such as the inclination of the lens, the late exposi-

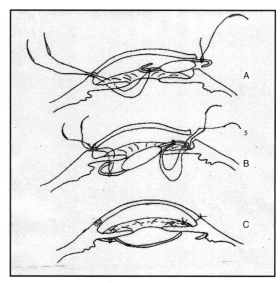

**Figure 9-2A, B, & C.** Lens fixation to the iris. Both haptics are sutured with 10-0 Prolene, double needle. The distal prolene perforate the iris from front to back and go out from the previous short corneal distal incision. Both sutures fix the haptics to the iris.

tion of the scleral sutures and occasionally endophthalmitis, the secondary IOL is fixated to the iris. We will describe the Nose technique.[11] It uses a 6.5- or 7-mm optic diameter IOL. The distal haptic is thread with one 10-0 Prolene (Ethicon Inc., Sommerville, NJ) suture with holes in the haptic and the proximal haptic hole using a similar 10-0 Prolene suture double-curved needle. We make a short corneal distal incision to facilitate the exit of the suture. The IOL is placed in the anterior chamber sliding it behind the iris. On the upper haptic, with the lens in the appropriate position, the iris stroma is perforated from back to front with both needles. The suture is tied on the iris. The same technique is used on the lower haptic. To finish, the superior limbal wound is sutured where we introduced the IOL. The inferior corneal incision is edematized (Figures 9-2A, B, C, and 9-3).

# IOL WITH SCLERAL FIXATION

This technique is preferred by the most experienced surgeons. The lens is placed far from the corneal endothelium, avoiding the iris chaffe and iris deformity produced by the fixed lens to the iris. They may be implanted in eyes with poor iris tissue or glaucoma. It is necessary to properly know the surgical anatomy of the limbal area and surrounding area. The haptic of the IOL should be sutured with 10-0 Prolene in the ciliary sulcus corresponding to the outside 0.5 mm posterior to the blue limbal zone. The needles should not be placed in the horizontal diameter to avoid the posterior long ciliary vessels. There are several scleral fixation

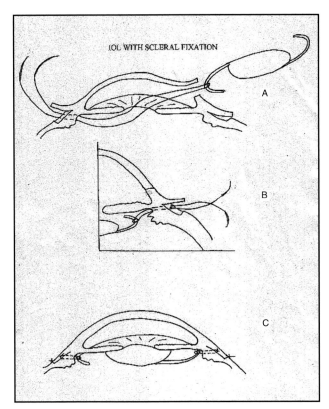

**Figure 9-4A, B, & C.** IOL with scleral fixation. (A) The eye is prepared with 2 lamellar sclerotomies, one distal and one proximal that are 2 to 3 mm of size, keeping the scleral flaps. (B) The same procedure is performed with the proximal haptic. (C) The scleral flaps are closed with 10-0 nylon and the limbal incision where the IOL was introduced is closed with 10-0 nylon.

techniques developed since Malbran first described it.[10] Essentially, after the pupil is dilated and previous local anesthesia, each haptic is fastened with double needle prolene 10-0 sutures. The eye is prepared with 2 lamellar sclerotomies, one distal and one proximal that are 2 to 3 mm of size, keeping the scleral flaps (Figure 9-4A). The IOL is introduced into the anterior chamber through a limbal or corneal incision and then the 2 needles of the distal haptic are passed behind the iris, perforating the sclera 0.5 mm behind the limbal zone, and exiting through the lamellar sclerectomy. The same procedure is performed with the proximal haptic (Figure 9-4B). The superior and inferior sutures are tightened smoothly, positioning the optical part of the lens in the correct position. The scleral flaps are closed with 10-0 nylon and the limbal incision where the IOL was

introduced is closed with 10-0 nylon (Figure 9-4C). This technique may have some complications as a tilt, decentration, or dislocation of the lens or vitreous hemorrhage, but in expert hands this technique gives satisfactory outcomes. It is important that the scleral suture be covered by conjunctiva; if not, the scleral suture could present a potential wick of bacterial entry in the vitreous cavity.[12]

## SUMMARY

Although there are advantages and disadvantages of the PCIOLs, an ACIOL in poor position brings more optical and clinical problems than a posterior chamber IOL in poor position.

## REFERENCES

1. Pande M, Noble BA. The role of intraocular lens exchange in the management of major implant-related complications. *Eye.* 1993;7:34-39.

2. Price FW Jr, et al. Changing trends in explanted intraocular lenses: a single center study. *J Cataract Refract Surg.* 1992; 18:470-474.

3. Kraff MC. A survey of intraocular lens explanations. *J Cataract Refract Surg.* 1986;12:644-650.

4. Doren G. Indications for and results of intraocular lens explanation. *J Cataract Refract Surg.* 1992;18:79-85.

5. Lyle WA, Jin JC. An analysis of intraocular lens exchange. *Ophthalmic Surgery.* 1992;23:453-458.

6. Sinskey RM. Indications for and results of a large series of intraocular lens exchanges. *J Cataract Refract Surg.* 1993; 19:68-71.

7. Price Jr FW. Explanation of posterior chamber lenses. *J Cataract Refract Surg.* 1992;18:475-479.

8. Coli A. Intraocular lens exchange for anterior chamber intraocular lens-induced corneal endothelial damage. *Ophthalmology.* 1993;100:384-393.

9. Carlson A. Intraocular lens complications requiring removal or exchange. *Survey of Ophthalmology.* 1998;42:417-440.

10. Boyd BJ. *World Atlas Series.* Panama: Highlights of Ophthalmology International; 1995:2:118-120.

11. Nose W. Personal Communication; 2001.

12. Schechter RJ. Suture-wick endophthalmitis with sutured posterior chamber intraocular lenses. *J Cataract Refract Surg.* 1990;16:755-756.

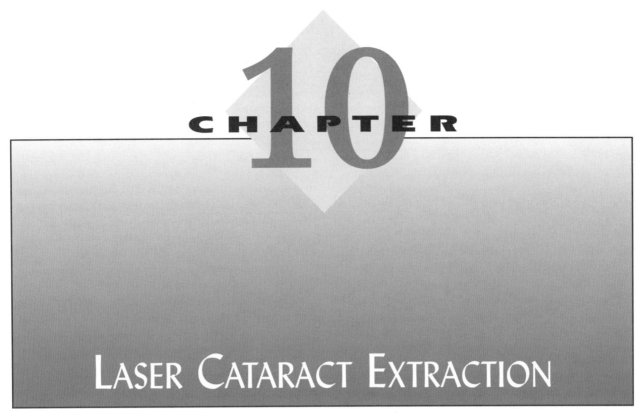

# LASER CATARACT EXTRACTION

*Jack M. Dodick, MD and Iman Ali Pahlavi, MD*

## INTRODUCTION

No surgical instrument has been as capable of inspiring awe in patients as the use of a laser (light-amplified stimulated emission of radiation). Often, patients are under the mistaken conviction that any small-incision modern surgery is, by definition, laser surgery. The development of laser surgery for the use of cataract extraction has been a process that has mirrored the development of ultrasound, or phacoemulsification, technology. Phacoemulsification languished for many years after its development due to the lack of a lens to take advantage of a foreshortened incision. Today, it is the procedure of choice among cataract surgeons.[1] Likewise, we have seen a similar resistance to the advent of ultra-small incision surgery. With the routine use of 1-mm lenses in Europe, however, interest in ultra-small incision cataract technology has peaked, as the approval of these lenses for use in the United States appears imminent. At the current time, there is only 1 laser that is FDA-approved for cataract surgery in the United States, and that is the Dodick Photolysis (ARC Laser Corp, Salt Lake City, UT) system.

There are several types of lasers that have historically been attempted to be used for cataract surgery. These lasers include the Erbium:YAG laser first investigated by Peyman and Katoh[2] and Tsubota.[3] The erbium technology unfortu-

nately developed the reputation of being extremely slow, and had been marketed under the term Phacolase MCL-29, Asclepion-Meditec (Germany). At the current time, this technology is no longer being pursued, but the false impression that all laser cataract extraction is slow remains. Francini[4] found using this technology that the average laser time was 9 minutes 23 seconds, with a total average energy of 62.74 Joules. In contrast, in a study published by Kanellopoulos et al[5] and involving 1000 patients, it was noted that for the majority of cases, laser time and phacoemulsification times were similar using the Dodick Photolysis (indirect Q-switched Nd:YAG laser) system. In addition, further confusion has ensued from the early development of the direct Nd:YAG laser system (Photon Paradigm Medical Industries, Salt Lake City, UT). This technology is no longer being pursued, according to a recent announcement. Interestingly, this technology was uni-manual, and thus required a wound size of 3 mm or greater nonetheless.

Dodick Photolysis involves the use of a indirect Q-switched Nd:YAG laser to emulsify cataracts. A laser beam is conducted through a 300-μm quartz-clad flexible fiber optic toward a titanium plate in the tip of the laser/aspiration handpiece. As the energy from the laser strikes the plate, a plasma wave is generated.[6] This plasma wave serves to emulsify the lens nucleus. Because this process does not involve the production of any heat (and renders burns impossible), the irrigating handpiece can be separated from the combination laser/aspiration tip, thus eliminating the cooling sleeve necessary for phacoemulsification. The current probes in use have an external diameter of 1.2 mm and an internal diameter of 0.75 mm, although smaller probe designs (0.9 mm external diameter) are currently being investigated.

The Dodick Photolysis system is a Venturi-pump system that generates aspiration with a range of 0 to 650 mmHg. The dynamic pressurized infusion system ranges from 0 to 200 mmHg. The laser output can be used with a pulse rate of 1 to 20 Hz, with an output of 8 or 10 mJ per pulse. Current surgical techniques involve the creation of 2 sub-1.4 mm paracentesis ports, one for the irrigation infusion and the other for the combination laser/aspiration probe. The handpieces are disposable, given the relative inexpensiveness of the quartz-clad fiber and the titanium targets, and the same handpieces may be used for the removal of cortical material, if so desired. This is an extremely important feature in Europe, where the public fear regarding prior diseases is mounting. In fact, the French government has released a health directive instructing surgeons that they *must* use disposable, single-use instruments whenever they are available, instead of the alternative.

The Photolysis unit comes with a Venturi phacoemulsification system that uses 2.75-mm phacoemulsification needles and either 1-piece or bimanual irrigation/aspiration handpieces for cortical removal. It also contains a superior high-speed vitrectomy unit that can use a 1-piece or split vitrector.

# INDICATIONS AND CONTRAINDICATIONS

One of the crucial aspects of the Dodick Photolysis system, as mentioned earlier, is that it produces no significant heat.[7] Thus, the laser probe requires no irrigation-cooling sleeve, unlike conventional phacoemulsification, which generates heat by the transformation of electrical energy into mechanical energy with the generation of the emulsifying shock waves.[8] Because there is no risk of corneal burns, the irrigation sleeve may be separated from the laser/aspiration probe, resulting in *true bimanual surgery*. Laser cataract extraction is appropriate where the surgeon would feel comfortable with phacoemulsification, and even in some cases where the surgeon would not. For example, in the case of frank phacodonesis, some surgeons would feel more comfortable pursuing conventional extracapsular cataract extraction instead of phacoemulsification. Similarly, the surgeon may choose to forgo laser cataract extraction in this scenario. However, it is important to note that there are no contraindications unique to Dodick Photolysis, as opposed to phacoemulsification.

Some of the advantages of photolysis include the decreased use of energy, which may be important in the preservation of contiguous structures of the eye, such as the cornea, iris, and retina, smaller incision size, which may be associated with safer, and more reproducible results. The only limit that the surgeon may note is an inability to successfully photolyse harder lenses early in the learning curve, somewhat similar to the experience in training in phacoemulsification. If a surgeon has difficulty removing a lens with photolysis, he or she can convert to the larger incision phacoemulsification, without any adverse consequences.

If iris is inadvertently aspirated during the process of photolysis, the results are far less disastrous than those that can occur with phacoemulsification. In addition, photolysis may be useful in cases of positive pressure, where the advantages of 2 ultra-small water-tight wounds are obvious. The biggest challenge for the beginning surgeon is learning to resist the temptation remove the nucleus from the capsular bag prematurely. Several techniques to facilitate nuclear removal have been described, and are outlined below.

# SURGICAL APPROACHES

The choice of anesthesia for this procedure is entirely up to the practitioner. Topical, local, or general anesthesia may all be safely used, without any difference between phacoemulsification and Photolysis. Specific techniques are outlined below:

*The classic technique* used for Photolysis is similar to early phacoemulsification, with the creation of a "bowl" prior to the removal of the lens from the capsular bag. Two 1.4-mm incisions are placed within the clear cornea. After the completion of a continuous circular capsulorrhexis (CCC), hydrodissection of the lens nucleus is performed. The bullet-shaped irrigation handpiece and the laser/aspiration handpiece are placed on the central anterior portion of the cataract. While using the irrigation handpiece to keep the nucleus down in the bag, the laser/aspiration handpiece touches down to ablate pieces of the cataract, lifting off periodically to allow the clearing of the port. Only once the central plate of the cataract has been ablated and the nucleus is substantially debulked can the residual shell be aspirated into the anterior chamber. This technique has several advantages, the most significant of which that this method does not require the development of additional skills while obtaining mastery of photolysis. It also allows the surgeon to continue to work centrally for the bulk of the ablation, as well as utilize the posterior capsule to provide mild counter-traction and keep the nucleus against the probe. The major disadvantage of this technique is that it is slightly slower than other techniques, and can only be utilized for nuclei up to 2+ in density.

*The Dodick technique* also involves the creation of two 1.4-mm incisions through which the cataract extraction is performed. After the creation of a continuous circular capsulorrhexis and hydrodissection of the lens nucleus, the lens is prechopped into 2 hemispheres using 2 Dodick-Kammen choppers in a horizontal chopping technique. One or both of the residual hemispheres can be then rechopped into quarters. The quadrants are then photolysed using the separate aspiration/laser and irrigation handpieces. Advantages to this technique are that the lens is broken into pieces early in the case, less energy is required (this is also true for pre-chopping using phacoemulsification), and a smaller capsulorrhexis may be used (which may provide for better centration of the intraocular lens). Disadvantages to this technique involve the learning curve necessary for mastering this skill.

*The Wehner technique* is unique in that it requires the creation of a large capsulorrhexis to allow the entire nucleus to be lifted into the anterior chamber using high aspiration with the port turned downward toward the nucleus. After the entire nucleus is raised out of the capsular bag with the laser/aspiration handpiece, the irrigation handpiece is placed beneath the nucleus with the irrigation probe directed posteriorly towards the posterior capsule. The nucleus is then brought down and "back-cracked" over the irrigation handpiece. The residual pieces are then photolysed or further lifted and "back-cracked" into quarters. To facilitate this process, a specialized irrigation handpiece, called a Wehner spoon, can be utilized. The Wehner spoon has a pointed end, which is angled upward toward the nucleus. Possible advantages to this technique are the potential protection of the posterior capsule as the irrigation port is directed downward towards it and away from the laser/aspiration handpiece. Potential disadvantages to this technique include the difficulty in passing the pointed, angled Wehner spoon into the eye, the need for a large capsulorrhexis, and the requirement to safely "back-crack."

*The Raut technique* can be used for nuclei up to "6+" in density. Dr. Rajeev Raut is an ophthalmologist in practice in Pune, India. He transitioned from extracapsular surgery to Photolysis without ever performing phacoemulsification, and he has developed a technique that permits him to perform surgery on extremely dense nuclei. In Dr. Raut's technique, hydrodissection is eliminated. The surrounding cortex is removed with aspiration after a CCC has been performed. He then uses the laser handpiece to "drill" a hole into the center of the nucleus. This hole is deep and narrow. Once he has completed this hole, he places the laser probe into the center of the hole. He then fires to generate an "earthquake" which shatters the lens into pieces, all of which can be easily aspirated.

*The Zerdab technique* is a technique created by Ivan Zerdab, who performs 80% to 100% of his cataracts with Photolysis. This is his "default" surgery. Dr. Zerdab is a left-handed surgeon, who effectively performs a vertical chop maneuver with Photolysis. He creates a radial paracentesis port for the combination laser/aspiration and a tangential

port for irrigation. His first hydrodissection is straight toward the nuclear core. Depending on his ability to infuse fluid into the innermost portion of the nucleus, he grades the nucleus from 1 to 4+. If the nucleus is hard, he proceeds to laser without further hydrodissection and hydrodelineation. If the nucleus is soft, he hydrodissects and hydrodelineates aggressively. After decompressing the central nucleus with laser pulses, he allows the nuclear rim to be aspirated upwards toward the cornea. He then uses an irrigating cannula with a Sinskey hook at the tip to perform vertical chopping maneuvers. He then removes the residual cortex using the Wehner spoon.

Just as every surgeon develops his own phacoemulsification style, so too are Photolysis techniques created. With the advances in probe strength and laser force, almost all cataracts can be removed with this technology.

## COMPLICATIONS AND MANAGEMENT

As mentioned earlier, there are no unique complications associated with Photolysis, and postoperative management is no different than with ultrasound. At the current time in the United States, we must still enlarge the wound to at least 2.75 mm to tolerate a foldable lens. In Europe, however, ultra-small IOLs are available, adding to the popularity of this procedure. Because of the ultra-small incision, stitches are less necessary than with conventional phacoemulsification. Many people worry about the status of the posterior capsule with this technology, since they are familiar with the Nd:YAG laser as used to perform capsulotomy after cataract extraction. It is impossible to laser the posterior capsule "open" during the surgery. The reason for this is that what is conducted from the mouth of the probe are plasma waves (the result of the laser energy striking the titanium plate), and not the YAG energy itself. Notably, it is possible to aspirate the posterior capsule, and thus cause a rent, much as this occurs using aspiration on the lens capsule during cortical clean-up.

## REHABILITATION

Rehabilitation is the same or faster than that seen with conventional phacoemulsification. An interesting article[9] published by Abraham Schlossman, MD, one of the fathers of modern ophthalmology, recounts his experience having Photolysis performed on him. He underwent 2 cataract surgeries in rapid succession, both with the same surgeon, same operating room, and the same IOL inserted. He reported a visual recovery that was hours in the Photolysis eye, as opposed to days with the phacoemulsification eye.

# Outcomes

In the largest published study to date, Kanellopoulos[5] et al studied 1000 patients in a multicenter study who had undergone laser cataract extraction measured photolysis patients in terms of improvement in visual acuity, total energy, mean operative time, and intraoperative and postoperative complications. The mean visual acuity improvement was from 20/70.2 to 20/24.4, and the mean energy used was 5.65 Joules per case. Average photolysis time was comparable to phacoemulsification times for the cataracts from 1 to 2+ in density, but the average time for 3+ lenses was 9.8 minutes. There were 16 cases of capsular ruptures and 2 cases of intraoperative hyphemae. In the postoperative period, there was 1 case of CME (partial anterior vitrectomy with sulcus IOL [PAV/sulcus IOL]), 1 case of pseudophakic bullous keratopathy (PAV/sulcus IOL), and 1 case of subluxated IOL (PAV/sulcus IOL). The authors concluded that photolysis was a safe and effective alternative to phacoemulsification in softer cataracts. It is important to note that, since this study's publication, newer techniques and development have resulted in similar operative times for cataracts up to 4+ in density whether removed by phacoemulsification or by Photolysis.

Huetz and Eckhardt,[10] in a separate clinical trial, reported 100 cases with photolysis with a 6-month follow up. Cataracts were divided into 3 groups (I-III) depending on the density of nuclear sclerosis (the LOCS III system). The mean total energy used in group I was 1.97±1.43 Joules, in group II was 3.37±1.59 Joules, and, in group III, 7.7±2.09 Joules. There was no significant difference in pachymetry in groups I and II preoperatively and postoperatively; however, group III experienced an average increase in pachymetry to 1.84% on postoperative day 2. At 6 months, there was no significant difference in pachymetry from preoperative values in all 3 of the groups.

# References

1. Learning DV. Practice styles and preferences of ASCRS members—1999 survey. *J Cataract Refract Surg.* 2000;26:913-921.

2. Peyman GA, Katoh N. Effects of an erbium: YAG laser in ocular ablation. *Int Ophthal.* 1987;10:245-253.

3. Tsubota K. Application of erbium: YAG laser in ocular ablation. *Ophthalmologica.* 1990;200:117-122.

4. Francini A, Galarati BZ. The Er:YAG laser emulsification: clinical results. Personal communication; 2001.

5. Kanellopoulos AJ, Dodick JM, Brauweiler P, Alzner E. Laser cataract surgery: a prospective clinical evaluation of 1000 consecutive laser procedures using the Dodick Photolysis neodymium:YAG system. *Ophthalmology.* 2001;108:649-654.

6. Dodick J, Christiansen L. Studies conducted in the early 1990s using high-speed photography to document the effects of laser cataract extraction. Personal communication; 1992.

7. Alzner E, Grabner G. Dodick laser phacolysis: thermal effects. *J Cataract Refract Surg.* 1999;25:800-803.

8. Kelman CD. Phacoemulsification and aspiration: a new technique of cataract removal, a preliminary report. *Am J Ophthalmol.* 1967;64:23-25.

9. Schlossman A. Dodick photolysis: a patient's perspective. *Ocular Surgery News.* September 2002.

10. Huetz WW, Eckhardt HB. Prospective clinical study with photolysis using the Dodick-ARC laser system for cataract surgery. Personal communication; 2001.

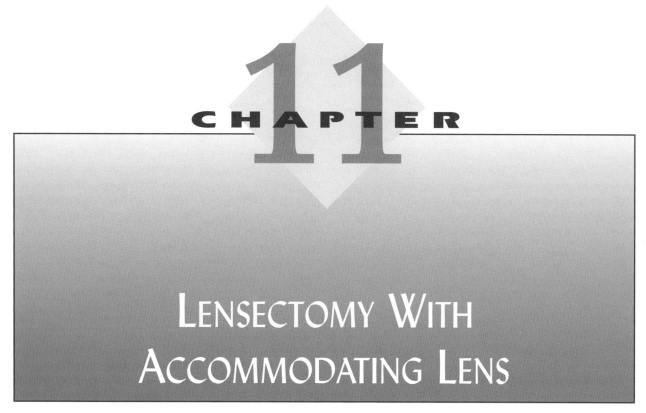

# CHAPTER 11

# LENSECTOMY WITH ACCOMMODATING LENS

*Roberto Zaldivar, MD; Susana Oscherow, MD; and Virginia Piezzi, MD*

## INTRODUCTION

Previously, ophthalmologists had successfully corrected ametropia, but were still trying to find a way to treat presbyopia in order to allow patients to read without glasses. Age-related accommodation loss has been studied and some theories have been proposed to explain and provide a solution to this inconvenience.

Following is a short review of eye physiology, highlighting the changes produced during accommodation:

1. The pupil is contracted during accommodation and convergence

2. The crystalline lens anterior pole moves forward, pushing the iris anteriorly, producing central flattening of the anterior chamber. The posterior pole does not change its position

3. The lens anterior surface becomes more convex while the posterior one increases its curvature slightly

4. As the posterior pole maintains its position and the anterior pole moves forward, central lens thickness increases

5. While lens thickness is increased, the lens diameter is reduced

6. Some changes on the lens capsule tension can be observed: the anterior capsule relaxes and moves forward relative to the posterior capsule

7. During accommodation, the crystalline lens is depressed by gravitational force

Changes inside the lens substantially modify its refraction power in addition to those produced by surface curvature changes when the ciliary body contracts. These internal variations are produced by changes in curvature of different lens portions that possess different refraction indices.[1]

The classical theory suggests that lens changes are produced by zonular relaxation that make the lens more spheric.

Dr. Ronald Schachar has suggested the possibility that zonular tension on the capsule adjusts and stretches the lens while keeping its elasticity. Embryologically, the lens derives from ectodermal tissue and it continues growing and developing throughout life. On the other hand, the sclera, ciliary body, and ciliary muscle develop from mesodermal tissue and stop growing at the end of puberty, keeping their size and circumference throughout adulthood. As the lens continues growing, it occupies more space, encroaching on the posterior chamber.

Another important element is ciliary body elasticity, or movement, which pushes the vitreous body forward, placing the lens more anteriorly. Another theory blames the loss of accommodation on a failure in the accommodation system—a rigid lens and a ciliary body unable to contract because of atrophy with loss of function.

The Tscherning theory suggests that the vitreous base advances against the lens' posterior periphery, modifying the lenticular shape.

In 1855, Helmholtz theorized that accommodation makes the lens posterior surface become more curved, meanwhile the anterior central portion of the surface becomes much more convex, which means that accommodation is produced by a change in lens shape.[2]

We must not forget that lens shape depends on capsular elasticity and zonular traction over the capsule. Finchman suggested that variations in the lens capsule thickness explained local variations in the curvature. In addition, he said that during accommodation, the thicker ring surrounding the central region of the anterior capsule contracts under diminished zonular traction, while the central capsule, which is thinner, bends forward in a sharper way (anterior physiological lenticonus).[3]

In other words, we can say that the Helmholtz theory modified by Finchman proposes that zonular relaxation makes the lens become more spherical, thereby allowing near vision. The loss of capacity for accommodation is probably due to hardening of the lens, because the ciliary body maintains its ability to function.

Based on this theory, Dr. Stuart Cumming began 10 years ago to investigate and develop a pseudophakic lens model that replaces the natural lens functions and characteristics:

1. Transparency, allowing single image formation on retina

2. Dioptric power

3. Accommodation

An IOL able to fulfill these premises would allow surgeons and patients the triple advantage sought nowadays in pseudophakic patients.

Before the Crystalens (C&C Vision, Aliso Viejo, Calif) accommodative IOL development and implementation, we tried to offer the presbyopic patient different alternatives in order to achieve maximum comfort in all their focal distances: far, intermediate, and near.

One alternative was the pseudophakic progressive AMO Array IOL (Allergan Medical Optics) that was created to offer distance visual acuity similar to monofocal IOL, better near visual acuity, with a slight loss in contrast sensitivity.[4,5]

However, authors reporting experience with the AMO Array IOL have found significant decreases in image quality and contrast sensitivity, along with night glare. The resulting image is comparable to the one produced by astigmatism, IOL decentration, posterior capsule opacification, and subclinical macular edema.[6]

Other authors recommend a foldable and angulated Bio Com Fold IOL (Morcher Gmbh, Germany) that was designed to move forward and backward during accommodative effort, but results could not be related to an increased accommodative amplitude.

Other techniques have been used in phakic patients to improve accommodation. One of them is the implantation of scleral expansion bands. Although the mechanism of action is unknown, these bands do not restore accommodation. Scleral expansion surgery does not restore accommodation in human presbyopia.[7]

Another example in phakic eyes is the anterior ciliary sclerotomy (ACS). Maloney recommends this technique for initial presbyopia or mid-distance correction in older patients, because it only restores 1.50 D of accommodation. The majority of surgeons using ACS found an initial improvement followed by a fast regression. Apparently, this technique does not permanently improve accommodation, either.[8]

In pseudophakic patients implanted with silicone plate haptic IOLs, we observed excellent postoperative results for near and distance vision in some patients, but over time this same excellent performance started diminishing, leaving only good distance vision. However, the reading capacity that patients achieved during the first post operative month intrigued us, and this made us interested in Dr. Cumming's 10-year project of designing an IOL capable of accommodating for near vision.

In this chapter we will describe our experience and results using the Crystalens accommodative IOL.

## PATIENTS AND METHODS

Twenty-four patients were implanted but only 19 came back to the control at the sixth month. From this sample (19 patients) seven were bilateral (14 eyes) and the rest, 12 patients (12 eyes), were unilateral. One of the monocular patients was excluded because of ARMD not seen before surgery due to the cataract. The final evaluated group was compounded by 25 eyes of 18 patients, 14 eyes bilateral and 11 unilateral.

At the second year we evaluated 11 patients: 16 eyes bilateral (8 patients) and 3 unilateral, so the final sample was 19 eyes.

We performed the following preoperative evaluations:

- ✧ Distance and near visual acuity with and without correction
- ✧ Subjective and objective refraction
- ✧ Applanation tonometry
- ✧ Biomicroscopy
- ✧ Dilated fundus examination
- ✧ Biometry to measure axial length
- ✧ Specular microscopy (Konan Noncon Robo-CA-ICO-NAN Inc., Hyogo, Japan)
- ✧ Corneal topography
- ✧ EAS photographs-slit lamp and retroillumination mode (EAS 1000, NIDEK, Gamagori, Japan).

Patients were followed up at 1, 6, 18 and 24 months. During the postoperative examinations we evaluated uncorrected distance visual acuity (UCDVA), uncorrected near visual acuity (UNVA), best-corrected distance visual acuity (BCDVA), distance-corrected near visual acuity (DCNVA), and distance-corrected intermediate visual acuity (DCIVA), monocular in all patients and binocular in patients with the CrystaLens accommodative IOL in both eyes. To measure all these parameters we use a technique that consists of asking the patient to read the smallest line possible, then read 1 row lower to see if he or she is able to manage it. If he or she cannot, we go immediately to the upper one again in order to let him or her see it, then we go down again to the line below. This procedure is necessary in order to gain maximum accommodation by having the patient continue reading.

Using this technique, we sometimes achieve different results. During the first 2 postoperative weeks, near vision results were not considered because patients had received atropine drops at surgery and 1 day postoperatively.

We also evaluated subjective and objective refraction, tonometry, biomicroscopy, and EAS photographs (slit lamp and retroillumination mode).

## PATIENT SELECTION

Currently we are using the Crystalens in patients with cataracts, low or moderate hyperopia, and emmetropic eyes as well. We can also use this IOL in high hyperopic patients without cataracts as a refractive procedure.

It is also considered a very good option for those patients who have visual activity requiring sight at different distances (far, intermediate, and near). The first 5 implants were performed in patients with a low requirement level for near vision activity.

When we first started implanting our patients with the Crystalens, we felt it was important not to generate patient expectations that might be too high. After evaluating the results and patient satisfaction in the first implanted patients, we saw that the results were excellent and we started to offer this IOL to patients with high-level requirements for near vision, among them CEOs, intellectuals, and a clock worker. We now believe that this IOL can be implanted in all patients that wish to have spectacle independence for near, intermediate, and distance vision.

## EXCLUSION CRITERIA

- ❖ Traumatic or congenital zonular weakness (eg, Marfan syndrome)
- ❖ Eyes that previously underwent other surgical procedures
- ❖ Anterior/posterior capsular rupture during surgery

The rest of the exclusion criteria does not differ from usual cataract surgery.

## SURGICAL TECHNIQUE

It is a similar technique used in any phacoemulsification procedure. Once surgery has been indicated we do a routine blood examination, coagulation study, and EKG (electrocardiogram) for surgical risk.

In our cases we usually measure the axial length with conventional biometry; however, the immersion method is preferred with manual K readings. We perform the IOL calculation using the Hoffer formula.

In bilateral surgical cases, the surgeries are performed on alternate days. However, C&C Vision recommends a cycloplegic refraction on the first eye at least 1 week postoperatively before selecting the lens power for the second eye.

The Crystalens is a plate-haptic IOL of a third-generation silicone called BIOSIL. It has the following characteristics: 4.5-mm optical zone, peripheral polyimide miniloops, 10.5-mm plate, 11.5-mm from miniloop-tip to miniloop-tip, and a hinge between the plate haptics and the optic, allowing flexibility and anterior/posterior movement of the optic. The optic has a square edge and its posterior location in the eye, excellent centration, and the fact that BIOSIL is a nonreflective material diminishes the complaints of halos and glare.

Two points in the design of this lens are important for its proper functioning: the loops and the hinge. It is very important to emphasize that a capsulorrhexis of no more than 5.5 mm should be done, through which the placement of the IOL can be carried out in 1 of 2 ways:

- ❖ Inserting it with specific forceps because the IOL hinge is near the optical zone. This IOL is very flexible but can be difficult to control inside the eye. However, if the appropriate maneuvers are used it is relatively simple to place
- ❖ Using an injector. (We are pioneers in this technique.) The technique is similar to that used with other foldable IOLs such as the phakic ICL

After placing a viscoelastic substance inside the cartridge we position the IOL carefully, being careful not to trap any part of the IOL, especially the loops (Figure 11-1).

Once the correct IOL position is verified, we insert the injector in the incision but not very deeply inside the anterior chamber. Slowly we start injecting the Crystalens until it is completely opened inside the bag.

The maneuvers must be done with special care because of the IOL length and shape. Sudden movements can break the capsule or damage the endothelium.

It is also necessary to take special care when the IOL enters the anterior chamber to make sure the hinge groove is on the front of the lens. However, with the appropriate technique and the practice of the procedure outside the eye, it becomes simple and efficient.

The injector technique needs an incision of 2.8 mm with all the advantages that this implies.

Among intraoperative considerations, it is very important to mention that when finishing the surgical procedure a drop of atropine is used, repeating it the first day of postoperative follow up. This atropine phase paralyzes the ciliary muscle for at least 1 week, permitting posterior positioning of the lens during the period of capsular fibrosis.

## REFRACTIVE RESULTS

A special emphasis on biometry, K readings, lens power selection and cataract surgical technique is important in order to maximize the results of the procedure. It is important that the patient postoperatively is emmetropic or with a maximum -0.50 D of myopia for distance vision. We avoid as best we can any induction of astigmatism. This way the patient can achieve independence from spectacles and can see at distance, intermediate, and near with the Crystalens.

A critical phase is the lens calculation. It is very important that the axial length be as accurate as possible in order to obtain a precise power calculation. Although other authors believe that the calculation is more precise with the use of the immersion biometry, we have had good results using standard A-Scan ultrasonography. We have an excellent biometrist who checks the axial length on each eye with 3 different biometers.

We analyzed data from patients with 6 and 24 months of follow up. We consider the 6-month data as the early control group and the 24-month data as the late control group. This discrimination was made to evaluate refractive changes in short and long term, paying special attention to posterior capsule changes.

With the first group (6 month) we were able to confirm that 25 eyes (100%) were able to achieve between J1 and J5 for near vision monocularly. UCNVA in 88% of these eyes was J3 or better. Our patients were happy and we considered this very acceptable vision for reading and also for all types of intermediate and distance visual work.

UCDVA in monocular vision patients was 20/40 or better in 84% of cases and the remaining 16% were between 20/50 and 20/60.

Analyzing distance vision, we discovered that 4 eyes presented less visual acuity than preoperatively. These patients presented -1.25 to -2.00 D of myopia.

The near and distance uncorrected vision in patients implanted binocularly improved over the monocular results, and these binocular patients achieved excellent results. In this group, 7 cases (14 eyes) (100%) were able to see J5 or better, and 6 of them (87%) were able to see J2 or better with both eyes, considered by us to be an excellent result. It

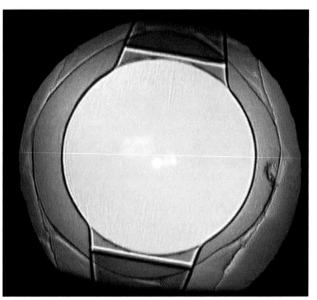

**Figure 11-1.** Crystalens: IOL centration postoperative.

also was very significant to us that 100% binocular patients were able to see 20/25 or better without glasses.

Comparing UCDVA with UCNVA in the same eye, we observed that 50% of those patients with 20/25 or better in distance vision reached J1 at near and the rest achieved J2.

One patient with less near vision (J5) presented posterior capsular fibrosis with halos and glare.

This situation was documented with photographs (scheimpflug camera). We concluded that pronounced posterior capsular fibrosis causes diminishment of accommodation.

In spite of the small 4.5-mm optical zone, patients did not complain of significant subjective symptoms of glare and halos.

Only 1 patient presented visual acuity loss. He suffered an ocular trauma and his iris was trapped in the wound. The iris was reconstructed and the wound was closed with a suture. The IOL maintained its position but the patient lost 2 lines of visual acuity (20/25 to 20/40). No other complications were detected.

At 2 years follow up, 19 eyes of 11 patients were examined, and 8 of these patients (16 eyes) were bilateral.

UCNVA in 15 eyes (79%) was J3 or better. UCDVA was 20/40 or better in 16 eyes (84%). The uncorrected vision in 13 eyes was 20/25 or better for distance and J1 in 9 eyes and J2 in 4 eyes for near.

The UCNVA was J2 or better in 100% of bilateral cases, and the UCDVA was 20/25 or better in 75% of cases.

Comparing both groups at 6 and 24 months we were able to observe that 22 eyes (88%) presented UCNVA of J3 or better at 6 months and 15 eyes (79.5%) at 2 years (Figure 11-2).

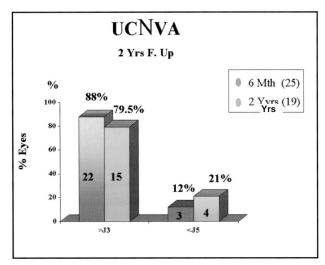

**Figure 11-2.** UCNVA: Comparison between both studied groups. It can be observed that at the sixth month 88% of the eyes could see J3 or better. 79.5% of them reached J3 or better at the second year.

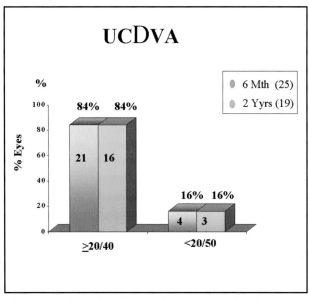

**Figure 11-3.** UCDVA: Comparison between both populations. Eighty-nine percent of both groups achieved 20/40 or better (21 eyes at sixth month and 16 at the second year). One hundred percent could see 20/50 or better.

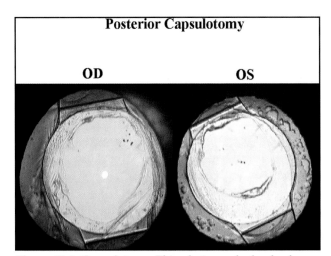

**Figure 11-4.** Capsulotomy. This photograph clearly shows different sizes of capsulotomies performed with Nd-Yag laser. Right eye capsulotomy shows a standard size but left eye is smaller. Right eye recovered distance and near visual acuity without correction (20/25 and J1 respectively). Left eye reached 20/40 and J5 without correction. Observe IOL's centration.

UCDVA was 20/40 or better in 84% of the eyes at both 6 months and 2 years (21 eyes at sixth month and 16 at second year) (Figure 11-3).

## POSTERIOR CAPSULE CHANGES

Without any doubt the posterior capsule opacification plays a very important role in the visual acuity of pseudopha-kic patients. We noticed that the capsule in contact with the Crystalens, made with Biosil (Jarrow, Los Angeles, Calif), a third-generation silicone, seems to create less fibrosis.

Since the beginning we tried to define the role of the capsule.

Before implanting the Crystalens, some questions regarding the lens design and function concerned us:

- ✧ When would opacification appear?
- ✧ How would it affect accommodation?
- ✧ What optic size would be adequate and safe according to the IOL design?
- ✧ Would accommodation be restored after capsulotomy?

The first opacifications appeared 1 year after surgery with some special characteristics: zones of major opacification alternating with lighter ones. The first case was a bilateral implant, and after capsulotomy we were able to observe that 1 eye had recovered near and distance vision, while the other eye did not improve to the same extent. The capsulotomy was smaller in the eye with the least recovery of near vision compared to the 1 in the other eye. The same problem was verified in other patients, so we concluded that capsulotomies have to be wide enough to recover the desired pseudoaccommodation (Figure 11-4), but not larger than the optic because this would allow the vitreous to get around the edge of the optic.

We did not observe any complications after capsulotomy in our patients. The IOLs remained well centered and accommodative function was restored.

# DISCUSSION

According to the Helmholtz theory, the ciliary body maintains its functionality over time, and the crystalline lens thickens; however, its hypertrophy over time blocks the natural function of the zonules, reducing and finally eliminating accommodation.

Cumming postulated the possibility of recovering the accommodative ability of the crystalline lens function by removing the cataractous lens and replacing it with an IOL capable of replicating the capsular movements created by the vitreous displacement during the accommodation process.

The displacement of the Crystalens accommodating lens by 1.0 mm has been calculated to produce accommodation of approximately 2.00 D, according to Dr. Stuart Cumming.

Silicone, the material used in this case, is capable of maintaining its flexibility over time. The shape and material of the loops allow firm fixation of the lens in the capsular bag. The hinge permits forward and backward movement of the IOL following contraction and relaxation of the ciliary muscle.

Due to a 4.5-mm optic with a square edge, the haptics, and all the characteristics mentioned above, plus the fact that the ciliary muscle is paralyzed during fibrosis, this lens has excellent centration.

# CONCLUSION

In our experience with cataract surgery, the limited number of methods by which we can allow the patient to gain near vision are:

⬧ Myopia induction, creating monocular vision. With this method, the patients generally are able to read with the nondominant eye. The patient must be informed preoperatively of the consequences of his postoperative condition. For example, we cannot use this technique in patients that require excellent distance visual acuity

⬧ Multifocal IOLs, which have improved lately, but still induce loss of contrast sensitivity with glare and halos

⬧ This new alternative, the Crystalens, produces accommodation, restoring the ability of the patient to see far, intermediate and near

Theoretically, the mechanism in this kind of IOL is as follows: After being placed in the bag, it locates in a very posterior position in the bag space up against the posterior capsule, against the vitreous. This, together with the hinged lens design, allows the IOLs forward movement when ciliary muscle contraction occurs, which increases of the vitreous pressure and causes the optic to move forward. Fibrosis of the anterior capsule facilitates its backward movement, with relaxation of the ciliary muscle.

We are able to conclude that after 2 years of follow up our patients implanted with the Crystalens do not need glasses for distance, intermediate, and near work. They are satisfied with the results. Only 2 are wearing a slight correction for near vision. The Crystalens is an effective method for near correction post lensectomy without compromising distance vision or inducing contrast sensitivity loss, glare and halos. Seventy-eight percent (78%) of patients can see 20/25 or better at distance and can see J2 at near without correction.

According to our preoperative IOL calculations we expected emmetropia in our patients. The results showed that all our patients achieved this or were slightly myopic. None of them were hyperopic.

Capsular fibrosis reduces accommodation over time but recovers after YAG laser capsulotomy. Comparing capsulotomy sizes, we have obtained better results with larger ones than with smaller ones; however, the capsulotomy should not be larger than 6.0 mm. Patients with a big capsulotomy (6.0 mm) did not present complications of IOL decentration or luxation.

It is essential to stress the importance of the ideal anterior capsulorrhexis size (5.5 mm) and the posterior capsule integrity before IOL injection through a shooter.

The position inside the bag regarding the axis of the lens is not important in order to achieve accommodative function; however, it is important to be certain that the optic is vaulted backward at the end of surgery and that if the capsulorrhexis is oval, the lens be placed such that the anterior capsule rim adequately covers the lens plate haptics.

In some patients with very low residual myopia, which allows very good UCDVA, UCNVA is also excellent. When comparing the monocular UCNVA with the distance-corrected near vision, it was a surprise that the near vision diminished with the distance correction. We were expecting similar results found in clinical trials, where the near vision improves over time. It was surmised that the small degree of myopia does not require the patient to use the ciliary muscle to focus at near, and therefore they were not required to accommodate for near vision. Based on this finding, the patients should not wear reading glasses postoperatively because they will not gain the benefit of accommodation if they are not requiring their ciliary muscle to provide near vision.

Although the Crystalens optical zone is relatively small, the patients do not complain of halos at night and are able to drive without problems. Complaints related to halos and glare were observed in some patients with capsular fibrosis.

Only 2 patients presented a marked decrease in near and distance vision, which was recovered after Nd:YAG laser capsulotomy.

The Crystalens centration is proper. The haptics design keeps it in position even after capsulotomy.

We consider the Crystalens as 1 of our first options in patients with cataract in which we try to recover near vision. We sincerely believe that this IOL is one of the most promising options for presbyopia in the future.

# REFERENCES

1. Moses R. Accommodation. In: Adler, Moses R, eds. *Physiology of the Eye—Clinical Application.* St. Louis, Mo: The CV Mosby Company; 1980:285-303.

2. Helmholtz H. *Treatise on Physiologic Optics.* New York: Dover Publication; Vol 1; 1962.

3. Finchman E. The mechanism of accommodation. *Br J Ophthalmol.* 1937;8:1-9.

4. Brydon K, Tokarwicz AC, Nichols B, et al. AMO Array multifocal lens versus monofocal correction in cataract surgery. *Cataract Refract Surg.* Jan 2000;26(1):96-100.

5. Steinert R, Aker B, Trentacost D, et al. A prospective comparative study of the AMO Array zonal progressive multifocal silicone intraocular lens. *Ophthalmology.* July 1999; 106(7):1243-1255.

6. Legeais JM, Werner L, Werner L, et al. Bio COM fold versus foldable silicone intraocular lens. *J Cataract Refract Surg.* February 1999; 25:262-267.

7. Steven M. *Ophthalmology.* May 1999;106(5):873-877.

8. Samalonis L. Sclerotomy and the correction of presbyopia. *Eye World.* February 2000.

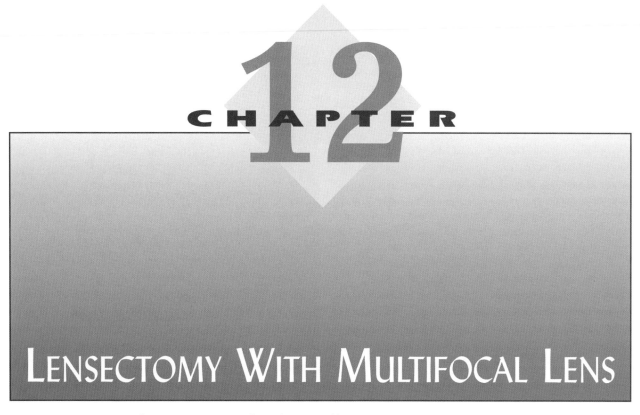

# CHAPTER 12

# LENSECTOMY WITH MULTIFOCAL LENS

*I. Howard Fine, MD; Richard S. Hoffman, MD; and Mark Packer, MD*

Excimer laser refractive surgery is growing in popularity throughout the world but has its limitations. Patients with extreme degrees of myopia and hyperopia are poor candidates for corneal refractive surgery and presbyopic patients must rely on reading glasses or monovision in order to obtain the full range of visual function. These limitations in laser refractive surgery have led to a resurgence of intraocular modalities for the correction of refractive errors.

Advances in small-incision cataract surgery have enhanced this procedure from one primarily concerned with the safe removal of the cataractous lens to a procedure refined to yield the best possible postoperative refractive result. As the outcomes of cataract surgery have improved, the use of lens surgery as a refractive modality in patients without cataracts has increased in popularity. The removal of the crystalline lens and replacement with a pseudophakic lens for the purposes of reducing or eliminating refractive errors has been labeled with many titles. These titles include clear lensectomy,[1,2] clear lens phacoemulsification,[3] clear lens replacement, clear lens extraction,[4-12] clear lens exchange, presbyopic lens exchange, and refractive lens exchange. Because these procedures may be performed in older patients with significant nuclear sclerosis but normal spectacle-corrected visual acuity, the term "clear lens" may not be appropriate to describe many older individuals undergoing lens exchange surgery. Similarly, a "clear lens exchange" in a young highly hyperopic patient may be performed for refractive purposes but not necessarily to address preexisting presbyopia and thus "presbyopic lens exchange" would not be an appropriate term for this group of patients. The term *refractive lens* exchange appears to best describe the technique of removing the crystalline lens and replacing it with a pseudophakic lens in any aged patient for the purpose of reducing or eliminating refractive errors and/or addressing presbyopia.

## MULTIFOCAL LENSES

Perhaps the greatest catalyst for the resurgence of refractive lens exchange has been the development of multifocal lens technology. High hyperopes, presbyopes, and patients with borderline cataracts who have presented for refractive surgery have been ideal candidates for this new technology. Multifocal IOL technology offers patients substantial benefits. The elimination of a presbyopic condition and restoration of normal vision by simulating accommodation greatly enhances the quality of life for most patients.

Historically, multifocal IOLs have been developed and investigated for decades. One of the first multifocal IOL designs to be investigated in the United States was the center-surround IOL now under the name NuVue (Bausch & Lomb, Rochester, NY). This lens had a central near add surrounded by a distance powered periphery. Other IOL designs include the 3M diffractive multifocal IOL (3M, St. Paul, Minn), which has been acquired, redesigned, and formatted for the foldable Acrysof acrylic IOL (Alcon, Fort Worth, Tex) Pharmacia has also designed a diffractive multifocal IOL, the Ceeon 811E (Monrovia, Calif), that has been implanted extensively outside of the United States. Alcon, Pharmacia, and Storz have also investigated 3-zone refractive multifocal IOLs that have a central distant component surrounded at various distances by a near annulus.[13]

The only multifocal IOL approved for general use in the United States is the Array (AMO, Santa Ana, Calif). The Array is a zonal progressive IOL with 5 concentric zones on the anterior surface (Figure 12-1). Zones 1, 3, and 5 are distance dominant zones while zones 2 and 4 are near dominant. The lens has an aspheric design and each zone repeats the entire refractive sequence corresponding to distance, intermediate, and near foci. This results in vision over a range of distances. The lens uses 100% of the incoming available light and is weighted for optimum light distribution. With typical pupil sizes, approximately half of the light is distributed for distance, one-third for near vision, and the remainder for intermediate vision. The lens utilizes continuous surface construction and consequently there is no loss of light through defraction and no degradation of image quality as a result of surface discontinuities.[14] The lens has a foldable silicone optic that is 6.0 mm in diameter with haptics made of PMMA and a haptic diameter of 13 mm. The lens can be inserted through a clear corneal or scleral tunnel incision that is 2.8 mm wide, utilizing the unfolder injector system manufactured by AMO.

## CLINICAL RESULTS

The efficacy of zonal progressive multifocal technology has been documented in many clinical studies. Early studies of the 1-piece Array documented a larger percentage of patients who were able to read J2 print after undergoing multifocal lens implantation compared to patients with monofocal implants.[15-17] Similar results have been documented for the foldable Array.[18] Clinical trials comparing multifocal lens implantation compared to monofocal lens implantation in the same patient also revealed improved intermediate and near vision in the multifocal eye compared to the monofocal eye.[19-20]

## CONTRAST SENSITIVITY

Many studies have evaluated both the objective and subjective qualities of contrast sensitivity, stereoacuity, glare dis-

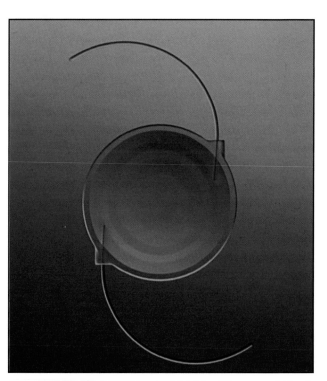

**Figure 12-1.** The AMO Array foldable silicone multifocal intraocular lens. (Reprinted with permission from Advanced Medical Optics.)

ability, and photic phenomena following implantation of multifocal IOLs. Refractive multifocal IOLs, such as the Array, have been found to be superior to diffractive multifocal IOLs by demonstrating better contrast sensitivity and less glare disability.[21] However, more recent reports comparing refractive and diffractive IOLs have revealed similar qualities for distance vision evaluated by modulation transfer functions but superior near vision for the diffractive lens.[22]

In regards to contrast sensitivity testing, the Array has been shown to produce a small amount of contrast sensitivity loss equivalent to the loss of 1 line of visual acuity at the 11% contrast level using Regan contrast sensitivity charts.[16] This loss of contrast sensitivity at low levels of contrast was only present when the Array was placed monocularly and was not demonstrated with bilateral placement and binocular testing.[23] Regan testing is perhaps not as reliable as sine wave grating tests that evaluate a broader range of spatial frequencies. Utilizing sine wave grating testing, reduced contrast sensitivity was found in eyes implanted with the Array in the lower spatial frequencies compared to monofocal lenses when a halogen glare source was absent. When a moderate glare source was introduced, no significant difference in contrast sensitivity between the multifocal or monofocal lenses was observed.[24] However, recent reports have demonstrated a reduction in tritan color contrast sensitivity function in refractive multifocal IOLs compared to monofocal lenses under conditions of glare. These differences were significant for distance vision in the lower spatial frequencies,

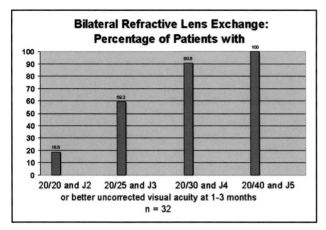

**Figure 12-2.** Clinical results of bilateral Array implantation following refractive lens exchange.

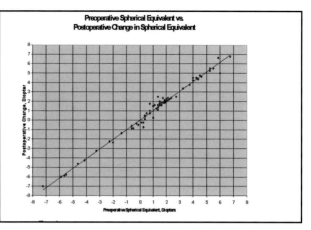

**Figure 12-3.** Scattergram demonstrating reduction of spherical equivalent in refractive lens exchange eyes.

and for near in the low and middle spatial frequencies.[25] A new aspheric multifocal IOL, the Progress 3 (Domilens, Lyon, France) also demonstrated significantly lower mean contrast sensitivity with the Pelli-Robson chart compared to monofocal IOLs.[26]

Ultimately, these contrast sensitivity tests reveal that in order to deliver multiple foci on the retina, there is always some loss of efficiency with multifocal IOLs when compared to monofocal IOLs. However, contrast sensitivity loss, random-dot stereopsis, and aniseikonia can be improved when multifocal IOLs are placed bilaterally compared to unilateral implants.[27] A recent publication evaluating a 3-zone refractive multifocal IOL demonstrated improved stereopsis, less aniseikonia, and greater likelihood for spectacle independence with bilateral implantation compared to unilateral implantation.[28]

## PHOTIC PHENOMENON

One of the potential drawbacks of the Array multifocal lens has been the potential for an appreciation of halos around point sources of light at night in the early weeks and months following surgery.[29-31] Most patients will learn to disregard these halos with time and bilateral implantation appears to improve these subjective symptoms. Concerns about the visual function of patients at night have been allayed by a driving simulation study in which bilateral Array multifocal patients performed only slightly worse than patients with bilateral monofocal IOLs. The results indicated no consistent difference in driving performance and safety between the 2 groups.[32] In a study by Javitt et al, 41% percent of bilateral Array subjects were found to never require spectacles compared to 11.7% of monofocal controls. Overall, subjects with bilateral Array IOLs reported better overall vision, less limitation in visual function, and less use of spectacles than monofocal controls.[33]

## REFRACTIVE LENS EXCHANGE

A small recent study reviewed the clinical results of bilaterally implanted Array multifocal lens implants in refractive lens exchange patients.[34] A total of 68 eyes were evaluated, comprising 32 bilateral and 4 unilateral Array implantations. One hundred percent of patients undergoing bilateral refractive lens exchange achieved binocular visual acuity of 20/40 and J5 or better, measured 1 to 3 months postoperatively. Over 90% achieved uncorrected binocular visual acuity of 20/30 and J4 or better, and nearly 60% achieved uncorrected binocular visual acuity of 20/25 and J3 or better (Figure 12-2). This study included patients with preoperative spherical equivalents between 7.00 D of myopia and 7.00 D of hyperopia with the majority of patients having preoperative spherical equivalents between plano and +2.50. Excellent lens power determinations and refractive results were achieved (Figure 12-3).

## PATIENT SELECTION

Specific guidelines with respect to the selection of candidates and surgical strategies that enhance outcomes with this IOL have been developed. AMO recommends using the Array multifocal IOL for bilateral cataract patients whose surgery is uncomplicated and whose personality is such that they are not likely to fixate on the presence of minor visual aberrations such as halos around lights. There is obviously a broad range of patients who would be acceptable candidates. Relative or absolute contraindications include the presence of ocular pathologies, other than cataracts, that may degrade image formation or may be associated with less than adequate visual function postoperatively despite visual improvement following surgery. Preexisting ocular pathologies that are frequently looked upon as contraindications include ARMD; uncontrolled diabetes or diabetic retinopathy;

uncontrolled glaucoma; recurrent inflammatory eye disease; retinal detachment risk; and corneal disease or previous refractive surgery in the form of radial keratotomy, photorefractive keratectomy, or laser assisted in-situ keratomileusis. However, a recent study has revealed comparable distance acuity outcomes in Array and monofocal patients with concurrent eye disease such as macular degeneration, glaucoma, and diabetic retinopathy.[35]

Utilization of these lenses in patients who complain excessively, are highly introspective and fussy, or obsess over body image and symptoms should be avoided. In addition, conservative use of this lens is recommended when evaluating patients with occupations that include frequent night driving and occupations that put high demands on vision and near work such as engineers and architects. Such patients need to demonstrate a strong desire for relative spectacle independence in order to be considered for a refractive lens exchange with Array implantation. Recent publications have found multifocal lens implantation to be a cost-effective option for low-income patients and patients in developing countries where the added expense of near vision spectacles would be prohibitive.[36,37] Additionally, multifocal IOL implantation was found to be a viable option for pediatric cataract patients, thus eliminating spectacle dependence in this susceptible group of patients.[38]

In our practice, patient selection has been reduced to a very rapid process. Once someone has been determined to be a candidate for refractive lens exchange, the patient is asked 2 questions. The first question is, "If an implant could be placed in your eye that would allow you to see both distance and near without glasses, under most circumstances, would that be an advantage?" Patients are then asked, "If the lens is associated with halos around lights at night, would it still be an advantage?" If they do not think they would be bothered by these symptoms, they receive a multifocal IOL. If concern over halos or night driving is strong then these patients may receive monofocal lenses with appropriate informed consent regarding loss of accommodation and the need for reading glasses or consideration of a different refractive surgical procedure.

Prior to implanting an Array, all candidates should be informed of the lens' statistics to ensure that they understand that spectacle independence is not guaranteed. Approximately 41% of the patients implanted with bilateral Array IOLs will never need to wear glasses, 50% wear glasses on a limited basis such as driving at night or during prolonged reading, 12% will always need to wear glasses for near work, and approximately 8% will need to wear spectacles on a full-time basis for distance and near correction.[32] In addition, 15% of patients were found to have difficulty with halos at night and 11% had difficulty with glare compared to 6% and 1% respectively in monofocal patients.

Finally, the patient's axial length and risk for retinal detachment or other retinal complications should be considered. Although there have been many publications documenting a low rate of complications in highly myopic clear lens extractions,[1,3,8,9,10] others have warned of significant long-term risks of retinal complications despite prophylactic treatment.[39,40] With this in mind, other phakic refractive modalities should be considered in extremely high myopes. If refractive lens exchange is performed in these patients, extensive informed consent regarding the long-term risks for retinal complications should naturally occur preoperatively.

## PREOPERATIVE MEASUREMENTS

The most important assessment for successful multifocal lens use, other than patient selection, involves precise preoperative measurements of axial length in addition to accurate lens power calculations. There are some practitioners who feel that immersion biometry is necessary for accurate axial length determination. However, applanation techniques in combination with the Holladay 2 formula yield accurate and consistent results with greater patient convenience and less technician time. A newer device now available, the Zeiss IOL Master (Meditec, Germany), is a combined biometry instrument for non-contact optical measurements of axial length, corneal curvature, and anterior chamber depth that yields extremely accurate and efficient measurements with minimal patient inconvenience. The axial length measurement is based on an interference-optical method termed partial coherence interferometry and measurements are claimed to be compatible with acoustic immersion measurements and accurate to within 30 microns. The Quantel Axis II immersion biometry unit is also a convenient and accurate device for axial length measurements. The device yields quick and precise axial length measurements using immersion biometry without requiring the patient to be placed in the supine position. Regardless of the technique being used to measure axial length, it is important that the surgeon use biometry that he or she feels yields the most consistent and accurate results.

When determining lens power calculations, the Holladay 2 formula takes into account disparities in anterior segment and axial lengths by adding the white-to-white corneal diameter and lens thickness into the formula. Addition of these variables helps predict the exact position of the IOL in the eye and has improved refractive predictability. The SRK T and the SRK II formulas can be used as a final check in the lens power assessment; and, for eyes with less than 22 mm in axial length, the Hoffer Q formula should be utilized for comparative purposes.

## SURGICAL TECHNIQUE

The multifocal Array works best when the final postoperative refraction has less than 1.00 D of astigmatism. It is thus very important that incision construction be appropriate

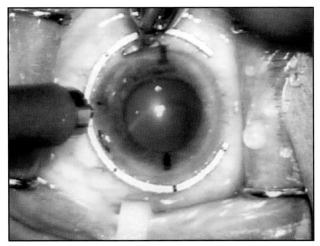

**Figure 12-4.** A fixation ring holds the globe as limbal relaxing incisions are placed just inside the surgical limbus in clear cornea using the preset 600 micron Nichamin Force blade.

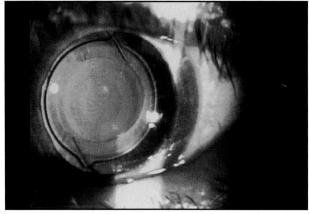

**Figure 12-5.** The Array multifocal intraocular lens in situ. Note the capsulorrhexis overlapping the edge of the lens optic.

with respect to size and location. A CCI at the temporal periphery that is 3 mm or less in width and 2 mm long is highly recommended.[41] Each surgeon should be aware of his or her usual amount of surgically-induced astigmatism by vector analysis. The surgeon must also be able to utilize one of the many modalities for addressing preoperative astigmatism. Although both T and arcuate keratotomies at the 7-mm optical zone can be utilized, there is an increasing trend favoring 600-μm deep LRIs (Figure 12-4) for the reduction or elimination of pre-existing astigmatism.[42,43]

In preparation for phacoemulsification, the capsulorrhexis must be round in shape and sized so that there is a small margin of anterior capsule overlapping the optic circumferentially (Figure 12-5). This is important in order to guarantee in-the-bag placement of the IOL and prevent anterior/posterior alterations in location that would affect the final refractive status. Hydrodelineation and cortical cleaving hydrodissection are very important in all patients because they facilitate lens disassembly and complete cortical cleanup.[44] Complete and fastidious cortical cleanup will hopefully reduce the incidence of posterior capsule opacification whose presence, even in very small amounts, will inordinately degrade the visual acuity in Array patients. It is because of this phenomena that patients implanted with Array lenses will require YAG laser posterior capsulotomies earlier than patients implanted with monofocal IOLs.

Minimally invasive surgery is very important. Techniques that produce effective phacoemulsification times of less than 20 seconds and average phacoemulsification powers of 10% or less are highly advantageous and can best be achieved with power modulations (burst mode or 2 pulses per second) rather than continuous phacoemulsification modes.[45,46] The Array is inserted easiest by means of the Unfolder injector system. Complete removal of all viscoelastic from the anterior chamber and behind the lens will reduce the incidence of postoperative pressure spikes and myopic shift from capsular block syndrome.

## COMPLICATIONS MANAGEMENT

When intraoperative complications develop they must be handled precisely and appropriately. In situations in which the first eye has already had an Array implanted, complications management must be directed toward finding any possible way of implanting an Array in the second eye. Under most circumstances, capsule rupture will still allow for implantation of an Array as long as there is an intact capsulorrhexis. Under these circumstances, the lens haptics are implanted in the sulcus and the optic is prolapsed posteriorly through the anterior capsulorrhexis. This is facilitated by a capsulorrhexis that is slightly smaller than the diameter of the optic in order to capture the optic in essentially an "in-the-bag" location. If full sulcus implantation is utilized then appropriate change in the IOL power will need to be made in order to compensate for the more anterior location of the IOL within the eye. When vitreous loss occurs, a meticulous vitrectomy with clearing of all vitreous strands must be performed.

It is important to avoid iris trauma since the pupil size and shape may impact the visual function of a multifocal IOL postoperatively. If the pupil is less than 2.5 mm, there may be an impairment of near visual acuity due to the location of the rings serving near visual acuity.[47] For patients with small postoperative pupil diameters affecting near vision, a mydriatic pupilloplasty can be successfully performed with the argon laser.[48] Enlargement of the pupil will expose the near dominant rings of the multifocal IOL, and restore near vision in most patients.

## TARGETING EMMETROPIA

The most important skill to master in the refractive lens exchange patient is the ultimate achievement of emmetropia. Emmetropia can be achieved successfully with accurate IOL power calculations and adjunctive modalities for eliminating astigmatism. With the trend toward smaller astigmatically neutral CCIs, it is now possible to more accurately address preexisting astigmatism at the time of lens surgery. The popularization of LRIs by Gills and Nichamin has added a useful means of reducing up to 3.50 D of preexisting astigmatism by placing paired 600-μm deep incisions at the limbus in the steep meridian. When against-the-rule astigmatism is present, the temporal groove of the paired LRIs can be utilized as the site of entry for the CCI. This is a simple and practical approach for reducing preexisting astigmatism at the time of surgery and because the coupling of these incisions is 1 to 1, no alteration in the calculated lens power is needed.

## REFRACTIVE SURPRISE

On occasion, surgeons may be presented with an unexpected refractive surprise following surgery. These miscalculations in lens power can be disappointing to both the surgeon and patient but happily the means for correcting these refractive errors are increasing. When there is a gross error in the lens inserted the best approach is to perform a lens exchange as soon as possible. When smaller errors are encountered or lens exchange is felt to be unsafe, various adjunctive procedures are available to address these refractive surprises.

One of the simplest techniques to address residual myopia following surgery is a 2-, 3-, or 4-cut radial keratotomy with a large optical zone. RK is still a relatively safe procedure with little likelihood for significant hyperopic shift with conservative incision and optical zone placement. When residual hyperopia is present following cataract surgery, CK is an option for reducing hyperopia and appears to work best in older patients and in patients with 1.00 D to 2.00 D of refractive error. Another option for reducing 0.50 D to 1.00 D of hyperopia involves rotating the IOL out of the capsular bag and placing it in the ciliary sulcus to increase the functional power of the lens. LASIK can also be performed to eliminate myopia, hyperopia, or astigmatism following surgery complicated by unexpected refractive results.

An interesting and simple intraocular approach to the postoperative refractive surprise involves the use of IOLs placed in the sulcus over the primary IOL in a piggyback fashion. STAAR Surgical (Monrovia, Calif) now produces the AQ5010V foldable silicone IOL that is useful for sulcus placement as a secondary piggyback lens. The STAAR AQ5010V has an overall length of 14.0 mm and is available in powers between -4.00 to +4.00 D in whole-diopter powers. In smaller eyes with larger hyperopic postoperative errors, the Staar AQ2010V is 13.5 mm in overall length and is available in powers between +5.00 to +9.00 D in whole-diopter steps. This approach is especially useful when expensive refractive lasers are not available or when corneal surgery is not feasible.

## POSTOPERATIVE COURSE

If glasses are required after surgery in a patient implanted with a multifocal IOL, the spherical correction should be determined by overplusing the patient to a slight blur and gradually reducing the power until the best acuity is reached. Patients are able to focus through the near portions of their IOL and thus it is possible to overminus a patient if care is not taken to push the plus power. When using this defocusing technique, it is critical to stop as soon as distance acuity is maximized to avoid overminusing the patient. The cylinder power should be the smallest amount that provides the best acuity. If add power is necessary, the full add power for the required working distance should be prescribed.

If patients are unduly bothered by photic phenomena such as halos and glare, these symptoms can be alleviated by various techniques. Weak pilocarpine at a concentration of 1/8% or weaker will constrict the pupil to a diameter that will usually lessen the severity of halos without significantly effecting near visual acuity. Similarly, brimonidine tartrate ophthalmic solution 0.2% (Alphagan, Allergan, Irvine, Calif) has been shown to reduce pupil size under scotopic conditions[49] and can also be administered in an attempt to reduce halo and glare symptoms. Another approach involves the use of overminused spectacles in order to push the secondary focal point behind the retina and thus lessen the effect of image blur from multiple images in front of the retina.[50] Polarized lenses have also been found to be helpful in reducing photic phenomena. Perhaps the most important technique is the implantation of bilateral Array lenses as close in time as possible in order to allow patients the ability to use the lenses together which appears to allow for improved binocular distance and near vision compared to monocular acuity. Finally, most patients report that halos improve or disappear with the passage of several weeks to months.

## FINAL COMMENTS

Thanks to the successes of the excimer laser, refractive surgery is increasing in popularity throughout the world. Corneal refractive surgery, however, has its limitations.

Patients with severe degrees of myopia and hyperopia are poor candidates for excimer laser surgery, and presbyopes must contend with reading glasses or monovision to address their near visual needs. The rapid recovery and astigmatically neutral incisions currently being used for modern cataract surgery have allowed this procedure to be used with greater predictability for refractive lens exchanges in patients who are otherwise not suffering from visually significant cataracts. The increased accuracy and safety of small-incision cataract surgery is now creating an incentive for borderline cataract patients to opt for surgery sooner than later for the refractive benefits of relative spectacle independence. Many of these patients are more than willing to proceed with refractive lens exchanges rather than wait for their cataracts to become visually significant to a level where private insurance or government insurance will cover the costs.

As this procedure becomes more popular, it will create a win-win situation for all involved. Firstly, patients can enjoy a predictable refractive procedure with rapid recovery that can address all types and severities of refractive errors in addition to addressing presbyopia with multifocal or accommodative lens technology. Secondly, surgeons can offer these procedures without the intrusion of private or government insurance and establish a less disruptive relationship with their patients. Finally, government can enjoy the decreased financial burden from the expenses of cataract surgery for the ever increasing ranks of aging baby boomers as more and more of these patients opt for lens exchanges to address their refractive surgery goals; ultimately reaching Medicare coverage as pseudophakes.

Successful integration of refractive lens exchanges into the general ophthalmologist's practice is fairly straightforward because most surgeons are currently performing small incision cataract surgery for their cataract patients. Essentially, the same procedure is performed for a refractive lens exchange differing only in removal of a relatively clear crystalline lens and simple adjunctive techniques for reducing corneal astigmatism. Although any style of foldable intraocular lens can be used for lens exchanges, multifocal intraocular lenses currently offer the best option for addressing both the elimination of refractive errors and presbyopia. Refractive lens exchange with multifocal lens technology is not for every patient considering refractive surgery but does offer substantial benefits especially in high hyperopes, presbyopes, and patients with borderline or soon-to-be clinically significant cataracts who are requesting refractive surgery. Appropriate patient screening, accurate biometry, lens power calculations, and meticulous surgical technique will allow surgeons to maximize their success with this procedure.

# REFERENCES

1. Colin J, Robinet A. Clear lensectomy and implantation of low-power posterior chamber intraocular lens for the correction of high myopia. *Ophthalmology.* 1994;101:107-112.

2. Siganos DS, Pallikaris IG. Clear lensectomy and intraocular lens implantation for hyperopia from +7 to +14 diopters. *J Refract Surg.* 1998;14:105-113.

3. Pucci V, Morselli S, Romanelli F, et al. Clear lens phacoemulsification for correction of high myopia. *J Cataract Refract Surg.* 2001;27:896-900.

4. Ge J, Arellano A, Salz J. Surgical correction of hyperopia: clear lens extraction and laser correction. *Ophthalmol Clin North Am.* 2001;14:301-13.

5. Fine IH, Hoffman RS, Packer P. Clear-lens extraction with multifocal lens implantation. *Int Ophthalmol Clin.* 2001; 41:113-121.

6. Pop M, Payette Y, Amyot M. Clear lens extraction with intraocular lens followed by photorefractive keratectomy or laser in situ keratomileusis. *Ophthalmology.* 2000;107:1776-1781.

7. Kolahdouz-Isfahani AH, Rostamian K, Wallace D, et al. Clear lens extraction with intraocular lens implantation for hyperopia. *J Refract Surg.* 1999;15:316-323.

8. Jimenez-Alfaro I, Miguelez S, Bueno JL, et al. Clear lens extraction and implantation of negative-power posterior chamber intraocular lenses to correct extreme myopia. *J Cataract Refract Surg.* 1998;24:1310-1316.

9. Lyle WA, Jin GJ. Clear lens extraction to correct hyperopia. *J Cataract Refract Surg.* 1997;23:1051-1056.

10. Lee KH, Lee JH. Long-term results of clear lens extraction for severe myopia. *J Cataract Refract Surg.* 1996;22:1411-1415.

11. Gris O, Guell JL, Manero F, et al. Clear lens extraction to correct high myopia. *J Cataract Refract Surg.* 1996;22:686-689.

12. Lyle WA, Jin GJ. Clear lens extraction for the correction of high refractive error. *J Cataract Refract Surg.* 1994;20:273-276.

13. Wallace RB. Multifocals: past and present. In: Wallace RB, ed. *Refractive Cataract Surgery and Multifocal IOLs.* Thorofare, NJ: SLACK Incorporated; 2001:179-186.

14. Fine IH. Design and early clinical studies of the AMO Array multifocal IOL. In Maxwell A, Nordan LT, eds. *Current Concepts of Multifocal Intraocular Lenses.* Thorofare, NJ: SLACK Incorporated; 1991:105-115.

15. Percival SPB, Setty SS. Prospectively randomized trial comparing the pseudoaccommodation of the AMO Array multifocal lens and a monofocal lens. *J Cataract Refract Surg.* 1993; 19:26-31.

16. Steinert RF, Post CT, Brint SF, et al. A progressive, randomized, double-masked comparison of a zonal-progressive multifocal intraocular lens and a monofocal intraocular lens. *Ophthalmology.* 1992;99:853-861.

17. Negishi K, Nagamoto T, Hara E, et al. Clinical evaluation of a five-zone refractive multifocal intraocular lens. *J Cataract Refract Surg.* 1996;22:110-115.

18. Brydon KW, Tokarewicz AC, Nichols BD. AMO Array multifocal lens versus monofocal correction in cataract surgery. *J Cataract Refract Surg.* 2000;26:96-100.

19. Vaquero-Ruano M, Encinas JL, Millan I, et al. AMO Array multifocal versus monofocal intraocular lenses: long-term follow-up. *J Cataract Refract Surg.* 1998;24:118-123.

20. Steinert RF, Aker BL, Trentacost DJ, et al. A prospective study of the AMO Array zonal-progressive multifocal silicone intraocular lens and a monofocal intraocular lens. *Ophthalmology.* 1999;106:1243-1255.

21. Pieh S, Weghaupt H, Skorpik C. Contrast sensitivity and glare disability with diffractive and refractive multifocal intraocular lenses. *J Cataract Refract Surg.* 1998;24:659-662.

22. Pieh S, Marvan P, Lackner B, et al. Quantitative performance of bifocal and multifocal intraocular lenses in a model eye: point spread function in multifocal intraocular lenses. *Arch Ophthalmol.* 2002;120:23-28.

23. Arens B, Freudenthaler N, Quentin CD. Binocular function after bilateral implantation of monofocal and refractive multifocal intraocular lenses. *J Cataract Refract Surg.* 1999;25:399-404.

24. Schmitz S, Dick HB, Krummenauer F, et al. Contrast sensitivity and glare disability by halogen light after monofocal and multifocal lens implantation. *Br J Ophthalmol.* 2000;84:1109-1112.

25. Pieh S, Hanselmayer G, Lackner B, et al. Tritan colour contrast sensitivity function in refractive multifocal intraocular lenses. *Br J Ophthalmol.* 2001;85:811-815.

26. Kamlesh S, Dadeya S, Kaushik S. Contrast sensitivity and depth of focus with aspheric multifocal versus conventional monofocal intraocular lens. *Can J Ophthalmol.* 2001;36:197-201.

27. Haring G, Gronemeyer A, Hedderich J, et al. Stereoacuity and aniseikonia after unilateral and bilateral implantation of the Array refractive multifocal intraocular lens. *J Cataract Refract Surg.* 1999;25:1151-1156.

28. Shoji N, Shimizu K. Binocular function of the patient with the refractive multifocal intraocular lens. *J Cataract Refract Surg.* 2002;28:1012-1017.

29. Dick HB, Krummenauer F, Schwenn O, et al. Objective and subjective evaluation of photic phenomena after monofocal and multifocal intraocular lens implantation. *Ophthalmology.* 1999;106:1878-1886.

30. Haring G, Dick HB, Krummenauer F, et al. Subjective photic phenomena with refractive multifocal and monofocal intraocular lenses. Results of a multicenter questionnaire. *J Cataract Refract Surg.* 2001;27:245-249.

31. Gills JP. Subjective photic phenomena with refractive multifocal and monofocal IOLs. Letter to the editor. *J Cataract Refract Surg.* 2001;27:1148.

32. Featherstone KA, Bloomfield JR, Lang AJ, et al. Driving simulation study: bilateral Array multifocal versus bilateral AMO monofocal intraocular lenses. *J Cataract Refract Surg.* 1999;25:1254-1262.

33. Javitt JC, Wang F, Trentacost DJ, et al. Outcomes of cataract extraction with multifocal intraocular lens implantation—functional status and quality of life. *Ophthalmology.* 1997;104:589-599.

34. Packer M, Fine IH, Hoffman RS. Refractive lens exchange with the Array multifocal lens. *J Cataract Refract Surg.* 2002;28:421-424.

35. Kamath GG, Prasas S, Danson A, et al. Visual outcome with the Array multifocal intraocular lens in patients with concurrent eye disease. *J Cataract Refract Surg.* 2000;26:576-581.

36. Sedgewick JH, Orillac R, Link C. Array multifocal intraocular lens in a charity hospital training program. A resident's experience. *J Cataract Refract Surg.* 2002;28:1205-1210.

37. Kaushik S, Kamlesh S. A clinical evaluation of an aspheric multifocal intraocular lens and its implications for the developing world. *Ophthalmic Surg Lasers.* 2002;33:298-303.

38. Jacobi PC, Dietlein TS, Konen W. Multifocal intraocular lens implantation in pediatric cataract surgery. *Ophthalmology.* 2001;108:1375-1380.

39. Rodriguez A, Gutierrez E, Alvira G. Complications of clear lens extraction in axial myopia. *Arch Ophthalmol.* 1987;105:1522-1523.

40. Ripandelli G, Billi B, Fedeli R, et al. Retinal detachment after clear lens extraction in 41 eyes with axial myopia. *Retina.* 1996;16:3-6.

41. Fine IH. Corneal tunnel incision with a temporal approach. In Fine IH, Fichman RA, Grabow HB, eds. *Clear-Corneal Cataract Surgery & Topical Anesthesia.* Thorofare, NJ: SLACK Incorporated; 1993:5-26.

42. Gills JP, Gayton JL. Reducing pre-existing astigmatism. In: Gills JP, ed. *Cataract Surgery: The State of the Art.* Thorofare, NJ: SLACK Incorporated; 1998:53-66.

43. Nichamin L. Refining astigmatic keratotomy during cataract surgery. *Ocular Surgery News.* 1993, April 15.

44. Fine IH. Cortical cleaving hydrodissection. *J Cataract Refract Surg.* 1992;18:508-512.

45. Fine IH. The choo-choo chop and flip phacoemulsification technique. *Operative Techniques in Cataract and Refractive Surgery.* 1998;1(2):61-65.

46. Fine IH, Packer M, Hoffman RS. The use of power modulations in phacoemulsification: choo choo chop and flip phacoemulsification. *J Cataract Refract Surg.* 2001;27:188-197.

47. Hayashi K, Hayashi H, Nakao F, et al. Correlation between pupillary size and intraocular lens decentration and visual acuity of a zonal-progressive multifocal lens and a monofocal lens. *Ophthalmology.* 2001;108:2011-2017.

48. Thomas JV. Pupilloplasty and photomydriasis. In Belcher CD, Thomas JV, Simmons RJ, eds. *Photocoagulation in Glaucoma and Anterior Segment Disease.* Baltimore, MD: Williams & Wilkins; 1984:150-157.

49. McDonald JE, El-Moatassem Kotb AM, Decker BB. Effect of brimonidine tartrate ophthalmic solution 0.2% on pupil size in normal eyes under different luminance conditions. *J Cataract Refract Surg.* 2001;27:560-564.

50. Hunkeler JD, Coffman TM, Paugh J, et al. Characterization of visual phenomena with the Array multifocal intraocular lens. *J Cataract Refract Surg.* 2002;28:1195-1204.

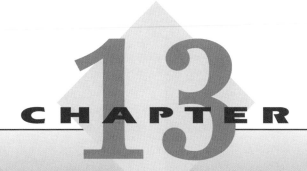

# CHAPTER 13

# PHACOLYTIC PHACOMORPHIC GLAUCOMAS

S. Fabian Lerner, MD

## INTRODUCTION

Different disorders of the lens may be associated with glaucoma. Cataract formation may be associated with open-angle or angle-closure glaucoma. This chapter will be focused on phacolytic and phacomorphic glaucomas. Ectopia lentis, simple or associated with other disorders, is not considered in this section.

## PHACOLYTIC GLAUCOMA TERMINOLOGY

In 1955, Flocks, Littwin, and Zimmerman proposed the term *phacolytic glaucoma* for the open-angle glaucoma associated with a leaking hypermature cataract.[1] They suggested that the mechanism of the glaucoma was the obstruction of the trabecular meshwork by macrophages and fluid escaped from the lens (Morgagnian fluid). This term was incorrectly applied later by others to all types of lens-induced glaucomas. In 1978, Epstein and coworkers reported that the leaking lens proteins may be the cause of the blockage of aqueous outflow.[2,3] Because of these studies, the term *lens protein glaucoma* has been suggested instead of phacolytic glaucoma.[4] This entity should be differentiated from *lens particle*

*glaucoma*, which occurs due to liberated lens debris or particles after cataract surgery, lens trauma or Nd:YAG laser posterior capsulotomy.[4]

## LENS PROTEIN GLAUCOMA— PATHOPHYSIOLOGY

Epstein et al have demonstrated that leaking proteins from the lens obstruct the trabecular meshwork, which may lead to the elevation of IOP.[2,3]

### Clinical Characteristics

The clinical picture is usually an old patient presenting with a unilateral red and painful eye. Visual acuity has been reduced typically for a long time due to a mature or hypermature cataract. Biomicroscopy shows conjunctival hyperemia, corneal epithelial edema, and an inflammatory reaction with flare in the anterior chamber. The lens has a mature or hypermature cataract (Figure 13-1). Sometimes 1 or more plaques of whitish material may be seen in the anterior capsule of the lens or floating in the anterior chamber. The IOP is high. Depending on the severity of the corneal edema and the inflammatory reaction, the angle may be seen. Gonioscopy reveals an open-angle. Another presentation of

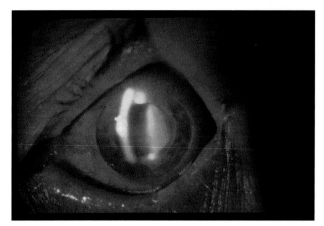

**Figure 13-1.** Lens protein glaucoma due to hypermature cataract.[2,3]

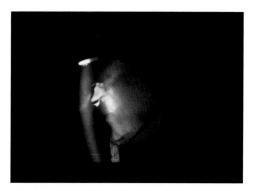

**Figure 13-2.** Lens particle glaucoma after trauma to the lens.[4]

phacolytic glaucoma may occur when the lens is dislocated in the vitreous. The signs and symptoms of this type of glaucoma are usually more subtle.

## Differential Diagnosis

Acute angle-closure glaucoma should be considered among the differential diagnoses in a patient presenting with unilateral pain, decreased vision, red eye, and high IOP. Gonioscopy makes the differential diagnosis as phacolytic glaucoma has an open angle. If corneal edema and anterior chamber inflammation preclude the observation of the angle, gonioscopic examination of the contralateral eye may help in the diagnosis.

The clinical history separates a traumatic glaucoma. The diagnosis may be more difficult in the presence of a hypertensive uveitis. Some signs that help to distinguish both entities are: the presence of a mature or hypermature cataract, the occasional presence of whitish material in the lens surface, or floating in the anterior chamber and the infrequency of keratic precipitates in the phacolytic glaucoma. Ultimately, a paracentesis with microscopic examination of the aqueous humor will show an amorphous proteinaceous fluid. Macrophages have also been described in the aqueous humor of patients with phacolytic glaucoma.[5]

## Treatment

Cataract extraction is the treatment of choice for phacolytic glaucoma. Medical treatment, however, should be administered to lower the IOP and reduce inflammation before proceeding to surgery. Reduction of IOP is achieved with the use of hyperosmotics, ß-blockers, oral and topical carbonic anhidrase inhibitors and/or α2-adrenergics. Topical glucocorticoids are administered to control inflammation. In a retrospective study, Mandal and Gothwal reviewed the vision and IOP outcomes of 45 consecutive patients presenting with phacolytic glaucoma that received an extracapsular cataract extraction (ECCE) with or without PCIOL

implantation.[6] Patients did not undergo implantation of PC IOL if they had satisfactory aphakic correction in the contralateral eye. With a minimum follow-up of 12 months, IOP was controlled in all patients (even the ones in which the visual acuity did not improve due to severe glaucomatous disc damage). Visual acuity improved in a significant percentage of patients (44% achieving 20/40 or better) who had very poor preoperative vision (barely light perception). Duration of more than 5 days and patients older than 60 years seemed to be risk factors for poor postoperative visual outcome.[7] McKibbin and coworkers reported vitreous loss as an intraoperative complication in 2 out of 4 phacolytic glaucomas (both eyes with vitreous loss also had pseudoexfoliation syndrome).[8] These authors did not recommend phacoemulsification due to corneal edema and/or intraocular inflammation. In a retrospective study of 135 eyes with phacolytic glaucoma, Braganza et al performed a combined trabeculectomy-cataract extraction procedure in those eyes in which the signs were present for more than 7 days or if IOP could not be controlled preoperatively under maximal tolerated medical therapy.[9] Although after 6 months eyes that received combined surgery had similar visual acuity and IOP than those that received only cataract extraction, the combined procedure provided better IOP control in the early postoperative period. The author recommends combined procedure for patients with long-standing or medically uncontrolled phacolytic glaucoma.

# LENS PARTICLE GLAUCOMA— PATHOPHYSIOLOGY

This glaucoma occurs due to liberated lens debris or particles after cataract surgery, lens trauma, or Nd:YAG laser posterior capsulotomy that block the trabecular outflow pathways[4] (Figure 13-2).

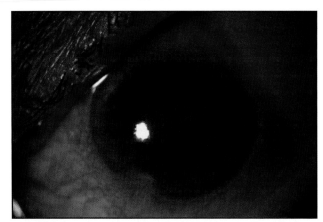

**Figure 13-3.** For practical purposes the glaucoma is produced by pupillary block with secondary angle-closure or by angle-closure without pupillary block.

## Clinical Characteristics

In contrast with phacolytic glaucoma, there is usually a previous cataract extraction, penetrating lens trauma, or Nd:YAG laser posterior capsulotomy. The interval between the insult and the elevation of the IOP ranges from a few days to several weeks. In the case of Nd:YAG capsulotomy, the interval is shorter as elevation of IOP may occur immediately following the procedure. The mechanism for the IOP elevation associated with Nd:YAG capsulotomy may be different than the blockage of the trabecular meshwork by lens particles.

Slit-lamp examination of phacolytic glaucoma usually shows lens fragments floating in the anterior chamber, which may also disclose inflammation with flare and cells. A hypopyon may also be present. Corneal edema may develop if the IOP is very elevated. Gonioscopy shows an open angle, and lens debris may also be seen. If severe and persistent inflammation is present, peripheral anterior synechiae may develop.

## Differential Diagnosis

The history and the presence of lens material in the anterior chamber usually help the clinician to make the diagnosis. Differential diagnoses include lens-protein glaucoma (which in fact may coexist with lens particle glaucoma), hypertensive uveitis, elevation of IOP due to vitreous in the anterior chamber, or use of corticosteroids.

## Treatment

Medical therapy with ß-blockers, oral and topical carbonic anhidrase inhibitors, and/or α2-adrenergics is indicated in order to reduce the IOP. Topical corticosteroids should be administered with caution to control inflammation as its use may delay the absorption of the lens debris. The pupil should be dilated. If medical therapy is not effective to control the situation, surgery is indicated to remove the lens

material. This indication should not be delayed as the operation may be more difficult in a later stage due to the fact that lens material may be sequestered within the capsular bag. Also, the elevated IOP and the inflammatory process are harmful for the eye if the course continues.

# PHACOMORPHIC GLAUCOMA— PATHOPHYSIOLOGY

In phacomorphic glaucoma the lens pushes the iris forward, closing the angle. This may be due to an enlargement of the lens itself, or to a pressure posterior to the lens. For practical purposes the glaucoma is produced by pupillary block with secondary angle-closure or by angle-closure without pupillary block.

## Clinical Characteristics

The typical picture is a very advanced cataract in which the lens becomes intumescent, pushing the iris forward. Flow of aqueous humor through the pupil may be impeded leading to a pupillary block or relative pupillary block mechanism. Aqueous humor in the posterior chamber further pushes the iris forward narrowing or closing the angle. Iris bombé may or may not be found depending on the pupillary block mechanism contributions to the situation.

Biomicroscopy shows a clinical picture similar to an acute angle-closure glaucoma (Figure 13-3). Corneal edema may be present, the anterior chamber is very narrow, the pupil is fixed and mid-dilated, and there is a mature, intumescent lens. IOP is elevated (usually higher than 40 mmHg). Gonioscopy shows a closed angle.

## Differential Diagnosis

Different types of angle-closure glaucoma such as pupillary block or malignant glaucoma (aqueous misdirection) should be considered as differential diagnoses of phacomorphic glaucoma. Pupillary block may also contribute to a phacomorphic glaucoma as an intumescent lens may block aqueous flow through the pupil. In the malignant glaucoma mechanism the misdirected aqueous creates a force that pushes the iris-lens diaphragm forward closing the angle, even in the presence of a patent iridectomy.

Phacomorphic glaucoma should be suspected in the presence of an intumescent lens. Differential diagnosis with angle-closure glaucoma is not always easy as thickness of the lens also contributes to the mechanism of angle closure.[10] Examination of the contralateral eye is helpful to compare anterior chamber depths, lens features, and opening of the angles.

Anomalies in the position of the lens, either congenital or acquired, should also be considered among the differential diagnoses. These include ectopia lentis simple or associated with other disorders such as homocystinuria, Weill-

Marchesani syndrome, or Marfan's syndrome, among other congenital anomalies. Acquired conditions include subluxation or luxation of the lens due to trauma or exfoliation syndrome. In the presence of subluxation of the lens, mild iridodonesis may be found due to loose zonules.

Ultrasound examination of the posterior segment is recommended in phacomorphic glaucoma due to opaque media. A phacomorphic glaucoma associated with a choroidal melanoma has been reported.[11]

## Treatment

Medical treatment with ocular hypotensive drugs should be attempted as the initial treatment. Pilocarpine should not be used as it may worsen a pupillary block mechanism and it may allow anterior lens movement.

Laser iridotomy has been recommended before subsequent cataract extraction.[12] Argon laser peripheral iridoplasty has also been advocated as the initial laser procedure to open the angle.[10]

Cataract extraction is the treatment of choice, and is best performed after the elevated IOP has been reduced by means of medical or laser treatment.[8] Special care should be taken when performing capsulorrhexis in these eyes.[13]

# PHACOANAPHYLACTIC GLAUCOMA

Phacoanaphylaxis is an uncommon inflammation that may occur after surgical or traumatic injury to the lens. It is usually a granulomatous uveitis and elevation of the IOP is rare. Different mechanisms may contribute to the development of elevated IOP, either with open angle (inflammation of the trabecular meshwork or corticosteroid glaucoma) or secondary closed angle (peripheral anterior synechiae or posterior synechiae with pupillary block). Differential diagnosis should be made with phacolytic glaucoma and with chronic types of uveitis such as sympathetic ophthalmia.

Treatment of the glaucoma depends on the mechanism of production. In all cases, inflammation should be treated with corticosteroids and surgical removal of the lens material should be performed.

Hypotensive drugs should be used in the open-angle glaucomas. Laser or surgical iridectomy is used to treat pupillary block. Iridoplasty, medical treatment, or trabeculectomy may be used as needed.

# REFERENCES

1. Flocks M, Littwin CS, Zimmerman LE. Phacolytic glaucoma: clinicopathologic study of 138 cases of glaucoma associated with hypermature cataract. *Arch Opthalmol.* 1955;54:37-47.

2. Epstein DL, Jedzniniak JA, Grant WM. Obstruction of aqueous outflow by lens particles and by heavy-molecular-weight soluble lens proteins. *Invest Ophthalmol Vis Sci.* 1978;17:272-277.

3. Epstein DL, Jedzniniak JA, Grant WM. Identification of heavy molecular weight soluble lens protein in aqueous humor in human phacolytic glaucoma. *Invest Ophthalmol Vis Sci.* 1978;17:398-402.

4. Epstein DL. Diagnosis and management of lens-induced glaucoma. *Ophthalmology.* 1982;89:227-230.

5. Goldberg MF. Cytological diagnosis of phacolytic glaucoma utilizing Millipore filtration of the aqueous. *Br J Ophthalmol.* 1967;51:847-853.

6. Mandal AK, Gothwal VK. Intraocular pressure control and visual outcome in patients with phacolytic glaucoma managed by extracapsular cataract extraction with or without posterior chamber intraocular lens implantation. *Ophthalmic Surg Lasers.* 1998;29:880-889.

7. Prajna NV, Ramakrishnan R, Krishnadas R, et al. Lens induced glaucomas—visual results and risk factors for final visual acuity. *Indian J Ophthalmol.* 1996;44:149-155.

8. McKibbin M, Gupta A, Atkins AD. Cataract extraction and intraocular lens implantation in eyes with phacomorphic or phacolytic glaucoma. *J Cataract Refract Surg.* 1996;22:633-636.

9. Braganza A, Thomas R, George T, et al. Management of phacolytic glaucoma: experience of 135 cases. *Indian J Ophthalmol.* 1998;46:139-143.

10. Liebmann JM, Ritch R. Glaucoma associated with lens intumescence and dislocation. In: Ritch R, Shields MB, Krupin T. eds. *The glaucomas.* St Louis: Mo: Mosby; 1996:2:1033-1053.

11. Al-Torbak A, Karcioglu ZA, Abboud E, Netland PA. Phacomorphic glaucoma associated with choroidal melanoma. *Ophthalmic Surg Lasers.* 1998;29:510-513.

12. Tomey KF, Al-Rajhi AA. Neodymium:YAG laser iridotomy in the initial management of phacomorphic glaucoma. *Ophthalmology.* 1992;99:660-665.

13. Rao SK, Padmanabhan P. Capsulorrhexis in eyes with phacomorphic glaucoma. *J Cataract Refract Surg.* 1998;24:882-884.

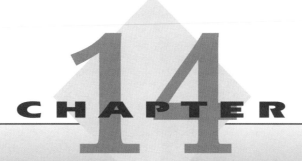

# CHAPTER 14

# CATARACT SURGERY IN PSEUDOEXFOLIATION SYNDROME

*William J. Rand, MD; Gabriel E. Velázquez, MD; and Barry A. Schechter, MD*

## INTRODUCTION

Pseudoexfoliation (PEX) syndrome is an ocular mystery. Many investigators over the years have attempted to clarify and identify its peculiar etiology, appearance, and propensity for ocular pathology.[1,2] Many associations have been established, complications treated, and manifestations documented. It has been found sporadically in many populations worldwide, yet its exact makeup and point of origin in the eye remain obscure.[3] PEX syndrome has the potential to create difficulties and catastrophic complications in cataract surgery. The study of PEX syndrome is important.

In this chapter we will describe in detail our current technique, designed to prevent and reduce the incidence of complications in cataract surgery for PEX patients. We will also offer a review of current information on this intriguing disease.

PEX syndrome is a systemic degenerative disorder that is characterized in the eye by deposits of an irregular meshwork of fibrillar eosinophilic material. This material may be found on the structures of the anterior and posterior chambers. This condition may be associated with cataract and glaucoma. The precise composition of the PEX material has not yet been identified. Studies suggest an important role of proteoglycans in the pathogenic pathway in PEX syndrome.[4-11]

PEX syndrome has been suggested to include a blood-aqueous barrier impairment associated with higher protein content in the aqueous humor. It has also been suggested that PEX syndrome may be associated with elevated serum amyloid levels,[12] but this has not been substantiated.[13]

In PEX syndrome, conjunctival biopsy may reveal the presence of PEX material, even though the conjunctiva does not display clinical manifestations.[14] PEX material has been documented on the ciliary processes and zonule,[15] but PEX syndrome is more commonly associated with deposition of material on the anterior lens surface, which is more readily visualized with dilated pupils.[16] Deposition is more marked in the midperiphery of the lens; with a translucent central zone surrounded by an intermediate clear zone (iris movement denudes the capsular surface of PEX material) (Figure 14-1). Deposition material is also frequently seen at the pupillary margin and is often associated with iris transillumination defects ("moth-eaten"' appearance).[17] Posterior synechiae are often associated with PEX syndrome. Broad posterior synechiae and miosis may prevent adequate viewing of the anterior lens capsule, making the clinical diagnosis of PEX syndrome difficult. In eyes with broad, circular posterior synechiae, the possibility of PEX syndrome should be considered.[18] Pigment and PEX material (flakes) are sometimes found on the corneal endothelium. A reduction in the number of endothelial cells may be present.[14,19,20]

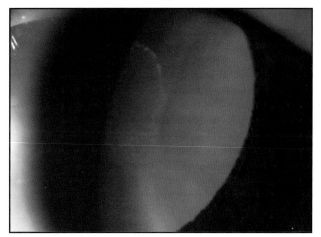

**Figure 14-1.** Photograph of patient with PEX material on anterior capsule.

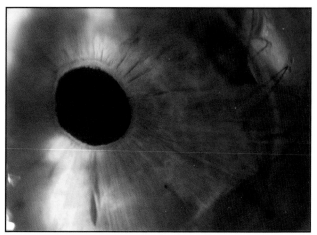

**Figure 14-2.** Photograph of patient with PEX syndrome and iris atrophy.

One of the major difficulties encountered with PEX is glaucoma. PEX glaucoma is likely secondary to the accumulation of PEX material in the trabecular meshwork.[21-23] The meshwork is frequently pigmented in a patchy fashion in contrast to the dense, homogeneous deposition seen in pigmentary dispersion syndrome.[16] Pigment dispersion syndrome should be included in the differential diagnosis for PEX syndrome as it is also associated with the deposition of material within the ocular tissues. Pigment dispersion syndrome and pigmentary glaucoma tend to occur in younger, myopic patients, with pressure spikes seen after exercise.[24] In contrast, PEX syndrome tends to occur in the sixth decade and beyond. In pigment dispersion syndrome, Krukenberg's spindle, a triangular-shaped adherence of pigment to the corneal endothelium is present due to the current flows of the aqueous humor. In PEX syndrome, white fibrillar material in no apparent pattern may be noted on the endothelium. In pigment dispersion syndrome, radial, midperipheral iris transillumination defects can be seen with retroillumination. In PEX syndrome, iris atrophy can also be seen, but it usually has a peripupillary distribution (Figure 14-2). In pigment dispersion syndrome, a peripheral iridotomy has been shown to change the dynamics and architecture of the lens-iris diaphragm, often affecting a cure.[25]

PEX glaucoma is likely secondary to the accumulation of PEX material, which blocks aqueous outflow in the trabeculum.[26,27] IOP tends to be higher than in eyes with primary open-angle glaucoma (POAG).[28,29] PEX glaucoma is associated with greater visual field loss and worse optic nerve cupping.[30,31]

PEX glaucoma tends to be less responsive to medical therapy than POAG[31-35] and surgical treatment is more commonly necessary.[31,36] In PEX glaucoma, argon laser trabeculoplasty is initially effective in lowering IOP,[37-39] but there is a significant loss of effect over long-term follow-up.[37] Filtering surgery for PEX glaucoma has similar results to

POAG.[40] In true exfoliation of the lens, which is secondary to trauma, chronic exposure to heat, or inflammation, elevated pressures are not typically seen.

The association of PEX syndrome with phacodonesis and spontaneous subluxation of the lens is due to zonular breaks at the insertion of the zonular fibers into the ciliary body epithelium and not at the insertion of the zonule into the lens capsule.[41,42] Some studies imply a genetic role at the cellular level in the pathogenesis of PEX syndrome.[43-46]

Different reports have given a wide range in the prevalence of PEX according to age and sex distributions, which may be due to genetic factors, differences in diagnostic technique, or differences in the populations studied.[47-53] The prevalence of PEX syndrome has been studied in Scandinavians and other Europeans,[48,54] Japanese,[15] Australian aborigines,[49] Australian non-aboriginal adults,[55] Navajo Indians,[56] natives of India[57] and Pakistan,[58] Bantu tribe of South Africa,[52] African-Americans,[59] and others.

PEX syndrome tends to be bilateral but is usually clinically asymmetric rather than unilateral. Upon clinical examination, many patients with PEX syndrome reveal only unilateral ocular involvement. This has been investigated by transmission electron microscopy and immunohistochemistry. When 1 eye demonstrates clinical evidence of PEX syndrome, alterations can be found in the anterior segment tissue of the fellow eye. Because PEX syndrome is associated with glaucoma and is an important risk factor for complications during cataract surgery, the potential involvement of both eyes in the PEX process is important.[60,61]

In PEX syndrome, involvement of the lens, zonule, ciliary body, iris, trabecular meshwork, and corneal endothelium may result in open-angle glaucoma, angle-closure glaucoma, phacodonesis, lens dislocation, and/or poor pupillary dilation. When performing cataract surgery in the presence of PEX syndrome, special consideration must be given to the increased risk of complications such as lens subluxation,[62] zonular dialyses or breaks,[63,64] posterior capsular rupture,[65] vitreous loss,[66,67] subluxation of the IOL,[64,68,69] uveitis,[70,71] hemorrhage, formation of posterior synechiae, and corneal endothelial decompensation.[72,73]

Even though PEX syndrome has traditionally been associated with increased risk, modern cataract surgery with appropriate surgical technique and preventative measures makes it possible to achieve good results, avoiding the increased complication rate attributed to PEX syndromes.

## INDICATIONS AND SPECIAL CONSIDERATIONS FOR CATARACT SURGERY IN PEX SYNDROME

Cataract surgery should be performed when reduced visual function impairs the quality of life sufficiently to warrant the risk of surgery. The increased risk of complications associated with PEX syndrome must be balanced against the experience and expertise of the operating surgeon. In the best of hands, when all resources are brought to bear, it is possible to reduce the risk of complications considerably. Most of the potential complications associated with PEX syndrome can be either prevented or readily managed during surgery, even when there is a complete dislocation of the lens. The surgeon should fully discuss with the patient the indications, risks, and benefits for the proposed cataract surgery. The decision to perform or delay the surgery and whether there is a benefit in referring the patient to a more experienced surgeon should be considered.

A comprehensive ophthalmic examination should include a complete history of current and past medical pathology including specific questions about systemic illnesses (ie, diabetes, systemic hypertension, ischemic heart disease, chronic pulmonary disease, renal disease, obesity, mental status) and all medications taken.[74] A careful personal and familial ocular history is also important (cataract surgery on the fellow eye, glaucoma, trauma, inflammatory episodes, amblyopia, infections, previous ocular surgery complications, and any topical medications).

Various aspects of visual function should be considered. Testing may include visual acuity at distance and near, visual field testing, color vision, contrast sensitivity, light adaptation, and depth perception. Cataracts may coexist with other causes of decreased visual function.[75,76] In the presence of significantly decreased visual acuity and a dense cataract, the ophthalmologist may evaluate entoptic phenomena, use the Potential Acuity Meter,[77,78] perform laser interferometry,[79] A- and B-scan ultrasonography, and/or visual electrophysiology (electroretinography-ERG and visually evoked potentials [VEP])[80,81] to determine the possibility of visual rehabilitation.

Brisk pupillary reflexes suggest good retinal function. The extent of pupillary dilation with mydriatics should be evaluated. If the pupils will not dilate widely, posterior adhesions may be present or the dilator muscle is weak. It should be anticipated that appropriate measures might be necessary to enlarge the pupil during surgery to allow adequate access to the lens. These may include stronger mydriatics, topical NSAIDs, epinephrine in the irrigating solution, lysis of posterior adhesions, pupillary expansion devices, iridectomy, stretching the pupil, or sphincterotomy.

Preoperative examination of the eyelids and lacrimal apparatus should identify cases of blepharitis, ectropion, entropion, lagophthalmos, keratoconjunctivitis sicca, and dacryocystitis. This will enable appropriate measures to be taken to reduce the risk of infection, keratitis, or wound-related complications. Corneal endothelial dystrophy, as seen frequently with PEX syndrome, might lead to clinically significant corneal decompensation. Iridodonesis and phacodonesis may herald a dislocated or subluxated lens and the surgeon should be prepared for the possibility of vitreous loss during surgery. Fundus examination with pupillary dilation should be performed to detect peripheral retina pathology.

If the patient has medically controlled glaucoma, it may be anticipated that IOP will remain under control with the same or less medications after surgery. If glaucoma control is poor, a combined trabeculectomy and cataract procedure should be considered. The combined procedure has greater associated risk than phacoemulsification with IOL implantation alone.[82]

Prior to scheduling surgery, all patients should be fully informed of risks and benefits, the alternatives and elective nature of their procedure. Options for optical correction, including the different types of implants and their desired postoperative refractive status—both eyes focused at distance, monovision, and multifocal IOLs should be considered. A final visual outcome of emmetropia to mild myopia is usually ideal, but the refractive error and overall status of the fellow eye should be considered carefully since anisometropia may not be well tolerated. Appropriate informed consent is obtained.[83,84]

## SURGICAL TECHNIQUE

### *Anesthesia: The Rand-Stein Analgesia Protocol*

Surgical technique and good results partially depend on good anesthesiology. The Rand-Stein Analgesia Protocol (RSAP) is an intravenous technique for providing profound ocular and body analgesia virtually without sedation. Anxiety and patient cooperation are managed separately with intravenous sedative medication. The control of pain, anxiety and patient cooperation are even more important in the presumed fragile ocular environment of PEX syndrome.

We have consistently used the RSAP on all of our cataract surgery patients.[85] We have not had an intraoperative conversion to local anesthesia in more than 15,000 cases. This technique can be expected to allow the PEX syndrome patient to undergo a controlled, painless, and anxiety-free cataract procedure using a sutureless corneal incision with virtually no probability of having to rely on or convert to local anesthesia.

Reviewing the literature, we find that general anesthesia is seldom used for cataract surgery. However, local (retrobulbar or peribulbar) anesthesia with intravenous sedation is still in common usage. Retrobulbar and peribulbar anesthesia techniques for cataract surgery are associated with potentially disfiguring, blinding, and life-threatening complications.[86-93] The very nature of a blind injection into the periocular tissues carries with it the potential for catastrophic retrobulbar hemorrhage, which can cause permanent blindness.[94] Many local anesthesia blocks fail to provide adequate ocular analgesia.[95]

Careful anesthesiology monitoring is indispensable to prevent and control complications in elderly patients as they often have serious associated systemic disease, such as coronary artery disease, hypertension, diabetes, and/or chronic lung disease.[96,97]

With phacoemulsification, the necessity for complete ocular akinesia has been eliminated. Topical anesthesia techniques significantly reduced the risk of surgically induced diplopia, amaurosis, ptosis, lid ecchymosis, and pain associated with injection anesthesia.[98] Topical anesthesia, however, is inadequate for providing profound internal analgesia for the eye and offers no remedy for the management of the uncooperative patient.[99,100] Approximately 10% of topical anesthesia patients require intraoperative conversion to local anesthesia with the eye already surgically opened.[101] Topical anesthetics and intracameral anesthetic agents have the potential to cause endothelial cell injury,[102] and they can damage the ocular surface in older patients with dry eye and blepharitis.[103] The RSAP eliminates the risks of topical and local anesthesia. The RSAP offers the benefits of reduced morbidity while providing control of the patient's ability to cooperate.

The RSAP uses low-dose intravenous Alfentanil HCl (Taylor Pharmaceuticals, Decatur, Ill) for its intense, rapid-onset analgesia without sedation.[104,105] Low-dose Methohexital Sodium (Eli Lilly, Indianapolis, Ill) provides a rapid-onset, ultra-short-acting sedative effect that precisely controls the patient's state of alertness. Preoperative Midazolam HCl (Abbott Laboratories, North Chicago, Ill) can be used optionally for preoperative anxiety.

Alfentanil HCl is reversible with Naloxone HCl (Abbott). Midazolam HCl is reversible with Flumazenil (Romazicon, Roche, Nutley, NJ). Methohexital sodium requires no reversal agent because of its ultra-short duration of action. Droperidol (American Regent Laboratories, Shirley, NJ) can

be used for its antiemetic function when nausea is present and an additional sedative effect is desired. We use Metoclopramide (Baxter Healthcare Corporation, Irvine, Calif) for nausea when no additional sedation is needed (Table 14-1).

# The Cataract Procedure in PEX Syndrome

Cataract surgery in PEX syndrome has the potential to become complicated and extensive due to inherent structural weakness. By utilizing a precision microsurgical approach, these complications can be significantly reduced, yielding consistently better postoperative results. Cataract surgery in PEX syndrome will frequently encounter small pupils, shallow anterior chambers, posterior adhesions, weak zonular support, partial subluxation, or complete dislocation of the crystalline lens. Final placement of the implant may be adversely affected by inadvertent stress exerted upon the zonular structures during surgery, resulting in subluxated or dislocated lens implants. This may be become apparent during the intraoperative, postoperative, or even in the long-term postoperative period. The principles that will be described here may be useful for performing better surgery for all surgical patients, but become more critical in the unstable ocular environment of PEX syndrome.

## Preoperative Considerations

In patients with PEX syndrome, intraoperative pupillary size can be expected to be significantly smaller compared to normal patients undergoing cataract surgery. Postoperatively, IOP and aqueous cell response is similar in both groups, but a significantly higher flare response has been observed in PEX syndrome patients.[106] Topical Ketorolac Tromehamine 0.5% (Acular, Allergan, Irvine, Calif) is an effective inhibitor of miosis during extracapsular cataract extraction and IOL implantation. It provides a stable mydriatic effect throughout surgery.[107]

## Prep and Drape

After instilling tetracaine hydrochloride drops (Alcon, Fort Worth, Tex), sterile prep and drape (Cataract Pack # 6974-03, Alcon) are performed. While the surgeon is scrubbing, analgesia and sedation are initiated in accordance with the RSAP guidelines.

## Speculum and Eye Wash

A speculum (Barraquer Adult Speculum, Bausch & Lomb Surgical, St. Louis, Mo) is placed. The eye is washed with BSS (Sterile Irrigating Solution, Alcon). 5% Iodine-Povidine (Applicare, Branfort, Conn) is placed in the conjunctival cul-de-sac for 30 seconds. Antibiotic drops, such as

# Rand-Stein Analgesia Protocol Summary

## *Preoperatively (In The Preoperative Area)*

*Midazolam HCl,* 1 mg IV in preoperative area after vitals signs confirmed stable. If needed, additional 1 mg IV, 10 to 15 minutes after first dose.
*Reversal agent:* Flumazenil, 2 cc (0.2 mg) IV

*Methohexital sodium,* 1 cc (10 mg) IV, PRN, 10 to 15 min before transfer to the operating room. Used only in cases with severe preoperative anxiety.
*Reversal agent:* None needed, short acting, less than 3 to 5 min, if inadvertent overdosage occurs, use simple. If SaO$_2$ falls below 90%, suspend administration and remind patient to breathe in and out deeply. If needed, Ambu ventilation until spontaneous respiration returns, usually 3 to 5 min.

*If prior history of nausea or vomiting,* (previous anesthesia), pretreat with:
*Droperidol,* 1 to 2 mg (75 mcg/Kg) IV, on arrival (for sedative/antiemetic effect), or
*Metoclopramide,* 10 mg, IV, on arrival (for a pure antiemetic effect, without sedation)

## In the Operating Room

*Tetracaine HCl,* 1 drop previous to washing, prepping, and draping the eye.

*Alfentanil HCl,* (500 mcg/cc) 4 to 6 doses of 125 mcg (1/4 cc), every 30 to 45 seconds. For inadequate analgesia or to prolong the analgesia effect: additional Alfentanil HCl, 125 mcg (1/4 cc) IV, every 30 to 45 seconds, until relief of pain. If SaO$_2$ falls below 90%, suspend administration and remind patient to breathe in and out deeply, as needed.
*Reversal agent:* Naloxone HCl, 0.2 to 0.4 mg (1/2 to 1 cc)

For intraoperative anxiety or persistent anxiety, squeezing, poor cooperation:
*Methohexital sodium,* 1 cc (10 mg) IV, every 2 minutes until relief of anxiety, and reassertion of control.

## *Postoperatively*

If nausea or vomiting during or after surgery:
*Metoclopramide,* 10 mg IV

**TABLE 14-1**

Gentamycin (American Pharmaceutical Partners. Los Angeles, Calif) and/or Cefalozin (Apothecon, Bristol-Myers Squibb, Princeton, NJ) are placed in the cul-de-sac, prior to the first incision, the counter-incision.

## *Surgical Incisions*

For the past 15,000 cataract surgeries with foldable lens implantation, we have utilized CCIs. Obviously, some PEX syndrome patients required sclerocorneal incisions, such as those in whom combined cataract surgery and trabeculectomy or larger, PMMA implants (retinal pathology) were indicated. We believe that CCIs are the procedure of choice for PEX syndrome patients. CCIs generate less inflammation, irritation, pain, and redness, because the conjunctiva is not traumatized. The conjunctiva is conserved for possibly needed glaucoma surgery in the future. CCIs generate minimal astigmatism in the axis where they are made (flattening this axis approximately 0.50 to 0.75 D in the authors' experience). The incision can be made in the steepest axis and the

counter-incision approximately 90 degrees away (Figure 14-3). We will describe the procedure for a right-handed surgeon in a slight with-the-rule astigmatism eye.

The procedure is designed to provide the gentlest tissue-handling possible of the ocular structures, preserving the integrity of structures that might be significantly weakened. Careful attention to the principles of precision microsurgery are strictly adhered to, including frequent refocusing of the microscope and a 3-D proprioceptive technique, which are continuously employed to significantly reduce stress on the cornea and zonules.

The procedure starts with a counter-incision at the 2- to 3-o'clock position through the posterior limbus, 1 mm in size. By cutting the tip off of an eye spear (Cellulose Sponge Spear, Hurricane Medical, Brandenton, Fla), approximately halfway down, the spear can be used as a blunt instrument. This avoids using a forceps that can cause a conjunctival hemorrhage. The sponge is placed on the limbus at 180 degrees from where the counterincision is to be made, min-

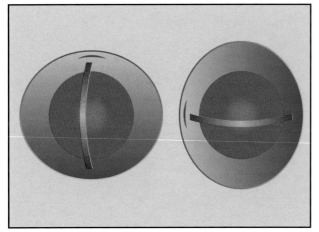

**Figure 14-3.** CCI should be on the steepest axis.

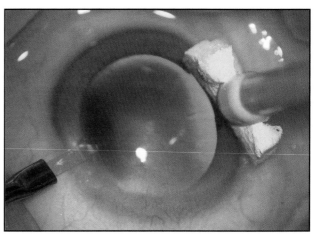

**Figure 14-4.** Photograph of the counterincision.

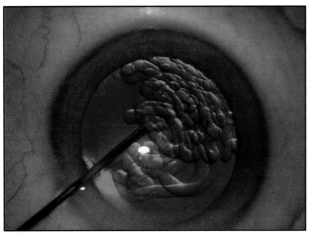

**Figure 14-5.** Photograph of viscoelastic filling the anterior chamber.

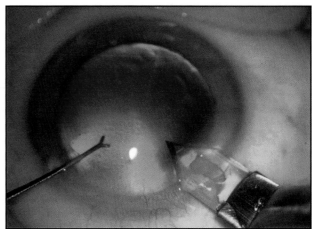

**Figure 14-6.** Photograph of the 3.2-mm CCI.

imizing conjunctival trauma while providing sufficient grip to prevent the eye from moving (Figure 14-4). The tip of a 1-mm (30-degree angle) Crystal keratome (HUCO Vision SA, St. Blaise, Switzerland) is placed at the posterior margin of the limbus and is advanced at an angle that will penetrate into the anterior chamber, making a corneal tunnel of approximately 2 mm in length and 1 mm in width. The anterior chamber is then filled with Viscoat (Alcon Ft. Worth, Tex) without overfilling. The viscoelastic solution protects the corneal endothelium and deepens the anterior chamber (Figure 14-5).

A Bechert Rotator (Bausch & Lomb Surgical, St. Louis, Mo) is then inserted into the counter-incision and braced against the edge of the incision to prevent the eye from moving. Placing the tip of a 3.2-mm (60-degree angle) Crystal keratome at the posterior margin of the limbus, approximately 90 degrees from the counterincision, pressure is applied pushing at an angle that will allow penetration into the anterior chamber after producing a corneal tunnel of

approximately 2 to 3 mm in length and 3.2 mm in width (Figure 14-6). Initially, the incision is engaged with a slight downward direction. Then the 3.2-mm Crystal keratome is quickly redirected so it becomes parallel to the plane of the cornea and enters the anterior chamber more or less horizontally. This consistently creates corneal incisions with self-sealing valves. Additional Viscoat may be injected into the anterior chamber, to protect the cornea during the capsulorrhexis.

## Posterior Adhesions and the Small Pupil:

If there are posterior adhesions of the iris, or if the pupil does not dilate well for any reason, this must be addressed before doing the capsulorrhexis. Two ideal instruments are the Bechert Rotator and the Kuglen Hook (Bausch & Lomb Surgical, St. Louis, Mo). These instruments can be inserted through the incisions and by "pulling" in opposite directions, they can effectively stretch the pupillary margins enlarging the pupillary aperture (Figure 14-7). Alternatively

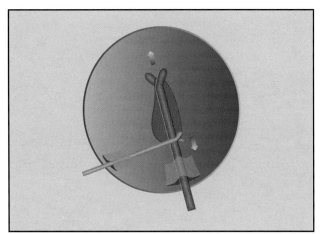

**Figure 14-7.** Liberating posterior adhesions.

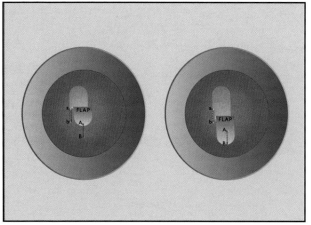

**Figure 14-8.** Cutting (shearing) the anterior capsule.

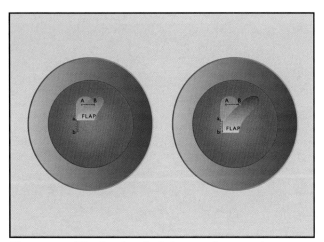

**Figure 14-9.** Ripping (tearing) the anterior capsule.

a pupil-stretching device can be used. We no longer use these devices because they are cumbersome and time consuming. If the pupil cannot be enlarged sufficiently using a bimanual stretching technique, we prefer to make a series of appropriate-sized radial sphincterotomies. Although not as cosmetically attractive, these sphincterotomies produce a much safer pupil access environment and assure much better postoperative retina visualization.

## Capsulorrhexis

The advantages of "in-the-bag" PCIOLs make the CCC the preferred method of capsulotomy. Especially important in PEX syndrome, the force is applied tangential to the zonule when creating a continuous circular tear. This reduces direct traction on the zonule and the risk of zonular dehiscence. The smooth edge capsulotomy with the absence of irregular anterior capsular tags or flaps reduces the risk of inadvertently pulling on the capsule, causing disinsertion. If a capsular tag becomes engaged in the automated tip during emulsification or during irrigation/aspiration of cortical

material, this can cause zonule and/or capsular dialysis and lead to vitreous loss. When a posterior capsular tear occurs (with or without vitreous loss), an intact anterior capsular ring can still provide excellent support for a PCIOL with the optic placed anterior to the capsulotomy and the haptics placed in the ciliary sulcus.

Utilizing different instruments, 2 basic physical principles can be applied during CCC—shearing (cutting) and ripping (tearing).[108] When cutting (shearing) the anterior capsule, the vector forces created by the instrument that generates traction (from A to B) on the capsular flap (CF) is parallel to the vector in which the cut is made (from A to B) (Figure 14-8).

When tearing (ripping) the anterior capsule, the vector of the force created by the instrument that generates traction (from A to B) on the capsular flap (CF) is not parallel to the vector in which the cut is made (from A to B) (Figure 14-9).

These 2 concepts have been explained in a 2-D plane ($x = 9$ to 3 and $y = 6$ to 12). In order for an appropriate capsulorrhexis to occur, all traction in the third dimension (anterior-posterior or Z) should be eliminated or carefully controlled. The anterior chamber should be adequately filled with viscoelastic solution to avoid displacement of the lens (too much viscoelastic will displace the lens posteriorly and not enough anteriorly). When the lens capsule is displaced anteriorly or posteriorly, the zonule will exert traction on the capsule. These forces should be neutralized to avoid an equatorial extension of the capsulorrhexis. The anterior capsule can also be pushed posteriorly against the anterior cortical masses; this generates vectorial forces that will alter the radius of curvature of the capsulorrhexis. Understanding of these principles can be useful to reduce the radius of curvature (in order to bring the capsulorrhexis towards the center and away from the periphery). If too much pressure is applied, the cystotome might tear the anterior capsule or even rupture the posterior capsule.

Our capsulorrhexis is created utilizing only a bent 22-gauge needle (Becton Dickinson and Company, Franklin

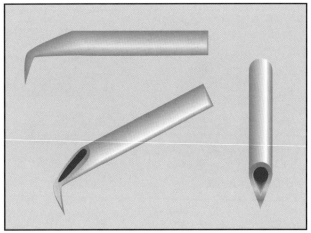

**Figure 14-10.** Bending a needle (cystotome) for capsulorrhexis.

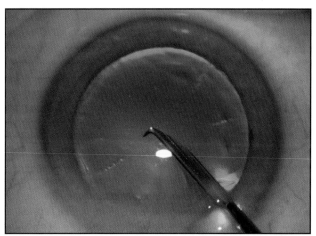

**Figure 14-11.** Photograph of a cystotome in the anterior chamber.

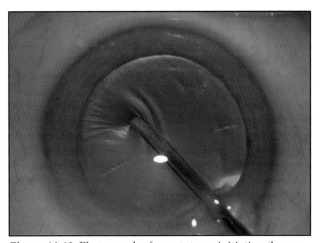

**Figure 14-12.** Photograph of a cystotome initiating the capsulorrhexis.

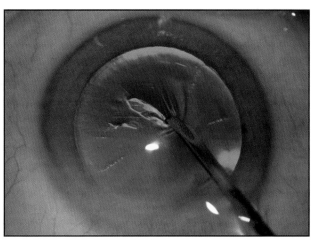

**Figure 14-13.** Photograph of the initial tear in a capsulorrhexis.

Lakes, NJ). Although we do not find it necessary, the CCC can also be done with Utratta Forceps (Bausch & Lomb Surgical, St. Louis, Mo). To bend the 22-gauge needle, the needle is grasped in the non-dominant hand with a Castroviejo Needle Holder—Heavy (Bausch & Lomb Surgical). The needle's tip is grabbed with another needle holder in the dominant hand and bent away from the bevel until approximately an 80- to 90-degree angle is created (Figure 14-10).

Our technique for capsulorrhexis[109] is as follows: The bent needle is placed in the lower left quadrant (approximately at 4:30) (Figure 14-11). Using a relatively quick sweeping motion (the needle is twisted or rotated while traction is exerted from 4:30 toward the 8- or 9-o'clock position), a triangular, anterior capsular tear is made from the 4:30 position until approximately the 6-o'clock position (Figures 14-12 and 14-13). The initial motion is to pull the capsulotomy tangentially when close to the site of tearing, but as the tear becomes more peripheral and away from

where the bent 22-gauge needle is grabbing the anterior capsule, the more radial a force needs to be exerted (toward the center of the anterior capsule).

The bent 22-gauge needle is then placed at the 6-o'clock area, near the tear, and gentle pressure is applied on the anterior capsule while the needle creates traction towards the 10- or 11-o'clock position. As previously described, traction initially is tangential to the capsulotomy, but traction shifts to a radial force (toward the center) as the tear extends peripherally. This brings the tear to the 9-o'clock position (Figure 14-14). Once again, the bent 22-gauge needle is repositioned near the tear at the 9-o'clock area, and pressure is applied on the anterior capsule while the needle creates traction towards the 12-o'clock position. As the tear becomes more peripheral and away from where the bent 22-gauge needle is grabbing the anterior capsule, the more radial force is exerted (toward the center of the anterior capsule) (Figures 14-15 and 14-16). The bent 22-gauge needle is then placed near the tear at the 12-o'clock position, and traction is gen-

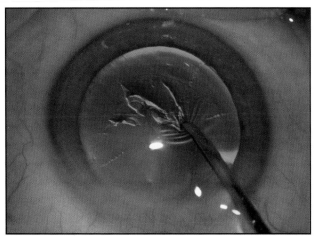

**Figure 14-14.** Photograph of the continuation of a capsulorrhexis.

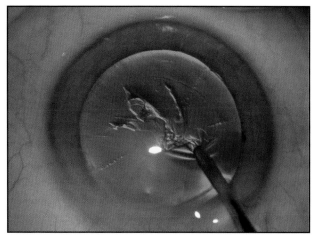

**Figure 14-15.** Each subsequent tear starts with traction tangential to the capsulorrhexis.

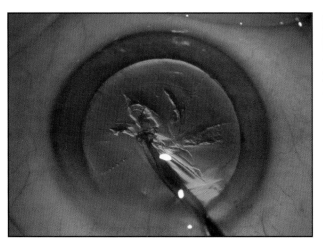

**Figure 14-16.** In each subsequent tear, traction shifts from tangential towards the center of the capsule (radial).

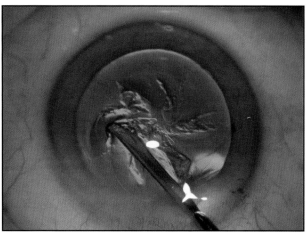

**Figure 14-17.** Photograph of the capsulorrhexis being finished.

erated toward 4-o'clock position (Figure 14-17). As previously described, this motion is continued by a more radial traction vector (toward the central capsule), and continued until the CCC is completed.

It is very important to observe the striae (stretch marks) formed on the anterior capsule because they will predict where the tear is going. This is even more important when the pupil dilates poorly, because capsulorrhexis can be created under the iris without direct visualization. This procedure requires expertise and shouldn't be attempted before mastering the above technique. To minimize the possibility of the capsulotomy flaring out, downward pressure is exerted onto the nucleus to keep the capsulotomy centripetal (turns inward, toward the center). When the capsulotomy size needs enlargement (a larger radius of curvature or to flare out), the needle is placed more superficially and ahead of the already torn portion of the capsule so that it extends outward

(centrifugal). In this manner, the capsulotomy can be kept reliably on course.

An important point is to apply only enough pressure to keep the needle from slipping off the capsule edge as it tears. If too much force is applied, the epinucleus becomes scuffed, the surgeon will not be able to identify the cut capsule edges and will loose control of the capsulotomy.

## Hydrodissection

The main purpose of the hydrodissection maneuver is to float the nucleus out of the bag to reduce the stress that can be transferred to the zonular elements. This is essential in reducing complications in cataract surgery for patients with PEX syndrome. Hydrodissection uses BSS under pressure to separate the capsule from the cortex and cortex from the nucleus. By separating the different layers of the lens, the nucleus can be floated out of the bag and freely rotated dur-

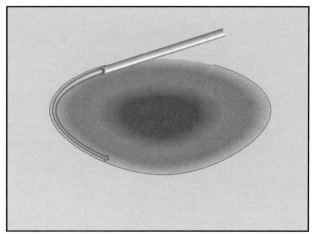

**Figure 14-18.** Hydrodissection between capsule and cortex.

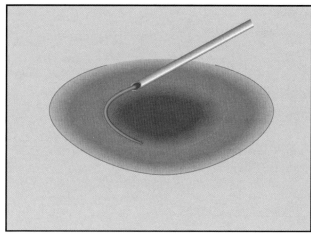

**Figure 14-19.** Hydrodissection between cortex and nucleus.

ing emulsification without stressing the fragile zonular system.

A 25-gauge hydrodissection cannula (Bausch & Lomb Surgical, St. Louis, Mo) is placed approximately 90 degrees with a tangent line to the edge of the CCC. The tip of the cannula is introduced just underneath the anterior capsule approximately 2 mm in the direction of the equator, as far as direct visualization permits. It should be placed at approximately 180 degrees from the counterincision. BSS is then continuously injected under pressure with the tip held firmly in contact with the underside of the anterior capsule flap, forcing the fluid to flow all the way around the lens. We want a free egress of fluid from the eye during this maneuver. It helps to wash out the viscoelastic situated between the area of the hydrodissection and the 3.2-mm incision, in order to prevent initial overfilling of the eye. The hydrodissection cleavage can take place between the capsule and cortex (Figure 14-18), or between the cortex and nucleus (Figure 14-19), accomplished by burying the cannula deeper within the lens substance. Either way, the nucleus is separated from the capsule and any force exerted upon the nucleus will no longer be transmitted directly to the zonule structure. Several hydrodissecting BSS injections might be needed in order to completely loosen the nucleus until it floats out of the bag, at least 180 degrees. When changing the position of the hydrodissection cannula, the surgeon should avoid Descemet's membrane and endothelial trauma.

## *Phacoemulsification (Nucleus Equatorial Reduction Technique)*

We prefer machine settings that are relatively aggressive for our phacoemulsification machine (Diplomax, American Medical Optics, North Andover, Mass). The ultrasound is set to 100% power, but it is flexibly controlled in a linear and pulsed ultrasound mode. The maximum aspiration rate is set to 34, also in linear mode. The maximum vacuum limit

is at the 150 level. These high levels provide maximum power and force, but remain entirely adjustable for appropriate intraoperative modulation. The bottle height is approximately 33 inches above the level of the patient's eye.

Viscoat is placed between the prolapsed nuclear equator and the corneal endothelium. Maintaining a protective film of thick viscoelastic material is necessary to protect the endothelium. Phacoemulsification starts by simply sculpting out the central nucleus to remove the central bulk of the lens. A vital consideration is that the surgeon must continuously maintain a constant depth of the anterior chamber with stable inflation of the posterior capsule. This prevents chamber collapse with its potential damage to the capsule, zonules, or cornea through inadvertent stress or contact with the surgical instruments. This is accomplished by making sure that the aspiration port of the phacoemulsification tip is always occluded with lens material whenever the aspiration mode (position 2 or 3 on the foot switch) is engaged.

During all manipulations, it is important to apply 3-D thinking to the surgical process. This can considerably reduce or eliminate much of the tissue distortion that can occur. It is common for less-experienced surgeons to regard their instruments as being fixed in a horizontal plane. If the phaco tip is directed downward, there is no need to commit the rest of the instrument to descend in the same plane. This can cause needless tissue distortion, trauma, and unnecessary stress. The instruments should be conceptualized to rotate around the incision as if it were a fulcrum, central to all movements in all 3 dimensions.

In the emulsification process, the phacoemulsification tip is initially held in an almost vertical position as it enters the eye and engages the nucleus. It then slides forward assuming a more horizontal direction as it advances toward the 6-o'clock position of the nucleus.

We perform several passes in order to debulk the center of the lens nucleus (Figure 14-20). Occasional air bubbles and

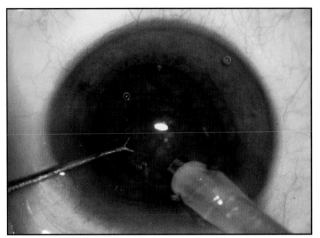

**Figure 14-20.** Photograph of the debulking of the nucleus.

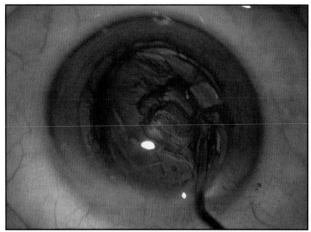

**Figure 14-21.** Photograph of the equatorial lens beginning to "float" with hydrodissection.

lens debris may be trapped in the protective layer of Viscoat. This material can be useful in confirming that the endothelium is well insulated and protected. It is not necessary to perfectly visualize all of the structures and lens material at all times, as long as we can be confident that the posterior capsule remains expanded with no potential for anterior chamber collapse and the cornea is adequately shielded. We can not overemphasize the key element of continually maintaining an occluded aspiration port on the ultrasonic probe while aspiration is engaged (position 2 and 3 on the foot pedal). Otherwise, fluid will be suctioned out of the eye faster than it can be infused and the posterior capsule will come forward, increasing the risk of capsule rupture and vitreous loss. Additional Viscoat can be periodically instilled to maintain the protective coating of viscoelastic material.

After the initial sculpting, the lens is floated up by hydrodissection. When hydrodissection is infused at about the 9-o'clock position, the equatorial nucleus will tend to dislocate and tilt upward at approximately the 3-o'clock position. The anterior equator of the left side of the nucleus will usually float up over the level of the capsulotomy and over the pupillary plane (Figure 14-21). In this position, the nucleus can readily be maneuvered with a Bechert Rotator placed through the counterincision. Additional hydrodissection may be necessary to refloat the nuclear tilt from time to time.

Once the lens has been tilted into the pupillary plane, it can be assumed that it has been sufficiently floated out of the bag and the zonules will no longer bear all of the pressure of the phacoemulsification process. The lens removal strategy is to sequentially reduce the equatorial diameter. As the equator-to-equator lens diameter is reduced, the ability of the lens to exert force on the intraocular structures is diminished. To avoid endothelial trauma, ultrasound fragmentation should always occur at or below the level of the pupil (iris). The nucleus is maintained at approximately the pupil-

lary plane with a Bechert Rotator holding up the lens through the counterincision as ultrasonic fragmentation is performed. The equatorial reduction technique gradually wears away the equator, as the lens is gradually rotated 360 degrees. The phacoemulsification tip slides sideways or is directed peripherally through the equatorial nucleus from the center outward, amputating a portion of the equator. Countertraction is applied by pushing the nucleus with the Bechert Rotator. The force applied may be used to produce a nuclear cracking to reduce the nucleus into smaller, more manageable pieces (Figures 14-22 and 14-23).

As the phacoemulsification tip advances peripherally, the Bechert Rotator controls the nucleus, "feeding" the phacoemulsification tip, while holding the nucleus at the pupillary plane. As the equator is reduced, the lens diameter shrinks, lessening the forces against the capsule (posterior and equatorial). The nucleus is slowly rotated in a bimanual fashion utilizing the Bechert Rotator and the phaco tip, until the entire equatorial nucleus has been removed. A mixture of lens material, air bubbles, and viscoelastic between the phaco tip and the cornea may partially impede visualization but this buffer zone protects the endothelium. A combination of feeding the lens material, bimanual nuclear cracking and short horizontal movements of the phaco probe can facilitate the nuclear removal process, all the time keeping force from impacting the lens zonule. The last nuclear fragments should be emulsified by holding them against the phaco tip, while reducing the ultrasound energy applied with the foot pedal. The use of low ultrasound energy reduces the tendency for the phaco probe to repel lens fragments and can actually be more efficient in removing the smaller particles. Nuclear fragments can be held against the phacoemulsification tip, to emulsify them or to crack them into smaller pieces. This can prevent fragments from being directed against the endothelium by the turbulence (Figure 14-24).

Sometimes, lens material will remain hidden under the iris or in the peripheral anterior chamber. We use a Bechert

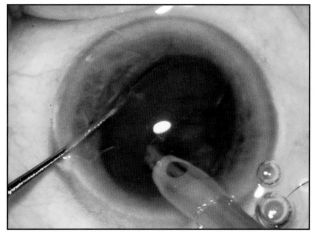

**Figure 14-22.** Photograph of the phacoemulsification tip emulsifying the equatorial nucleus.

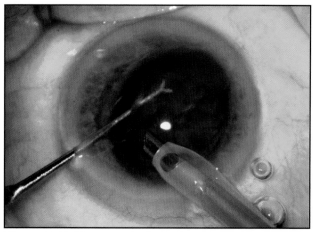

**Figure 14-23.** Photograph of a Bechert Rotator pushing the nucleus so the phacoemulsification tip slides peripherally to emulsify the equatorial nucleus.

Rotator to move the iris, stretching the pupil to the angle while the I/A tip is still irrigating in the anterior chamber to search out and reveal any nuclear or cortical fragments that may remain.

## Management of the Cortex: Irrigation and Aspiration

It is quite common in PEX cataracts to have significant amounts of thick cortex. Much of the thicker cortical material can be removed with the phacoemulsification tip using I/A only, without ultrasound or with very short, low power bursts to increase the flow of lens material into the phaco probe (Figure 14-25). The remaining cortical material is removed with a 0.3-mm I/A tip, maximum aspiration rate at 36 (linear mode), maximum vacuum limit at 100 and a bottle height of approximately 33 inches above the level of the patient's eye.

When pulling on cortex in a radial fashion, significant zonular stress can be created. A significant zonule stress reduction can be effected by capitalizing on our ability to expand the space between the anterior and posterior capsule at the equator of the lens. This is where the equatorial cortex is anchored. To remove the cortex without stressing the zonules, we initially engage the cortex by inserting the I/A tip into the cortex at the equator of the capsule with the aspiration port pointing upward. As the aspiration begins and the tip becomes occluded, we then push the phaco tip downward, toward the optic nerve. This pushes the posterior capsule down and away from the anterior capsule, widening the space between the anterior and posterior capsules. The equatorial cortex will virtually deliver itself without the need to pull radially, sparing significant zonular stress (Figure 14-26).

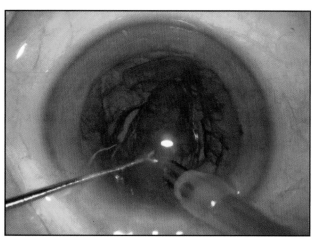

**Figure 14-24.** Photograph of the phacoemulsification tip emulsifying the last fragments of nucleus.

## Management of the Posterior Capsule:

Vacuuming of the posterior capsule can be performed with a 0.3-mm I/A tip, maximum aspiration rate at 14 (linear mode), maximum vacuum limit at 40 and a bottle height of approximately 33 inches above the level of the patient's eye, if zonular integrity is sufficient. If capsular striae enter the aspiration port and remain fixed and do not readily move as the capsule is rasped clean, the aspiration and movement should be stopped and the probe removed under irrigation only. It may be necessary to back-flush the aspiration line to free the capsule from the aspiration port.

If there is danger of capsular rupture or zonular dehiscence, it is better to leave the capsule somewhat clouded because this can be handled with a YAG laser later on. Intentionally leaving some capsule debris on the equatorial or central aspect of the capsule can provide a measure of

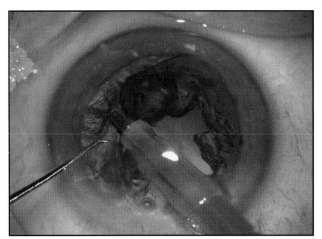

**Figure 14-25.** Photograph of the phaco tip performing aspiration of the cortex.

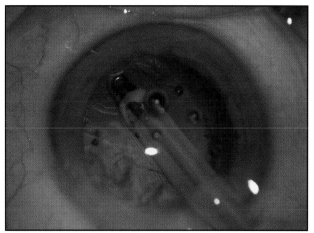

**Figure 14-26.** Photograph of the I/A tip.

support in very fragile capsules. The integrity of the capsule and zonular structures is the primary concern for proper implant fixation.

Capsule expansion rings can be effective in bridging the areas of weak zonules. We find them generally unnecessary, but they will become widely available in the future. Further experience may result in a greater role of these devices in PEX cataract surgery.

## IOL Implantation

When considering which PCIOL to use, the implant material is important. We prefer silicone lenses. These lenses are relatively weightless and are inherently less stressful on the posterior capsule on insertion. Silicone lenses have been associated with a significantly lower degree of posterior capsular opacification. One study reported that the mean percentage area of posterior capsular opacification for hydrogel lenses was 63%; for PMMA, 46%; and for silicone, 17%. Less posterior capsule opacification was associated with less Nd:YAG laser capsulotomies.[110]

When inserting a flexible silicone lens implant, care should be exerted to avoid the stress of inappropriate rotation of the implant as it is placed. As the implant unfolds, the lead haptic or the unfolding optic can cause traction on the capsule structures. In PEX cataract, it is especially important to prevent insertional haptic incarceration in the flaccid posterior capsule, which can literally rip the capsule and zonules off of their insertion points.

The technique is to insert the implant with only horizontal insertion force, negating all vertical forces. To accomplish this, we rotate the implant cartridge selectively in order to deliver the implant without any vertical insertion force. The implant is advanced far enough for the lead haptic to come to lie horizontally over the iris at the 2- to 3-o'clock position (down and to the left in the surgeon's view) (Figure 14-27).

This is accomplished by turning the inserter upside-down, rotated clockwise approximately 180 degrees. As the implant is further unfolded, it will leave the optic upside down unless an immediate 180 degrees counterclockwise twist of the inserter is made to deliver the lens and the following haptic right side up, in the horizontal plane. If the iris is not used to hold the lead haptic during this maneuver, it is possible for the lead haptic to turn vertical and incarcerate itself in the fragile PEX capsule. The iris can securely hold the lead haptic in place and prevent it from twisting until the optic is correctly delivered horizontally. The lead haptic will advance to where it delivers itself into the capsule bag in most cases, or at least it will come to lie over the inferior iris, where it can be directly inserted in the bag (Figure 14-28). The implant is then manipulated until visual verification confirms that the lead haptic is in the capsular bag inferiorly.

To complete the insertion and place the following haptic in the bag, we use a bimanual insertion technique. Through the counterincision, the nondominant hand utilizes a Kuglen hook to grab the anterior capsule and lift it upward toward the incision site. A Bechert Rotator is then utilized to rotate the implant only slightly, while directing the implant downward, into the posterior capsule. There is little rotation, only enough to allow the haptic to slide over the bag. The essential force is downward toward the optic nerve. In this manner, the following haptic will deliver itself into the bag with little or no rotational stress on the zonules (Figure 14-29). A common mistake is to rely only on horizontal movements, pushing the implant far to the side. This can place severe stress upon the zonules and capsule structures. It is not necessary to actually visualize the implant going into the bag. If the Kuglen hook holds the anterior capsular bag while the implant is being eased downward with slight rotation, the haptic will almost invariably end up in the right place.

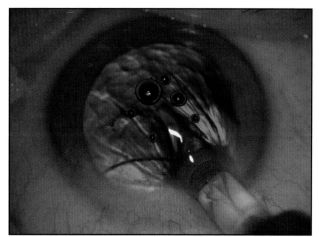

**Figure 14-27.** Photograph of the first haptic of a posterior chamber IOL over the iris as it is being inserted into the anterior chamber.

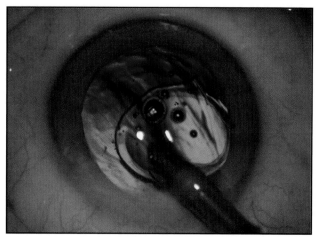

**Figure 14-28.** Photograph of the IOL with the first haptic placed inferiorly.

## Clean-up and Final Inspection

The viscoelastic is removed from the anterior chamber with the I/A tip (same settings as aspirating cortex). If the capsular structures are exceptionally fragile, some Viscoat may be left in the anterior chamber. If so, the patient can be given oral acetazolamide (Diamox, Lederle Pharmaceutical div. American Cyanamid Company, Pearl River, NY) 500 mg, which can be repeated 10 to 12 hours later.

Before terminating the surgery, a 25-gauge air needle with BSS irrigates the anterior chamber above the iris plane to wash out any loose viscoelastic material and to provide a small turbulence in the anterior chamber which can liberate any possible hidden fragments of nuclear or cortical material.

The placement of a small bolus of Viscoat under the inner aspect of the 3.2-mm incision assures a better initial seal and prevents leakage during the early postoperative period (Figure 14-30). Using the 30-gauge cannula, the anterior chamber is refilled with BSS to the proper tension. The epithelial site of the 3.2-mm incision is pressured with a cellulose spear and an adequate seal is confirmed (Figure 14-31). Before removing the lid speculum, a corneal shield (Surgilens, Bausch & Lomb Surgical, St. Louis, Mo) soaked in Gentamycin and/or Cefazolin solution can be placed over the cornea (Figure 14-32).

## Recovery

Using the RSAP, patients are expected to be alert at the end of the surgery and are transferred to the recovery room by wheelchair. They are monitored for 30 minutes. A light snack is offered and instructions are given. The patient is discharged by the anesthesiologist and allowed to return home.

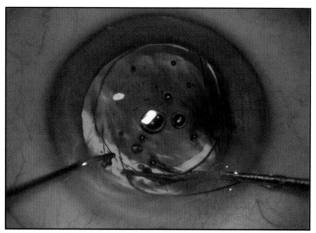

**Figure 14-29.** Photograph of the insertion of second haptic of an IOL.

# POSTOPERATIVE MANAGEMENT

Postoperative management is very liberal. The patient can go home without a patch on the eye. A shield is worn for only 1 night. By the next day, patients are allowed to golf, play tennis, or return to work. Only restrictions against contamination such as avoiding rubbing or swimming are imposed.

If too much viscoelastic remains in the anterior chamber, IOP can become elevated. We can often anticipate this and pretreat with Acetazolamide. For the few patients in whom the pressure goes up unexpectedly, causing pain or discomfort, the patient can be brought back to the office. At the slit lamp, a small amount of fluid is allowed to escape by exerting a slight downward pressure on the scleral portion of the counterincision with a sterile disposable needle. This allows a safe and gradual reduction of pressure without rapid depressurization, and without violating the sterility of the incision.

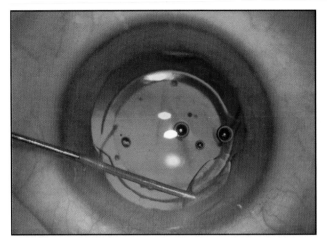

**Figure 14-30.** Photograph of Viscoat sealing the 3.2-mm incision.

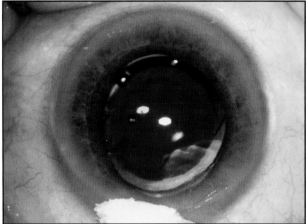

**Figure 14-31.** Photograph of a 3.2-mm incision with no leakage.

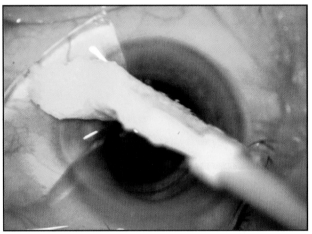

**Figure 14-32.** Photograph of a corneal shield with antibiotic being placed over the cornea at the end of the procedure.

Follow-up visits are scheduled on the next day after the procedure, and at the 1- and 3-week periods. Special attention is given to the possibility of elevated IOP and/or inflammation.

## COMPLICATIONS

Complications associated with PEX syndrome can be medically or surgically treated. PEX glaucoma has already been discussed. We will review some complications of cataract surgery in patients with PEX syndrome.

Patients with PEX syndrome and cataracts tend to have poorly dilating pupils, synechiae and tenuously supported capsular bags. The combination of these findings significantly increases the intraoperative and postoperative risk in these patients.

In PEX syndrome, a shallow anterior chamber may be associated with zonular instability and the cataract surgeon should be aware of a higher risk of intraoperative complications. In eyes with pseudoexfoliation, an anterior chamber depth of less than 2.5 mm was associated with a risk of 13.4% for intraoperative complications compared to an overall incidence of intraoperative complications of 6.9% and an incidence of 2.8% for an anterior chamber depth of 2.5 mm or more.[111]

The odds ratio for intraoperative complications such as capsular tears, zonular break, and vitreous loss was estimated to be 5.1 for patients with PEX compared to normal patients. PEX was associated with a statistically significant increase in intraoperative complications during cataract surgery ($p < 0.0001$).[112]

PCIOLs are susceptible to dislocation secondary to insufficient capsular or zonular support, or following trauma, in PEX syndrome (Figure 14-33). A dislocated PCIOL may be repositioned or removed and replaced with an appropriate IOL. Repositioning the dislocated PCIOL into the ciliary sulcus is generally considered the best option. There are many techniques to reposition and obtain adequate stability of the dislocated PCIOL including scleral fixation of the dislocated IOL. Endoscopy, though not always available, allows viewing of the retropupillary area and verification of precise haptic placement. Sometimes repositioning of a PCIOL cannot easily be accomplished. Removing it and replacing it with an ACIOL is an option that is frequently less traumatic and involves less risk, but elevated IOP may be more pervasive[113] (Figure 14-34). Care must be taken during all steps of the phacoemulsification procedure not to use excessive force which could easily rupture the zonule, cause a "dropped nucleus," or plainly lead to vitreous loss which is associated with a higher risk of endophthalmitis. In our practice, when vitreous is lost, broad spectrum oral antibiotics are prescribed to obtain adequate vitreous antimicrobial concentrations, such as ofloxacin (Floxin, Ortho-McNeil Pharmaceutical, Raritan, NJ) 400 mg twice daily by mouth for 1 week.

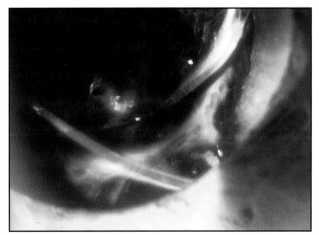

**Figure 14-33.** Photograph of a subluxated posterior chamber IOL in a patient with PEX syndrome.

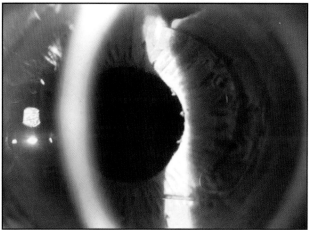

**Figure 14-34.** Photograph of an anterior chamber IOL and a corneal transplant in a patient with PEX syndrome.

Even when the capsule is compromised, an IOL can be placed in the bag. Despite perfect placement, long-term difficulties can be encountered. Patients with PEX syndrome may have a higher risk for dislocation of endocapsular PCIOLs. A study reported a mean time from IOL implantation to dislocation of 85 months after surgery. They were treated with IOL exchange.[114] In a patient with PEX, 12 years after cataract surgery, liberated lens cortical material after spontaneous dislocation of a PCIOL was associated with lens particle glaucoma in patients.[115] Despite the association of PEX syndrome with subluxated in-the-bag IOLs after cataract extraction, risks can be reduced by not using a foldable IOL, using IOLs with larger optics, and early Nd:YAG anterior capsulotomy.[116]

Due to focal zonular lysis in PEX syndrome, the capsular bag may "shrink" in areas, making it difficult to place an implant in-the-bag. Implanting a CTR before phacoemulsification of the nucleus has been suggested as an appropriate method to reduce the risk of zonular separation. In some studies, it increased the rate of endocapsular IOL fixation, and improved postoperative UCVA.[117] In patients with PEX syndrome that undergo phacoemulsification with CCC, cataract extraction, and IOL implantation (even with an endocapsular ring), anterior capsule fibrosis with complete occlusion of the capsule opening (causing significant visual loss) can occur. After a Nd:YAG laser anterior capsulotomy, visual acuity can be restored. Endocapsular ring implantation does not prevent anterior capsule contraction syndrome but can prevent IOL decentration.[118]

Pressure spikes can easily occur, sometimes as a result of pupillary dilation liberating fibrillar material; therefore, IOP control is extremely important. Pressure should be monitored carefully in the immediate postoperative period. Over the long term, patients tend to do well. Six and 12 months after phacoemulsification with an IOL implant, patients with PEX syndrome have a greater postoperative IOP reduc-

tion than patients with POAG and cataract control groups.[119] IOP decreased after phacoemulsification cataract surgery in the presence of PEX similarly as in normal eyes.[120] If a more severe glaucoma is present, a combined clear cornea phacoemulsification, IOL implant, and trabecular aspiration in patients with PEX glaucoma may be a safe and effective way to control IOP with fewer postoperative medications than clear cornea phacoemulsification with IOL implant alone. A statistically significant decrease in postoperative IOP has been found.[121] Considering IOP elevation in PEX glaucoma is due to obstruction of the intertrabecular spaces by exfoliation material, Jacobi et al[122] recommended bimanual trabecular aspiration with a 400-μm-in-diameter intraocular aspiration probe. Trabecular debris and pigment is cleared with a suction force of 100 to 200 mmHg under light tissue-instrument contact. Irrigation of the anterior chamber is performed via a separate irrigation cannula. There is a slight regression in effect over time, attributed to liberation of exfoliative debris.

Endothelial cell loss has been found in PEX syndrome patients. This coupled with the poor lens support, and possibly elevated IOP may lead to an increased risk of corneal decompensation. Concomitant Fuch's dystrophy, also more commonly found in the elderly population (as is PEX syndrome) may compound the loss of endothelial cells and lead to pseudophakic bullous keratopathy.

Phacoemulsification cataract surgery is considered safe for most eyes with PEX, even though significantly more complications, such as capsular/zonular tear or vitreous loss may occur intraoperatively. Also, there may be an increased inflammatory response postoperatively, associated with increased flare in the aqueous humor.[123] This finding may suggest a reason for adding an NSAID to the postoperative regimen of steroids to reduce the potentially increased incidence of CME.

# ACKNOWLEDGEMENTS

We want to acknowledge the valuable help from Howard Goodman, MD and to Mr. Mooky Ben-David for their contributions to the photographic material used in this chapter.

# REFERENCES

1. Lindberg JG. Kliniska undersokningar over depigmentering av pupillarranden och genomylysbarkef av iris vid fall av alderstarr samit i normala ogon hos gamla personer. MD thesis. Diss Helsingfors; 1917.

2. Vogt A. Ein neues Spaltlampenbild des Pupillargebietes: Hellblauer Pupilearsaumfilz mit Hautchenbildunz aus der Lisenvorderkapsel. *Klin Monatsbl Augenheilkd.* 1925;75:1.

3. Dark AJ, Streeten BW. Pseudoexfoliation syndrome. In: Garner A, Klintworth GK, eds. *Pathobiology of Ocular Disease: A Dynamic Approach.* Part B. New York: Marcel Dekker; 1982:1303.

4. Winkler J, Lunsdorf H, Wirbelauer C, Reinhardt DP, Laqua H. Immunohistochemical and charge-specific localization of anionic constituents in pseudoexfoliation deposits on the central anterior lens capsule from individuals with pseudoexfoliation syndrome. *Graefes Arch Clin Exp Ophthalmol.* 2001 Dec;239(12):952-60.

5. Dark AJ, Streeten BW, Cornwall CC. Pseudoexfoliative disease of the lens: a study in electron microscopy and histochemistry. *Br J Ophthalmol.* 1977;61:462

6. Davanger M. The pseudoexfoliation syndrome: a scanning electron microscopic study. I. The anterior lens surface. *Acta Ophthalmol.* 1975;53:809.

7. Davanger M. A note on the pseudoexfoliation fibrils. *Acta Ophthalmol.* 1978;56:114.

8. Davanger M. Studies on the pseudoexfoliation material. *Graefes Arch Clin Exp Ophthalmol.* 1978;208:65.

9. Streeten BW, Gibson SA, Dark AJ. Pseudoexfoliative material contains an elastic microfibrillar-associated glycoprotein. *Trans Am Ophthalmol Soc.* 1986;84:304.

10. Ringvold A. A preliminary report on the amino acid composition of the pseudoexfoliation material. *Exp Eye Res.* 1973; 15:37.

11. Ringvold A, Husby G. Pseudoexfoliation material—an amyloid-like substance. *Exp Eye Res.* 1973;17:289.

12. Berlau J, Lorenz P, Beck R, et al. Analysis of aqueous humour proteins of eyes with and without pseudoexfoliation syndrome. *Graefes Arch Clin Exp Ophthalmol.* 2001 Oct; 239(10):743-6.

13. Ritch R, Schlotzer-Schrehardt U. Exfoliation syndrome. *Surv Ophthalmol.* 2001;45(4):265-315.

14. Speakman JS, Ghosh M. The conjunctiva in senile lens exfoliation. *Arch Ophthalmol.* 1976;94:1757.

15. Mizuno K, Muroi S. Cycloscopy of pseudoexfoliation. *Am J Ophthalmol.* 1979;87:513.

16. Prince AM, Ritch R. Clinical signs of the pseudoexfoliation syndrome. *Ophthalmology.* 1986;93:803.

17. Ohrt V, Nehen JH. The incidence of glaucoma capsulare based on a Danish hospital material. *Acta Ophthalmol.* 1981;59:888.

18. Mardin CY, Schlotzer-Schrehardt U, Naumann GO. "Masked" pseudoexfoliation syndrome in unoperated eyes with circular posterior synechiae: clinical-electron microscopic correlation. *Arch Ophthalmol.* 2001 Oct;119(10):1500-3.

19. Wirbelauer C, Anders N, Pham DT, Wollensak J. Corneal endothelial cell changes in pseudoexfoliation syndrome after cataract surgery. *Arch Ophthalmol.* 1998 Feb;116(2):145-9.

20. Vannas A, Setala K, Ruusuvaara P. Endothelial cells in capsular glaucoma. *Acta Ophthalmol.* 1977;55:951.

21. Benedict O, Roll P. The trabecular meshwork of a nonglaucomatous eye with the exfoliation syndrome. *Virchow's Arch.* 1979;384:347.

22. Sampaolesi R, Argento C. Scanning electron microscopy of the trabecular meshwork in normal and glaucomatous eyes. *Invest Ophthalmol Vis Sci.* 1977;16:302.

23. Rodrigues MM, Spaeth GL, Sivalingam E, Weinreb S. Value of trabeculectomy specimens in glaucoma. *Ophthalmic Surg.* 1978;9:29.

24. Richardson TM. Pigmentary glaucoma. In: Ritch R, Shields MB, eds. *The Secondary Glaucomas.* St. Louis, Mo: CV Mosby; 1982; 84-98.

25. Lieberman JM. Pigmentary glaucoma: new insights. *Focal Points: Clinical Modules for Ophthalmologists.* San Francisco: American Academy of Ophthalmology. 1998;16(2).

26. Pohjola S, Horsmanheimo A. Topically applied corticosteroids in glaucoma capsulare. *Arch Ophthalmol.* 1971;85:150.

27. Gilles WE. Corticosteroid-induced ocular hypertension in pseudoexfoliation of the lens capsule. *Am J Ophthalmol.* 1970;70:90

28. Aasved H. Intraocular pressure in eyes with and without fibrillopathia epitheliocapsularis. *Acta Ophthalmol.* 1971;49:601.

29. Hartsen E, Sellevold OJ. Pseudoexfoliation of the lens capsule. III Ocular tension in eyes with pseudoexfoliation. *Acta Ophthalmol.* 1970;48:446.

30. Layden WE. Exfoliation syndrome. In: Ritch R, Shields MB, eds. *The Secondary Glaucomas.* St. Louis: CV Mosby; 1982; 115.

31. Aasved H. The frequency of optic nerve damage and surgical treatment in chronic simple glaucoma and capsular glaucoma. *Acta Ophthalmol.* 1971;49:589.

32. Layden WE, Shaffer RN. Exfoliation syndrome. *Am J Ophthalmol.* 1974;78:835.

33. Tarkkanen A. Treatment of chronic open-angle glaucoma associated with pseudoexfoliation. *Acta Ophthalmol.* 1965;43:514.

34. Aasved H, Seland JH, Slagsvold JE. Timolol maleate in treatment of open angle glaucoma. *Acta Ophthalmol.* 1979;57: 700.

35. Bilka S, Saunte E. Timolol maleate in the treatment of glaucoma simplex and the glaucoma capsulare: a three-year follow-up study. *Acta Ophthalmol.* 1982;60:967.

36. Aasved H. The frequency of fibrillopathia epitheliocapsularis (so-called senile exfoliation or pseudoexfoliation) in patients with open-angle glaucoma. *Acta Ophthalmol.* 1971;49:194.

37. Ritch R, Podos S. Laser trabeculoplasty in the exfoliation syndrome. *Bull NY Acad Med.* 1983;59:339.

38. Pohjanpelto P. Late results of laser trabeculoplasty for increased intraocular pressure. *Acta Ophthalmol.* 1983;61:988.

39. Thomas JV, Simmons RJ, Belcher D III. Argon laser trabeculoplasty in the presurgical glaucoma patient. *Ophthalmology.* 1982;89:187.

40. Jerndal T, Kriisa V. Results of trabeculectomy for pseudoexfoliative glaucoma. *Br J Ophthalmol.* 1974;58:927.

41. Bartholomew RS. Lens displacement associated with pseudocapsular exfoliation: a report on 19 cases in the Southern Bantu. *Br J Ophthalmol.* 1970;54:744.

42. Bartholomew RS. Phakodonesis. A sign of incipient lens displacement. *Br J Ophthalmol.* 1970;54:663.

43. Damji KF, Bains HS, Amjadi K, et al. Familial occurrence of pseudoexfoliation in Canada. *Can J Ophthalmol.* 1999 Aug;34(5):257-65.

44. Kozobolis VP, Detorakis ET, Sourvinos G, Pallikaris IG, Spandidos DA. Loss of heterozygosity in pseudoexfoliation syndrome. *Invest Ophthalmol Vis Sci.* 1999 May;40(6):1255-60.

45. Pohjanpelto P, Hurskainen L. Studies in relatives of patients with glaucoma simplex and patients with pseudoexfoliation of the lens capsule. *Acta Ophthalmol.* 1972;50:255.

46. Jerndal T, Svedbergh B. Goniodysgenesis in exfoliation glaucoma. *Adv Ophthalmol.* 1962;(Suppl)71:1.

47. Hiller R, Sperduto RD, Krueger DE. Pseudoexfoliation, intraocular pressure and senile lens changes in a population-based survey. *Arch Ophthalmol.* 1982;100:1080.

48. Aasved H. The geographical distribution of fibrillopathia epitheliocapsularis, so-called senile exfoliation or pseudoexfoliation of the anterior lens capsule. *Acta Ophthalmol.* 1969; 47:792.

49. Taylor HR, Hollows FC, Mann D. Pseudoexfoliation of the lens in Australian aborigines. *Br J Ophthalmol.* 1977;61:473.

50. Kozart DM, Yanoff M. Intraocular pressure status in 100 consecutive patients with exfoliation syndrome. *Ophthalmology.* 1982;89:214.

51. Aasved H. Mass screening for fibrillopathia epitheliocapsularis, so-called senile exfoliation or pseudoexfoliation of the anterior lens capsule. *Acta Ophthalmol.* 1971;49:334.

52. Bartholomew RS. Pseudocapsular exfoliation in the Bantu of South Africa. II. Occurrence and prevalence. *Br J Ophthalmol.* 1973;57:41.

53. Taylor HR. The environment and the lens. *Br J Ophthalmol.* 1980;64:303.

54. Meyer E, Haim T, Zonis S, et al. Pseudoexfoliation: epidemiology, clinical and scanning electron microscopic study. *Ophthalmologica.* 1984;188:141.

55. McCarty CA, Taylor HR. Pseudoexfoliation syndrome in Australian adults. *Am J Ophthalmol.* 2000 May;129(5):629-33.

56. Faulkner HW. Pseudoexfoliation of the lens among the Navajo Indians. *Am J Ophthalmol.* 1972;72:206.

57. Sood NN, Ratnaraj A. Pseudoexfoliation of the lens capsule. *Orient Arch Ophthalmol.* 1968;6:62.

58. Khanzada AM. Exfoliation syndrome in Pakistan. *Pakistan J Ophthalmol.* 1986;2:7.

59. Gradle HS, Sugar HS. Glaucoma capsulare. *Am J Ophthalmol.* 1947;30:12.

60. Hammer T, Schlotzer-Schrehardt U, Naumann GO. Unilateral or asymmetric pseudoexfoliation syndrome? An ultrastructural study. *Arch Ophthalmol.* 2001;119(7):1023-31.

61. Mardin CY, Schlotzer-Schrehardt U, Naumann GO. Early diagnosis of pseudoexfoliation syndrome: a clinical electron microscopy correlation of the central, anterior lens capsule. *Klin Monatsbl Augenheilkd.* 1997;211(5):296-300.

62. Sugar HS. *The Glaucomas.* New York: Paul B. Hoeber; 1957: 329-331.

63. Skuta GL, Parrish RK II, Hodapp E, et al. Zonular dialysis during extracapsular cataract extraction in pseudoexfoliation syndrome. *Arch Ophthalmol.* 1987;105:632.

64. Guzek JP, Holm M, Coter JB, et al. Risk factors for intraoperative complications in 1000 extracapsular cataract cases. *Ophthalmology.* 1987;94:461.

65. Awan KJ, Humayun M. Extracapsular cataract surgery risks in patients with exfoliation syndrome. *Pakistan J Ophthalmol.* 1986;2:79.

66. Lee V, Bloom P. Microhook capsule stabilization for phacoemulsification in eyes with pseudoexfoliation-syndrome-induced lens instability. *J Cataract Refract Surg.* 1999;25(12):1567-70.

67. Menkhaus S, Motschmann M, Kuchenbecker J, Behrens-Baumann W. Pseudoexfoliation (PEX) syndrome and intraoperative complications in cataract surgery. *Klin Monatsbl Augenheilkd.* 2000;216(6):388-92.

68. Raitta C, Setala K. Intraocular lens implantation in exfoliation syndrome and capsular glaucoma. *Acta Ophthalmol.* 1986;64: 130.

69. Tarkkanen AHA. Exfoliation syndrome. *Trans Ophthalmol Soc UK.* 1986;105:233.

70. Schumacher S, Nguyen NX, Kuchle M, Naumann GO. Quantification of aqueous flare after phacoemulsification with intraocular lens implantation in eyes with pseudoexfoliation syndrome. *Arch Ophthalmol.* 1999;117(6):733-5.

71. Abela-Formanek C, Amon M, Schauersberger J, Schild G, Kruger A. Postoperative inflammatory response to phacoemulsification and implantation of 2 types of foldable intraocular lenses in pseudoexfoliation syndrome. *Klin Monatsbl Augenheilkd.* 2000;217(1):10-14.

72. Naumann GO, Schlotzer-Schrehardt U, Kuchle M. Pseudoexfoliation syndrome for the comprehensive ophthalmologist. Intraocular and systemic manifestations. *Ophthalmology.* 1998;105(6):951-68.

73. Abbasoglu OE, Hosal B, Tekeli O, Gursel E. Risk factors for vitreous loss in cataract surgery. *Eur J Ophthalmol.* 2000;10(3):227-32.

74. Leydhecker W, Gramer E, Kriegstein GK. Patient information before cataract surgery. *Ophthalmologica.* 1980;180:241.

75. Jaffe NS, Jaffe MS, Jaffe GF. *Cataract Surgery and Its Complications.* 5th ed. St. Louis, Mo: CV Mosby; 1990.

76. Weinstein GW, Odom JV, Hobson RR. Visual acuity and cataract surgery. In Reinecke RD, ed. *Ophthalmology Annual 1987.* Norwalk, CT: Appleton-Century-Crofts; 1987.

77. Minkowski JS, Palese M, Guyton DL. Potential acuity meter using a minute aerial pinhole aperture. *Ophthalmology.* 1983;90:1360.

78. Asbell PA, Chiang B, Amin A, et al. Retinal acuity evaluation with the potential acuity meter in glaucoma patients. *Ophthalmology.* 1985;92:764.

79. Faulkner W. Laser interferometric prediction of postoperative visual acuity in patients with cataracts. *Am J Ophthalmol.* 1983;95:626.

80. Vrijland HR, van Lith GH. The value of preoperative electro-ophthalmological examination before cataract extraction. *Doc Ophthalmol.* 1983;55:153.

81. Weinstein GW. Clinical aspects of the visual evoked potential. *Ophthalmic Surg.* 1978;9:56.

82. Layden WE. Pseudophakia and glaucoma. *Ophthalmology.* 1982;89:875.

83. Rubin ML. A case for myopia. *Surv Ophthalmol.* 1991;35:307.

84. Morgan LW, Schwab IR. Informed consent in senile cataract extraction. *Arch Ophthalmol.* 104:42, 1986.

85. Rand WJ, Stein SC, Velazquez GE. Rand-Stein Analgesia Protocol for Cataract Surgery. *Ophthalmology.* 2000;107:889-895.

86. Gomez RS, Andrade LO, Costa JR. Brainstem anaesthesia after peribulbar anaesthesia. *Can J Anaesth.* 1997;44:732-4.

87. Corboy JM, Jiang X. Postanesthetic hypotropia: a unique syndrome in left eyes. *J Cataract Refract Surg.* 1997;23:1394-8.

88. Rosenblatt RM, May DR, Barsoumian K. Cardiopulmonary arrest after retrobulbar block. *Am J Ophthalmol.* 1980;90:425-7.

89. Nicoll JMV, Acharya PA, Ahlen K, et al. Central nervous system complications after 6000 retrobulbar blocks. *Anesth Analg.* 1987;66:1298-302.

90. Abraham SE, Hogan QH. Complications of nerve blocks. In: Benumof JL, Saidman LJ, eds. *Anesthesia and Perioperative Complications.* St. Louis: CV Mosby Year Book; 1992:67.

91. Hamilton RC. Brain stem anesthesia following retrobulbar blockade. *Anesthesiology.* 1985;63: 688-90.

92. Edge KR, Davis A. Brainstem anaesthesia following a peribulbar block for eye surgery. *Anaesth Intensive Care.* 1995;23:219-21.

93. Hamilton RC. Brain-stem anesthesia as a complication of regional anesthesia for ophthalmic surgery. *Can J Ophthalmol.* 1992;27:323-5.

94. Puustjarvi T, Purhonen S. Permanent blindness following retrobulbar hemorrhage after peribulbar anesthesia for cataract surgery. *Ophthalmic Surg.* 1992;23:450-2.

95. McGoldrick KE. Ophthalmic and systemic complications of surgery and anesthesia. In: McGoldrick KE, ed. *Anesthesia for Ophthalmic and Otolaryngologic Surgery.* Philadelphia: WB Saunders Co; 1992.

96. Donlon JV. Anesthesia for the eye, ear, nose, and throat. In: Miller RG, ed. *Anesthesia.* New York: Churchill Livingstone; 1986;1837-58.

97. Forrest JB, Lam L, Woo J, Rifkind A. Oxygen desaturation in elderly patients during cataract surgery. *Can J Anaesth.* 1990; 37:50.

98. Nielsen PJ. Immediate visual capability after cataract surgery: topical versus retrobulbar anesthesia. *J Cataract Refract Surg.* 1995;21:301-4.

99. Johnston RL, Whitefield LA, Giralt J, et al. Topical versus peribulbar anesthesia, without sedation, for clear corneal phacoemulsification. *J Cataract Refract Surg.* 1998;24:407-10.

100. Rosenthal KJ. Deep, topical, nerve-block anesthesia. *J Cataract Refract Surg.* 1995;21:499-503.

101. Dinsmore SC. Drop, then decide approach to topical anesthesia. *J Cataract Refract Surg.* 1995;21:666-71.

102. Judge AJ, Najafi K, Lee DA, et al. Corneal endothelial toxicity of topical anesthesia. *Ophthalmology.* 1997;104:1373-9.

103. Lindstrom R. *Ocular Surgery News.* June 1, 1998.

104. White PF, Coe V, Shafer A, et al. Comparison of alfentanil with fentanyl for outpatient procedures. *Anesthesiology.* 1986; 64:99-106.

105. Scott JC, Ponganis KV, Stanski DR. EEG quantitation of narcotic effect: the comparative pharmacodynamics of fentanyl and alfentanil. *Anesthesiology.* 1985;62:234-41.

106. Shastri L, Vasavada A. Phacoemulsification in Indian eyes with pseudoexfoliation syndrome. *J Cataract Refract Surg.* 2001;27(10):1629-37.

107. Srinivasan R, Madhavaranga. Topical ketorolac tromethamine 0.5% versus diclofenac sodium 0.1% to inhibit miosis during cataract surgery. *J Cataract Refract Surg.* 2002;28(3):517-20.

108. Seibel BS. *Phacodynamics: Mastering the Tools and Techniques of Phacoemulsification Surgery.* Thorofare, NJ: SLACK Incorporated; 1993.

109. Rand WJ, Velazquez GE. Continuous circular capsulorrhexis. *Franja Ocular.* 1999;1(3):10-14.

110. Hollick EJ, Spalton DJ, Ursell PG, Meacock WR, Barman SA, Boyce JF. Posterior capsular opacification with hydrogel, polymethylmethacrylate, and silicone intraocular lenses: two-year results of a randomized prospective trial. *Am J Ophthalmol.* 2000;129(5):577-84.

111. Kuchle M, Viestenz A, Martus P, Handel A, Junemann A, Naumann GO. Anterior chamber depth and complications during cataract surgery in eyes with pseudoexfoliation syndrome. *Am J Ophthalmol.* 2000;129(3):281-5.

112. Scorolli L, Scorolli L, Campos EC, Bassein L, Meduri RA. Pseudoexfoliation syndrome: a cohort study on intraoperative complications in cataract surgery. *Ophthalmologica.* 1998;212(4):278-80.

113. Chan CK, Agarwal A, Agarwal S, Agarwal A. Management of dislocated intraocular implants. *Ophthalmol Clin North Am.* 2001 Dec;14(4):681-93.

114. Jehan FS, Mamalis N, Crandall AS. Spontaneous late dislocation of intraocular lens within the capsular bag in pseudoexfoliation patients. *Ophthalmology.* 2001;108(10):1727-31.

115. Lim MC, Doe EA, Vroman DT, Rosa RH Jr, Parrish RK 2nd. Late onset lens particle glaucoma as a consequence of spontaneous dislocation of an intraocular lens in pseudoexfoliation syndrome. *Am J Ophthalmol.* 2001;132(2):261-3.

116. Breyer DR, Hermeking H, Gerke E. Late dislocation of the capsular bag after phacoemulsification with endocapsular IOL in pseudoexfoliation syndrome. *Ophthalmologe.* 1999; 96(4):248-51.

117. Bayraktar S, Altan T, Kucuksumer Y, Yilmaz OF. Capsular tension ring implantation after capsulorrhexis in phacoemulsification of cataracts associated with pseudoexfoliation syndrome. Intraoperative complications and early postoperative findings. *J Cataract Refract Surg.* 2001;27(10):1620-8.

118. Moreno-Montanes J, Sanchez-Tocino H, Rodriguez-Conde R. Complete anterior capsule contraction after phacoemulsification with acrylic intraocular lens and endocapsular ring implantation. *J Cataract Refract Surg.* 2002;28(4):717-9.

119. Merkur A, Damji KF, Mintsioulis G, Hodge WG. Intraocular pressure decrease after phacoemulsification in patients with pseudoexfoliation syndrome. *J Cataract Refract Surg.* 2001;27(4):528-32.

120. Wirbelauer C, Anders N, Pham DT, Wollensak J, Laqua H. Intraocular pressure in nonglaucomatous eyes with pseudoexfoliation syndrome after cataract surgery. *Ophthalmic Surg Lasers.* 1998;29(6):466-71.

121. Georgopoulos GT, Chalkiadakis J, Livir-Rallatos G, Theodossiadis PG, Theodossiadis GP. Combined clear cornea phacoemulsification and trabecular aspiration in the treatment of pseudoexfoliative glaucoma associated with cataract. *Graefes Arch Clin Exp Ophthalmol.* 2000;238(10):816-21.

122. Jacobi PC, Dietlein TS, Krieglstein GK. Bimanual trabecular aspiration in pseudoexfoliation glaucoma: an alternative in nonfiltering glaucoma surgery. *Ophthalmology.* 1998; 105(5):886-94.

123. Drolsum L, Haaskjold E, Sandvig K. Phacoemulsification in eyes with pseudoexfoliation. *J Cataract Refract Surg.* 1998; 24(6):787-92.

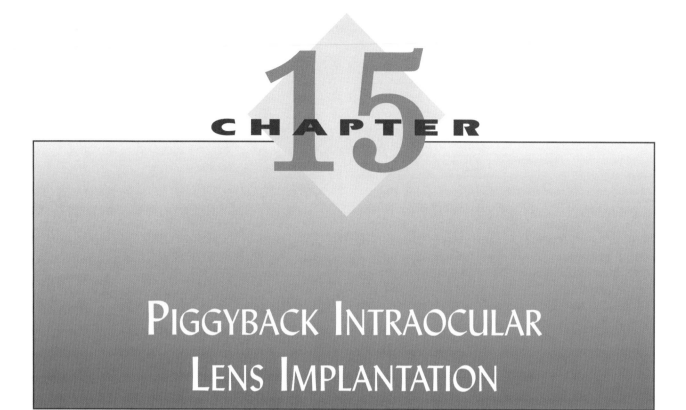

# Chapter 15

# Piggyback Intraocular Lens Implantation

*James P. Gills, MD and Myra Cherchio, COMT*

For cataract patients with extreme refractive errors, implanting 2 IOLs in 1 eye, piggyback style, provides an opportunity to treat the refractive error along with the cataract. The piggyback lens implantation strategy (Figure 15-1) can be used to treat high hyperopia,[1-5] extremely high myopia,[6] and high astigmatism (using toric lenses). In many cases, clear lens replacement with piggyback lenses is the ideal procedure for those who are beyond the range of many other procedures.

Although the piggyback implantation technique is essentially the same for any patient, different patient populations present unique issues that require special attention. For example, high hyperopes often present with disproportional anatomy that causes challenges to power calculations, while high astigmats receiving torics require meticulous attention to the axis of implantation.

## Piggybacks in High Hyperopes

### Measurements and Calculations

The highly hyperopic patient presents the surgeon with 2 potential problems. The first is the possibility of surgical complications that may arise from the structural nature of the hyperopic eye. The second is implanting adequate power

while maintaining good optical quality and an accurate refraction. Calculating the correct IOL power in highly hyperopic patients presents unique challenges due to the difficulties in obtaining accurate measurements in short eyes, and the limitations of most IOL formulas.[7]

Accurate measurement of axial length in hyperopic eyes is especially important because any error is greatly magnified in proportion to the length of the eye. Yet it is in short eyes that accurate measurements are most difficult to obtain. Ultrasound axiometers are calibrated with average velocities for normal length eyes. These velocities are incorrect for short eyes, causing significant measurement errors.[8] However, this problem can be corrected by applying the correct tissue velocity to the aqueous, lens, and vitreous.

Performing applanation biometry is frequently difficult in short-eye cases with shallow anterior chambers because it can be difficult to distinguish the initial "bang" echo from the iris and establish perpendicularity. Decreasing the ultrasound gain may be necessary when this occurs so each echo can be visualized; however, doing so can make the scan more difficult to perform. The most significant problem with applanation biometry is that the cornea is easily indented even in the hand of the most skilled ultrasound technician. Even the slightest indentation can cause significant measurement errors, which are magnified when the eye is short.[8-10]

Acquiring axial length measurements through non-contact biometry, whether immersion or the IOL Master (Zeiss

Meditec, Germany) provides superior results in these cases.[11,12] First, it is impossible to indent the cornea and shorten the axial length. Thus, by their very nature, these methods are more reliable than applanation. Immersion biometry allows visualization of the corneal echoes, ensuring perpendicularity and improving accuracy. In order to obtain the most accurate measurement, the skilled ultrasound technician will watch for consistency of echo height, axial length, lens thickness, and anterior chamber depth readings.

Optimizing axial length measurements does not guarantee the desired outcome. In a study by the author performed with Dr. Jack Holladay,[8] several hyperopic patients were examined and more detailed anatomical measurements were taken. Most of the short-eye cases had normal anterior segment dimensions (corneal diameter, keratometry, and anterior segment length) but shortened posterior segments. Only about 20% of eyes with axial length less than 21 mm had disproportionately small anterior segment sizes.[7]

Based on these observations, we can conclude that many third-generation power formulas systematically generate hyperopic errors in power calculation among extreme hyperopes because they assume the anterior segments are proportionate the shortened posterior segment.[7] Thus they predict the IOL position to be too anterior, resulting in hyperopic error in approximately 80% of the cases.

Holladay has reported that prediction accuracy in short eyes is significantly improved with the Holladay II formula, which incorporates additional measurements to take into account the unusual anatomy found in most high hyperopes.[7] He reported a decrease in mean absolute error among short eye cases from about 4.50 D with other formulas to a little less than 1.00 D with the Holladay II formula. He also found that about 4% of eyes with average axial lengths have anterior segment sizes that are large or small relative to the posterior segment. These patients may also benefit from the use of an IOL formula based on more measurements.

Furthermore, when the piggyback technique is used in high hyperopes, power calculations must be adjusted again. By measuring the distance from the iris to the IOL vertex, Holladay and Gills[8] determined that the anterior-most lens is in the usual position while the posterior-most lens is pushed back, causing additional hyperopic error. Apparently the anterior lens pushes the posterior lens further back due to the elastic nature of the capsular bag. Thus, additional power must be factored into the equation. The Holladay II formula provides such adjustments.[7] For these reasons, the Holladay II is the formula of choice for calculating piggyback IOLs. We have found improved accuracy in our piggyback cases after switching to this formula.[13]

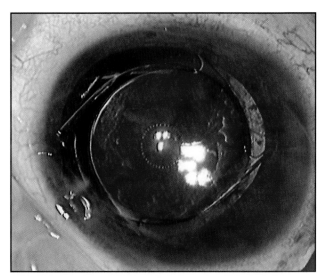

**Figure 15-1.** Piggybacked IOLs.

## Surgical Technique

All patients undergoing lens extraction surgery receive a thorough explanation of the type of anesthesia to be used, what to expect during surgery, and the risks involved. This is especially important for high hyperopes because compliance during surgery is critical. Topical anesthesia can be used for these patients, just as for cases with average axial lengths. However, managing complications is certainly more difficult under topical anesthesia, and high hyperopes are at greater risk for certain complications such as shallow anterior chambers; iris prolapse; pupillary block while the pupil is dilated, which can result in a hard eye; and choroidal effusion or fluid misdirection. Many surgeons may prefer regional anesthesia for these cases.

Piggybacking IOLs requires close attention to phacoemulsification technique, both because of the higher risk associated with the population that usually receives piggyback IOLs, and because of the potential long-term complications that can arise with 2 IOLs implanted in the bag. We perform meticulous cortical clean-up, and polish the posterior capsule, which reduces the risk of intralenticular cellular growth.

For myopic or hyperopic primary piggyback cases, we use 2 PMMA single-piece biconvex IOLs with an optic size of 5.5 mm. Both IOLs are placed in the capsular bag. PMMA IOLs require the use of a self-sealing scleral-tunnel incision. CCIs are avoided in these cases to reduce the risk of infection associated with wound leak. The incision is placed at the steep meridian to correct preexisting astigmatism. In some cases limbal or CRIs are also performed to correct preexisting astigmatism.[7]

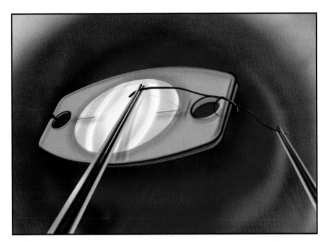

**Figure 15-2.** Suturing piggybacked toric lenses together eliminates the possibility of counter-rotation.

# CORRECTING HIGH ASTIGMATISM WITH PIGGYBACK TORIC IOLS

While astigmatism greater than 5.00 D is rare, it can be visually disabling, typically limiting the quality of vision. Patients with very high astigmatism often have associated corneal pathology, making the astigmatism more challenging to correct, and the result more unpredictable with incisional procedures alone. Before the availability of toric IOLs, the amount of surgical correction required to correct high astigmatism involved multiple limbal and CRIs, which often caused corneal distortion and visual aberrations. We have had excellent results correcting high astigmatism by implanting 2 toric IOLs, even if the patient would not have otherwise required piggyback implantation for high hyperopia. By implanting 2 toric lenses piggyback style, corneal disturbance can be significantly reduced, providing safer, less invasive surgery.

Because the maximum correction with a single toric lens is 2.40 D with the 3.50 D toric IOL, we utilize 2 toric lenses to correct astigmatism greater than 5.00 D. Implanting two 3.50-D toric IOLs back to back theoretically doubles the effective correction. Patients with less than 5.00 D of astigmatism may receive a single toric IOL, astigmatic keratotomy, strategic wound placement and size, or a combination of procedures, depending on the individual. Correcting higher levels of astigmatism typically requires more than 1 technique. However, reducing high astigmatism to a manageable level with piggyback toric IOLs makes residual astigmatism simpler to correct.

A concern with any toric implantation is rotation of the lens. A rotation up to 30 degrees will reduce the effective astigmatism correction, and a rotation greater than 30 degrees will actually worsen the astigmatism.[14] Rotation in toric piggybacks is even more problematic, because the effect of off-axis rotation will be doubled. Even worse is the possibility of the lenses counter-rotating.

We have implanted piggyback toric lenses in a relatively small number of patients with few problems of postoperative rotation, and no counter-rotations. The risk of rotation with 2 toric lenses is smaller than if 1 is used, because the piggyback system fills the bag.

The potential risk of counter-rotation can be completely avoided by suturing the IOLs together through the fixation holes. Because the cylindrical component is incorporated on the anterior surface of the toric lens, we suture the lenses back to back (rather than front to back) to decrease the possibility of dimpling the optic. If the optics were compressed, there could be a reduction of the effective cylinder correction.

Suturing the lenses together necessitates a larger incision, which can actually be useful in correcting some of the incision if it is placed at the steep axis. The impact of the incision on the corneal astigmatism must then be taken into account when calculating the amount of desired correction. To suture toric lenses together, the edges of the lenses are held with a soft lens grabber. The IOLs are secured with tying forceps and 9-0 nylon, using 1 throw and 1 knot through the fixation holes at each end (Figure 15-2).

## Determining the Axis

When evaluating the preoperative axis of astigmatism, manual keratometry and corneal topography frequently differ, due to the different ways the instruments acquire the readings. We identify the steep axis preoperatively with corneal topography and manual keratometry. In the event of a discrepancy, the surgical keratometer is the final arbiter. Using the surgical keratometer before, during, and after insertion of the IOL ensures the most accurate placement of the toric lens, astigmatic keratotomy and cataract incision. We have found the surgical keratometer to be a vital tool in the operating room and believe it to be even more accurate than corneal topography. Precise identification of the steep axis is especially critical for patients receiving piggyback toric lenses, since the effect caused by a slight off-axis placement is doubled.

Correct orientation of the lens is determined during surgery using the surgical keratometer. The axis marked on the lens is aligned with the steep axis identified with the surgical keratometer.

## Correcting Rotation of the Piggyback Toric System

If the toric lenses are placed off axis, or if they rotate postoperatively, they can be rotated back into position. IOLs usually do not rotate on their own once capsular fusion takes

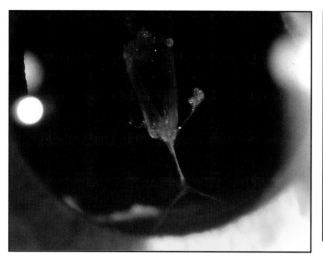

**Figure 15-3.** Interlenticular opacification (ILO), or cellular ingrowth, into the piggyback lens interface.

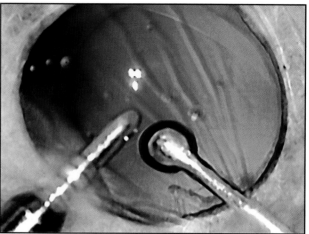

**Figure 15-4.** Polishing the capsule removes more lens epithelial cells and may reduce the incidence of ILO.

place,[15] and are difficult to rotate surgically after 2 weeks postoperatively, as breaking the adhesions risks zonular disruption.

When we surgically rotate toric lenses, we routinely use a 30-gauge needle on a syringe with Xylocaine (AstraZeneca, Waltham, Mass). We first anesthetize the cornea with topical Alcaine (Alcon, Fort Worth, Tex) and Xylocaine jelly. Using the 30-gauge needle, we enter the anterior chamber at the desired axis of rotation. We then remove a small amount of aqueous and reinject with Xylocaine to prevent the patient from jerking during the lens rotation. Before the lenses are rotated into the correct position, they are freed 360 degrees with a gentle rocking motion, loosening any adhesions. The tip of the needle is simply placed along the edge of the lenses, and both lenses are easily rotated into position.

# COMPLICATIONS AND RISKS

## *Intralenticular Opacification*

Intralenticular opacification (ILO), a long-term complication of piggyback lenses, has been reported.[16-19] ILO is cellular growth between piggybacked lenses that is often characterized as Elschnig pearl formation, and may even result in a fibrous membrane formation between the lenses. ILO has been reported primarily in acrylic lenses with long-term follow up, although it has also been seen to a lesser degree in PMMA and silicone piggybacks.[16-19]

Gayton[19] has reported an incidence of ILO of 43% among his acrylic piggybacks and 22% among his PMMA piggybacks. He has reported a number of cases with thick, opaque membranes that have severely impacted vision and required surgical removal. Moreover, both Gayton[18] and Shugar[16] have reported a shift in refraction among cases with significant ILO.

We conducted a study of all our piggyback cases with at least 2-year possible follow-up and examined them at slit lamp to determine the extent of the problem in our practice. We examined 50 eyes of 34 patients, 22 eyes with piggybacked PMMA lenses, 19 with silicone, and 9 with 1 PMMA and 1 silicone lens.

We found 3 eyes, or 6%, showed signs of ILO, 2 with piggybacked PMMA (Figure 15-3), and 1 with mixed PMMA and silicone. In these 3 cases, we saw only mild interface growth, with no impact on visual function, no shift in refraction, and no symptoms of glare or shadows. We found no cases of ILO in double-silicone piggybacks, even with both in the bag.

We found a much lower incidence and severity of ILO in our practice than reported by Gayton[18] or Shugar,[16] which may be due either to a difference in IOL material, because we do not use acrylic, or to a difference in surgical technique. Dr. Apple has implicated incomplete removal of epithelial cells as a possible cause of ILO.[16,19] Because we routinely polish the capsule in all our cataract cases (Figure 15-4), we effect a more complete removal of lens epithelial cells at surgery, which may have significantly lowered our incidence of ILO.

While we believe that polishing the capsule is an important step for all lens extraction cases, meticulous attention to removal of all epithelial cells is especially crucial in piggyback cases. While the causes of this complication are not yet well understood, and methods of treatment still under study, careful polishing of the capsule and removal of all lens epithelial cells may significantly lower the incidence and severity of the problem.

# Conclusion

The piggyback lens implantation technique provides the opportunity to correct or reduce extreme refractive errors in cataract and refractive surgery patients. When using the piggyback technique in high hyperopes, the often unusual anatomy of short-eye patients presents unique challenges in power calculation and surgical technique. In high astigmats, the piggyback technique used with toric lenses can theoretically correct up to 5.00 D of cylinder, while suturing the lenses together avoids any possibility of counter-rotation. The risk of the long-term complication of interlenticular opacity, or cellular growth between the lenses, is reduced with the use of PMMA and silicone lenses, and meticulous cleaning of the capsule.

# References

1. Gayton JL, Sanders VN. Implanting two posterior chamber intraocular lenses in a case of microphthalmos. *J Cataract Refract Surg.* 1993;19:776-777.

2. Gayton JL, Raanan MG. Reducing refractive error in high hyperopes with double implants. In: Gayton JL, ed. *Maximizing Results.* Thorofare, NJ: SLACK Incorporated; 1996;139-148.

3. Gills JP, Gayton JL, Raanan MG. Multiple intraocular lens implantation. In: Gills JP, Fenzl R, Martin RG, eds. *Cataract Surgery: State of the Art.* Thorofare, NJ; SLACK Incorporated; 1998.

4. Shugar JK, Lewis C, Lee A. Implantation of multiple foldable acrylic posterior chamber lenses in the capsular bag for high hyperopia. *J Cataract Refract Surg.* 1996;22:1368-1372.

5. Gills JP. The implantation of multiple intraocular lenses to optimize visual results in hyperopic cataract patients and under-powered pseudophakes. *Best Papers of Sessions, 1995 Symposium on Cataract IOL and Refractive Surgery Special Issue;* 1996.

6. Gills JP, Fenzl RE. Minus power intraocular lenses to correct refractive error in myopic pseudophakia. *J Cataract Refract Surg.* 1999;25(9):1205-8.

7. Holladay JR. Achieving emmetropia in extremely short eyes. Presented at the 1996 Annual Meeting of the American Academy of Ophthalmology; Chicago, IL.

8. Holladay JR, Gills JP, Leidlein JL, Cherchio M. Achieving emmetropia in extremely short eyes with two piggyback posterior chamber intraocular lenses. *Ophthalmology.* 1996; 103:1118-1123.

9. Sanders, DR, Retzlaff JA, Kraff MC. A-scan biometry and IOL implant power calculations. In: *Focal Points: Clinical Modules for Ophthalmologists.* San Francisco, CA; American Academy of Ophthalmology; 1995;13(10)1-14.

10. Holladay JT, Prager TC, Ruiz RS, Lewis JW. Improving the predictability of intraocular lens power calculations. *Arch Ophthalmol.* 1986;104:539-541.

11. Shammus HJF. A comparison of immersion and contact techniques for axial length measurement. *Am Intraocular Implant Soc J.* 1984;10:444.

12. Rajan MS, Keilhorn I, Bell JA. Partial coherence laser interferometry vs conventional ultrasound biometry in intraocular lens power calculations. *Eye.* 2002;16(5):552-6.

13. Fenzl RE, Gills JP, Cherchio M. Refractive and visual outcome of hyperopic cataract cases operated on before and after implementation of the Holladay II formula. *Ophthalmology.* 1998;105(9):1759-64.

14. Sanders DR, Grabow HB, Shepherd J. The toric IOL. In: Gills JP, Martin RG, Sanders DR, eds. *Sutureless Cataract Surgery: An Evolution Toward Minimally Invasive Technique.* Thorofare, NJ: SLACK Incorporated; 1992.

15. Patel CK, Ormonde S, Rosen PH, Bron AJ. Postoperative intraocular lens rotation: a randomized comparison of plate and loop haptic implants. *Ophthalmology.* 1999;106:2190-6.

16. Gayton JL, Apple DJ, Peng Q, et al. Interlenticular opacification: clinicopathological correlation of a complication of piggyback posterior chamber intraocular lenses. *J Cataract Refract Surg.* 2000;26(3):330-6.

17. Shugar JK, Schwartz T. Interpseudophakos Elschnig pearls associated with late hyperopic shift: a complication of piggyback posterior chamber intraocular lens implantation. *J Cataract Refract Surg.* 1999;25:863-7.

18. Shugar JK, Keeler S. Interpseudophakos intraocular lens surface opacification as a late complication of piggyback acrylic posterior chamber lens implantation. *J Cataract Refract Surg.* 2000;26:448-55.

19. Gayton JL, Apple DJ, Van Der Karr M, Sanders V. Refractive stability and long-term interlenticular membrane formation of piggybacked intraocular implants. *J Cataract Refract Surg.* In press.

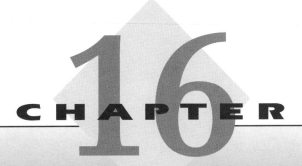

# CHAPTER 16

# SURGICAL IMPLANTATION OF TELESCOPIC INTRAOCULAR LENSES

*Christina Canakis, MD and Gholam A. Peyman, MD*

## INTRODUCTION

The ability of telescopes to produce magnification of images renders them a suitable means of improving visual function in patients with severely compromised central vision, as occurs most commonly in age-related macular degeneration (ARMD), diabetes, and myopia. In 1609, by enclosing the combination of a strong concave and a less powerful convex lens in a hollow tube, separated by a distance equal to the difference between their focal lengths, Galileo created his first telescope.

The magnification of a Galilean system is given from the formula:

$$\frac{\text{Dioptric strength of the eyepiece}}{\text{Dioptric strength of the objective}}$$

External devices based on the principles of the Galilean telescope were introduced later in ophthalmology as low-vision aids but generally have been found difficult to use in everyday tasks.[1,2] Models with some or all components designed for intraocular implantation have been developed with the purpose of limiting their size, easing their use, and producing a more physiological function compared to the external devices. As these models are not currently commercially available, we will describe their development and focus on those currently in clinical trials or models that hold promise for the future.

### *Anatomy*

#### ANTERIOR CHAMBER HIGH-MINUS IMPLANTS

Choyce described the first partially intraocular telescope in a paper read before the Section of Ophthalmology, Royal Society of Medicine (London), in October, 1962, and later reported on 4 patients in 1964.[3] In 1 patient, simultaneous intracapsular cataract extraction was performed, whereas in the other 3 patients, the crystalline lens was left in place. His concept involved insertion of a -30.00-D or -40.00-D concave eyepiece or ocular lens into the eye as the optic part of an anterior chamber implant (Figure 16-1), combined with a convex objective lens 13 mm in front of the cornea (ie, at spectacle distance).

#### POSTERIOR CHAMBER HIGH-MINUS IMPLANTS

In 1986, Donn and Koester proposed an ocular telephoto system that created a Galilean telescope by means of a strong negative IOL (-40.00 D to -100.00 D) that replaced the human crystalline lens, combined with a strong positive spectacle lens (+13.00 D to +27.00 D).[4] The magnification and visual field for a given implant could be altered by changing the power and vertex distance of the spectacle lens. Donn and Koester contended that such a system would offer

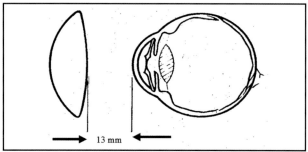

**Figure 16-1.** Choyce anterior chamber intraocular implant acts as the eye piece of a Galilean telescope. (Courtesy of Choyce P. *Intraocular Lenses and Implants*. London: HK Lewis; 1964;156-161.)

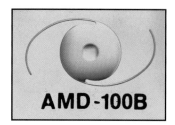

**Figure 16-2.** With spectacle lenses, the Koziol-Peyman posterior chamber lens maintains normal pseudophakic vision.

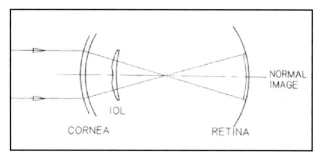

**Figure 16-3.** The teledioptric lens (AMD-100B) is a bifocal intraocular lens with a 1.9-mm high minus (-54.00 D) central zone. (Reprinted from *J Cataract Refract Surg*, 14, Peyman GA, Koziol J. Age-related macular degeneration and its management, 421-430, copyright [1988], with permission from Elsevier Science.)

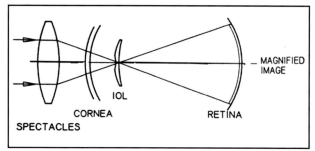

**Figure 16-4.** With the spectacle lens, the Koziol-Peyman posterior chamber lens forms a Galilean telescope producing a magnified image on the retina. (Reprinted from *J Cataract Refract Surg*, 14, Peyman GA, Koziol J. Age-related macular degeneration and its management, 421-430, copyright [1988], with permission from Elsevier Science.)

advantages over the model introduced by Choyce in terms of optical aberrations and visual field; however, their assumptions were challenged.[5]

The system's main drawback is that removal of the spectacle lens causes the eye with the IOL to be functionally blind with a refractive error at the cornea of approximately +60.00 D of hyperopia.

### TELEDIOPTRIC AND CATADIOPTRIC POSTERIOR CHAMBER IMPLANTS

Eyes implanted with high-minus IOLs experience extreme hyperopia without wearing the spectacle lens, with profound loss of visual acuity and peripheral vision. To eliminate this problem, Peyman and Koziol introduced the teledioptric and catadioptric systems.[6,7]

The teledioptric system consists of the teledioptric IOL with a spectacle lens. The teledioptric lens (AMD-100B, Allergan Medical Optics, Irvine, Calif; Figure 16-2) is a bifocal IOL derived from a modification of the AMO PC-25NB lens (Allergan Medical Optics). It has a diameter of 6.5 mm and a length of 13.5 mm in a PMMA 1-piece design with both plus and minus portions, suitable for posterior chamber implantation. The plus portion retains the characteristics of normal pseudophakic vision, provides a full visual field, and preserves the existing central vision (Figure 16-3).

The 1.9-mm high-minus (-54.00 D) central zone acts as the ocular of a Galilean telescope when used in conjunction with high-plus spectacles. The teledioptric spectacles are worn to produce a magnified image for distant and near vision (Figure 16-4). They are bielement, aspheric lenses with a power ranging between +18.00 D and +28.00 D.

The catadioptric lens is designed for posterior chamber implantation and uses mirrored surfaces to produce image magnification without the need for an external spectacle lens. This lens has a very high resolution and theoretically maintains a visual field of approximately 80 degrees, large enough to permit comfortable ambulation (Figure 16-5). The lens is made from PMMA; however, the coating of the mirrored surfaces consists of materials that must be tested for use in humans.

### FULLY IMPLANTABLE MINIATURIZED TELESCOPE

Partially external telescopes are sensitive to the distance between the eyeglass and the eye, with the off-center movements of the eyeball creating a tilt between the external converging lens and the internal diverging one, causing aberrations that distort the optical performance of the system. To overcome such problems, Lipshitz et al described an IOL into which an entire small telescope was incorporated.[8] With some improvements on the original model, the implantable

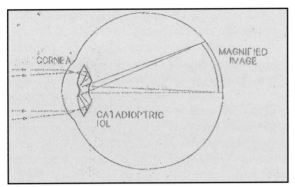

**Figure 16-5.** The catadioptric lens produces a magnified image on the retina without the use of additional plus lenses. (Reprinted from *J Cataract Refract Surg*, 14, Peyman GA, Koziol J. Age-related macular degeneration and its management, 421-430, copyright [1988], with permission from Elsevier Science.)

miniaturized telescope (IMT) has been manufactured and tested by VisionCare Ltd (Yehud, Israel), and is currently undergoing clinical trial.[9]

A miniature Galilean telescope is installed into a glass cylinder sealed on both sides to contain dehydrated air under a pressure of 1 atmosphere. The tube, which is 4.4 mm in length and 3 mm in diameter, is embedded in a carrying device that functions as a 7-mm x 4.75-mm 1-piece modified C-loop rigid all PMMA IOL, 13.5 mm in total length.[10,11] Flotation forces enable this device to fit in the capsular bag with a weight in the aqueous humor of 46 mg (approximately the weight of 4 conventional IOLs), as opposed to 95.8 mg in air. The IMT bulges into the anterior chamber through the pupil, maintaining a distance of approximately 2 mm from the cornea. It provides magnification 3X at a focusing distance of 50 cm; the power can be increased up to 6X or 8X with the addition of external spectacles. The resulting 6.6-degree visual field corresponds to 20 degrees on the retina.

Initially, the carrying device was made of a black PMMA formulation intended to prevent stray light from entering the eye, in an attempt to reduce glare in the visually compromised recipient eyes. The IMT allows funduscopy with a magnification inadequate for detailed examination. In the event of a sudden decrease in vision or of complications, ultrasonography can provide clues to the cause. Because the IMT also hinders the examination of peripheral retina and the performance of Nd:YAG laser posterior capsulotomy, the peripheral part of the carrying device in more recent models is fabricated from clear PMMA; however, the application of therapeutic techniques may remain difficult. The sacrifice of visual field for magnification is still the major problem limiting the wide application of this model, even in clinical trials.

## PHAKIC TELEDIOPTRIC IMPLANTS

The requirement for lens extraction prior to placement of the aforementioned implants is a disadvantage in the absence of a significant cataract. In addition to the general risks of such surgery, there is a possible link with deterioration of macular degeneration.[12-16]

To avoid this problem, Peyman and Koziol expanded the concept of their original posterior chamber teledioptric lens to encompass a universal phakic or pseudophakic teledioptric IOL design. In his 2001 innovator lecture, *A Telescopic IOLs and New Perspectives in Refractive Surgery* at the American Society of Cataract and Refractive Surgery Symposium in San Diego, Peyman described a teledioptric lens system (TLS) consisting of a modified Artisan (Ophtec, The Netherlands) or angle-fixed Kelman anterior chamber IOL, implantable in the presence of either a crystalline lens or a pseudophakos. For the latter case, Peyman and Koziol designed a flexible 1-piece Hydrogel IOL with a 1.5-mm central minus (-80.00 D) portion surrounded by a plano plate that can be implanted as a piggyback lens. This model awaits evaluation in a planned clinical study after obtaining FDA approval.

## *Preoperative Evaluation*

Preoperative evaluation by a team of ophthalmologists and low-vision experts is indispensable in identifying those patients who will benefit from and tolerate the implantation of a miniaturized telescope. The following procedures and measurements should be done preoperatively.

1. Near and distant visual acuity should be measured, along with near and distant BCVA with and without an external low-vision aid. In the presence of cataract, a potential acuity measurement offers useful information.

2. Slit-lamp examination of the anterior segment should be performed to rule out contraindications for lens placement. The anterior chamber depth should be measured when in doubt. The pupillary diameter should be measured before the eye is dilated for a fundus examination.

3. The patient's current medications, especially topical preparations that could potentially affect the size of the pupil, should be determined.

4. IOP measurements should be made to rule out glaucoma.

5. A dilated fundus examination is necessary to assess the stability of macular disease and any alterations of the peripheral retina.

6. Simulation with external telescopes is advisable. Initially the telescopic implants were designed to replace external devices in those individuals who had experienced difficulties with their use; however, it

seems more reasonable to use them in those patients who already have shown tolerance to the optical performance of external telescopes, but who do not use them because of their lack of convenience, poor cosmesis, or because tremor or paralysis preclude the use of hand-held devices. A near-vision telescope system allows a working distance that is longer than that which would be provided by the equivalent spectacle lens but at the expense of a significantly reduced field of view. The patient should be educated to expect a period of adaptation to the alterations in the physiology of visual perception, which can be so profound as to warrant IOL explantation. The evaluation of patient motivation is essential. The patient must recognize the risks and postoperative requirements of a surgical procedure, and intend to replace external low-vision aids at that cost.

7. Baseline visual field testing, intravenous fluorescein angiography, and reading speed can also provide opportunity for postoperative comparison. These evaluations may be included in the preoperative testing to help in drawing useful conclusions while procedures are still experimental. For the same purpose, keratometry, corneal topography, corneal endothelial cell count, and a questionnaire about performance of various daily activities may be added.

8. For models utilizing the implantable anterior chamber lens technology, the horizontal white-to-white or sulcus-to-sulcus diameter will be required as well.

# INDICATIONS AND CONTRAINDICATIONS

## General Indications

The primary indication for implantation of a telescopic system is central vision loss. The magnification provided by a telescopic system compensates for the loss of resolution suffered by such patients, permitting recognition of objects at greater distances than would be possible with unaided vision. Initially such systems were advocated for patients with ARMD with or without cataract, but other ocular conditions with central vision loss such as retinal vascular disorders, optic neuropathy, congenital toxoplasmosis, and diabetic maculopathy are also suitable. Eyes chosen for surgery should not have other active diseases, except for cataract and maculopathy, and the risks and benefits should be assessed especially carefully in patients who do not have ARMD. Diabetics have higher rates of postoperative fibrin and inflammation, especially in the presence of rubeosis iridis, as well as of posterior capsule opacification. The option of

intraocular telescopic systems should be restricted to dry, nonproliferative cases, and should be highly personalized. The ideal candidate has bilateral, stable, dry ARMD, or inactive disciform ARMD in the eye planned for surgery. In this eye, the improved visual acuity with an external telescope should be better than the BCVA of the fellow eye.

The patients' goals should be to improve their quality of life, specifically with tasks such as reading, face recognition, and watching television. The safety of driving with telescopic intraocular implants has not been proven with any of these models; achieving vision sufficient for a driver's license is unlikely.

## Indications (Specifics)

### INCLUSION CRITERIA
The specific inclusion criteria used with the Koziol-Peyman posterior chamber TLS[7] include:
- ❖ Age older than 60 years
- ❖ Clinical signs of both cataract and ARMD resulting in visual disability
- ❖ Unsuccessful prior treatment with alternative methods of low-vision aid, such as high-plus lenses and/or telescopic magnifiers
- ❖ A BCVA of 20/70 or worse in the better eye and a potential acuity meter reading of 20/50 to 20/200 in the better eye
- ❖ High level of motivation
- ❖ Availability for extensive follow up
- ❖ Informed consent

The inclusion and exclusion criteria for IMT implantation were determined by Vision Care Ophthalmic Technologies Ltd,[10] and include:
- ❖ The ability to read and sign an informed consent form
- ❖ Age older than 60 years
- ❖ The lack of contraindications to surgery under local anesthesia
- ❖ A BCVA in the surgical eye of 20/80 to 20/200 and in the fellow eye of no better than 20/80
- ❖ No ocular disease except cataract, ARMD, or inactive toxoplasmosis scars
- ❖ Bilateral dry ARMD
- ❖ Cataract

With FDA approval of the Peyman-Koziol phakic TLS pending, recruitment of patients with a BCVA of 20/50 to 20/200 in the surgical eye is contemplated.

### EXCLUSION CRITERIA
Contraindications for implantation of a miniaturized telescope are:
- ❖ Insufficient motivation
- ❖ Unstable visual deficit. In cases of progressive disease, some models may preclude the proper application of

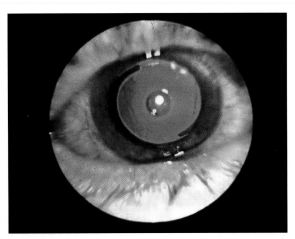

**Figure 16-6.** Postoperative view of an AMD-100B posterior chamber implant.

diagnostic modalities or therapeutic treatments such as lasers

The anatomic contraindications include:

*General*

✦ Fuch's endothelial dystrophy

✦ Low endothelial cell counts (less than 2,000 cells/mm² corneal endothelium). Although phacoemulsification surgery can be performed with lower cell counts with appropriate precautions, it should be avoided with these still-experimental lenses

✦ Glaucoma

✦ Uveitis and/or synechiae (anterior or posterior)

✦ Pupillary distortion or inappropriate pupillary diameter

*Specific*

✦ An anterior chamber depth (central distance from corneal endothelium to anterior crystalline lens) less than 2.8 mm is a contraindication for anterior segment models or the IMT. Once the IMT is implanted, the anterior part of the optic extends anteriorly for approximately 1 mm through the pupil. The device is designed to be stabilized approximately 2 mm posterior to the corneal endothelium

# SURGICAL TECHNIQUES

## Anesthesia

With the evolution of modern cataract surgery, intraocular telescopic systems can be implanted under local anesthesia with or without sedation. The surgeon may choose topical, retrobulbar, peribulbar, subtenon, or general anesthesia, taking into account the specific model to be implanted. The patient does not have to contribute actively in any step of the surgery.

## General Procedure

The routine steps of preparing the eye for cataract surgery are implemented, including dilating the pupil, applying antibiotic drops and proparacaine or tetracaine drops for local anesthesia cases, instillation of 5% povidone-iodine solution in BSS, and draping the eye in a sterile fashion.

Either a limbal or a scleral tunnel approach can be used with the latter providing a shorter healing period and less astigmatism. Viscoelastics protect the endothelium and should be used appropriately.

For implantation of the models that will replace the crystalline lens, phacoemulsification is the preferred method of lens extraction. The benefits of a continuous curvilinear anterior capsulorrhexis include stabilization and centration of the implant and possible decrease in posterior capsule opacification, if performed properly. The surgeon should seek to maintain iridal and zonular integrity. The lens capsule and iris are the structures that support the posterior chamber implants and are absolutely required to be intact if insertion of the relatively bulky IMT is contemplated.

Meticulous cortical clean-up and posterior capsule polishing are necessary to minimize the risk of posterior capsule opacification, which may be difficult to manage with the IMT.

Apart from the usual subconjunctival and topical antibiotics and steroids at the end of the procedure, the use of other agents depends on the model implanted (see below).

## Procedure (Specific)

POSTERIOR CHAMBER TLS OF KOZIOL-PEYMAN

✦ The teledioptric IOL[7] can be implanted with either planned extracapsular lens extraction or phacoemulsification followed by a posterior chamber implantation. The incision is appropriately enlarged to accommodate the 6.5-mm optic (Figure 16-6)

✦ One or more sphincterotomies ensure that the pupil will remain larger than the 1.9-mm central minus zone. A larger pupil (5 mm) reduces contrast more than a smaller pupil (3 mm). With a 3-mm pupil, the resolution efficiency matches that of an external telescope

IMPLANTATION OF IMT

✦ The technique in the IMT study includes a 180-degree conjunctival peritomy followed by cauterization and making a 3.2-mm limbal incision at the 12-o'clock position. Alternatively, a scleral tunnel can be constructed 3 to 4 mm posterior to the limbus. After intracameral injection of Healon GV[7] (Pfizer, New York, NY), a 7-mm CCC is made; hydrodissection and phacoemulsification are then performed.

✦ Thorough hydrodissection, cortex removal, and posterior capsule polishing are steps necessary to prevent posterior capsule opacification. The surgical treatment of postoperative posterior capsule opacification was the only option with the early IMT model

✧ The incision is enlarged to approximately 10 mm or an arc of 140 degrees to 160 degrees and the IMT is implanted in the capsular bag under viscoelastic. During manipulations the IMT should be held by the central flat part of the carrying device instead of the haptics. The glass cylinder should not be manipulated. Following insertion of the first haptic, insertion of the second haptic will require a downward movement of the central part of the device because the rigid loops preclude the implantation of the second haptic simply by a dialing maneuver. The haptics are oriented in the 6- to 12-o'clock meridian; this positioning is suggested by the manufacturer for optimal balance of the loop forces in the capsular bag and for stabilization

✧ A superior peripheral iridectomy is recommended to prevent postoperative pupillary block glaucoma

✧ The viscoelastic is removed by I/A and the wound is closed with interrupted 10-0 nylon sutures. The integrity of the wound should be confirmed and hypotony avoided to prevent postoperative IOL B corneal touch. Subconjunctival injection of 2 mg dexamethasone and 40 mg gentamicin follows

✧ The postoperative regimen includes dexamethasone and tobramycin drops QID tapered over 2 months, 1 drop of pilocarpine 2% in the morning, and 1 drop of phenylephrine 2.5% at bedtime for 10 days

IMPLANTATION OF PEYMAN-KOZIOL PHAKIC TLS

The phakic posterior chamber implants in the proposed study will be implanted following the rules of implantable contact lens insertion.

✧ A peripheral iridectomy to prevent postoperative pupillary block glaucoma will be made intraoperatively with forceps and scissors or with the vitrector at the end of the procedure following pharmacological miosis. The iridectomy should be located perpendicular to the longitudinal axis of the lens to avoid occlusion by IOL footplates

✧ The diameter of the pupil will have to be maintained at a postoperative size larger than the central minus portion of the IOL

# COMPLICATIONS AND MANAGEMENT

## *Intraoperative Complications*

The implantation of a telescopic system entails the general risks of anesthesia and extracapsular cataract extraction or phacoemulsification surgery. Appropriate use of viscoelastics will ensure optimal protection of the corneal endothelium from bulkier-than-usual models. The surgeon must become familiar with the model to be implanted to avoid lens damage from incorrect handling. Iris trauma was reported as the sole complication in the implantation of the AMD-100B and is a possibility where surgical iridotomy is required.

## *Postoperative Complications*

✧ Over a period of 18 months, 2 attacks of mild iritis occurring at 2 and 6 months in a patient implanted with an IMT were controlled with topical steroids and cycloplegics

✧ A peculiar complication was reported with the IMT: small droplets were noted in the air-filled optical cylinder that were later attributed to defective manufacturing missed at inspection.[11] After 12 months, this first generation IMT was explanted and uneventfully replaced with a single-piece all PMMA lens

✧ There were no cases of decentrated or tilted implants

✧ Posterior capsule opacification is difficult to manage in the presence of an IMT. Surgical capsulotomy was the only option with the first-generation models. Posterior capsule opacification is unlikely to impair the visual axis as the posterior part of the device creates a barrier effect to the migration of lens epithelial cells by pushing backward toward the posterior capsule

✧ Decompensation of the corneal endothelium was not encountered; however, longer follow-up is required

## *Functional Complications*

✧ *Vestibuloocular conflict:* With the partially implanted or external telescopes, the large intraocular magnification of images creates a vestibuloocular conflict in which the rotation of the head causes the object seen through the eye with the telescope to seem to move faster than the objects seen with the fellow eye. The vestibuloocular reflex automatically generates eye movements to compensate for head movements in order to maintain a stable retinal image during head rotation. These movements are equal in magnitude and opposite in direction in normal eyes (gain = 1); however, in the case of such telescopes, the demand for adaptation is different between the 2 eyes. This phenomenon, apart from causing discomfort or motion sickness, creates substantial image motion in the eye with the magnified image, disrupting its stability and decreasing sensitivity. Similarly, a target has different angular distance from fixation of the fellow eye and the eye with the aid, making fixation with that eye difficult. With the IMT, there is no relative movement between the eye and the telescope and the images are scanned with eye movements rather than head movements (vestibuloocular reflex gain = 1). This is more natural and advantageous in space and direction perception as well as clarity of vision in both eyes during eye movements, head movements, and tracking of moving targets.[17] Despite this theoretical advantage, the IMT did not solve this problem in the clinical study; the patients were better able to watch television but the increased velocity of objects in the field of vision was so bothersome that 2 patients preferred their unoperated eye for this task

✧ Experimental data have shown that dislocation of the anterior-posterior axis or minor tilt does not have any significant impact on the quality of vision and the modulation transfer factor of the implants. These complications have not been reported in any patients

✧ The monocular implantation of a telescopic system disrupts the stereo depth perception

✧ There is monocular restriction of the field of vision

## REHABILITATION

As in cataract surgery in which a non-foldable implant is inserted, postoperative refraction, astigmatism correction, and suture removal will be required. Patients with refractive error prior to surgery will need their presurgical correction postoperatively. Because it may be difficult to refract the patient after implantation of the IMT, the manufacturer developed a formula to estimate the postoperative refraction:[11]

$$\text{Refraction in Diopters} = (48.33 - 377/K) + (28.9 - 1.23A) + (7.28 - 3.1B)$$

where K = corneal keratometry in mm, A = axial length in mm, and B = distance between the corneal endothelium and the anterior surface of the IMT in mm.

The unavoidable functional complications of a telescopic system dictate a postoperative adaptation period and the need for education and continuous encouragement of the patient. Intolerance to this new condition of vision may lead to request for IOL explantation; therefore, the expectations of each candidate should be carefully evaluated preoperatively.

The spectacle lens of a TLS should be adjusted to the intended magnification and working distance for specific tasks of each patient. In the case of the IMT, use of low-plus (+1.00 to 3.50 D) eyeglasses enables the patient to read from 20 to 30 mm with a magnification of up to 8X. Low-minus eyeglasses enable reading at a distance of 2 to 3 m.

## OUTCOMES

### Teledioptric Implant AMD-100B

#### LABORATORY TESTING

*In vitro* testing was performed to determine the optical limitations and performance expectations of the TLS; its resolution was less than that of a combined standard IOL and external telescope because of the interface at the image plane between the images formed by each of the optical elements (analogous to a lesser degree to the decreased contrast provided by multifocal IOLs).

Laboratory data determined that optimal performance was achieved with a 1.9-mm central negative zone and that, with a 3-mm pupil, the resolution efficiency was similar to that of an external telescope. A larger pupil reduced contrast more.

#### CLINICAL RESULTS

IOL implantation was safe and easy; 56% of patients underwent phacoemulsification while the remaining 44% had planned extracapsular cataract extraction. The lens implantation was described as being of average difficulty by 92% of the investigators and less difficult than average by 8%. Sphincterotomy was performed in 82% of patients and an iridectomy or iridotomy in 12%. Six percent underwent both sphincterotomy and iridectomy/iridotomy.

Postoperative vision worsened in 12% of patients within 1 year of surgery; with potential acuity measurement, it was consistent with a decrease in the BCVA as a result of disease progression. Postoperatively, distance and near best-corrected vision improved in 68% of eyes and distance and near vision improved in 64% with the teledioptric spectacles during the first year. These percentages dropped to 22% and 30% after 1 year because of disease progression. In 22% of patients, there was a dramatic improvement in visual acuity (3 lines or more); the same patients reported an improvement in lifestyle and tasks such as reading, watching television, or pursuing a hobby.

Low-vision specialists recalled 20 patients for complete reevaluation. The distance visual acuities were measured with both the teledioptric spectacle lens and a 2.5X Selsi telescope. A tangent screen was used to test the visual field. With teledioptric spectacles, the resulting mean visual field was 24.1 degrees or 2.6 times larger than that achieved with the external telescope with a field of 9.3 degrees. The visual acuity with the teledioptric spectacles was better than the previous BCVA in 86% of patients during the first year after surgery and in 46% after 1 year. Acuities were similar with the teledioptric spectacles and the external telescope.

Forty-six percent of patients were satisfied with their vision with the teledioptric spectacles, 53% were satisfied with their vision without them, and 61% would recommend this surgery to a friend.

Although standard low-vision aids can be used anytime after teledioptric lens implantation, this system alone was limited to a 2.5X magnification, inadequate to accommodate disease progression or severe initial disease. The authors suggested improvements in their system that would allow 4X magnification. Clinical data of the improved design are not available.

Despite the positive results reported on preliminary testing in the United States with the bifocal IOL/spectacle system developed by Allergan, the AMD-100B lens was not brought to the market. A similar system is under testing in Europe by Morcher GmbH (Morcher IOL Type 59 Macular IOL, Stuttgart, Germany).

## *Implantable Miniaturized Telescope (IMT)*

### SAFETY RESULTS

Stabilization, centration, and prevention of tilt were evaluated in this relatively bulky lens. Data from this study enabled the developers to reduce the telescope length and adapt the location within the device, allowing greater distance between the implant and the corneal endothelium.[9] The lens could then be inserted through an incision of 120 to 150 degrees. Four of the 9 patients participating in this study were able postoperatively to watch television and to have the visual function for orientation in space.

### EFFICACY RESULTS

As of February 1999, 3 patients were willing to participate in this clinical trial and underwent implantation.[9,10] This study was conducted in Turkey with the purpose of evaluating the efficacy of the IMT in patients with macular degeneration.

During the 18-month follow-up period, all devices had remained well centered in the capsular bag with no tilting, anterior-posterior displacement, or iris irregularity. The distance between the corneal endothelium and the implant was at least 1.5 mm in the immediate postoperative period, later increasing to 2.0 mm. No case of CME, glaucoma, or corneal deterioration was encountered and the A with the rule astigmatism of the limbal incision was not greater than 0.50 D.

Distance and near vision improvement was noted in all patients; however, this achievement was not translated to a significant improvement in performing daily activities by 18 months postoperatively. The other main problems of external telescopes still remained unsolved: the narrow visual field and the need for intensive training and continuous encouragement postoperatively to help the patient to adapt to the significant changes in visual perception.

More patients are being recruited in clinical testing of this lens in Europe; a clinical trial is currently being conducted at 3 US sites: the University of California Irvine, Calif; Baylor College of Medicine, Houston, Tex; and Associated Eye Care, Stillwater, Minn.

# FUTURE DEVELOPMENTS

The existing models are still experimental but can provide acceptable modulation transfer function, visual field, and optical aberrations. Further improvement may be achieved by adapting foldable phakic IOL technologies and by advances in lens material, design, and surgical implantation. Ideally, the insertion of a telescopic implant should be easily reversible if the need emerges.

# REFERENCES

1. Newman JD. Telescopic systems. In: Faye EE, Hood CM, eds. *Low Vision.* Springfield, Ill: Charles C Thomas; 1975:17-30.

2. Bettman JW, McNair GS. A contact-lens-telescopic system. *Am J Ophthalmol.* 1939;22(1):27-33.

3. Choyce P. Galilean telescope using the anterior chamber implant as eye-piece: a low-visual-acuity aid for macular lesions. In: Choyce P, ed. *Intraocular Lenses and Implants.* London: HK Lewis; 1964:156-161.

4. Donn A, Koester CJ. An ocular telephoto system designed to improve vision in macular disease. *CLAO Journal.* 1986;12(2):81-85.

5. Bailey IL. Critical view of an ocular telephoto system. *CLAO Journal.* 1987;13(4):217-221.

6. Peyman GA, Koziol J. Age-related macular degeneration and its management. *J Cataract Refract Surg.* 1988;14(4):421-430.

7. Koziol JE, Peyman GA, Cionni R, et al. Evaluation and implantation of a teledioptric lens system for cataract and age-related macular degeneration. *Ophthalmic Surg.* 1994;25(10):675-684.

8. Lipshitz I, Loewenstein A, Reingewirtz M, Lazar M. An intraocular telescopic lens for macular degeneration. *Ophthalmic Surg Lasers.* 1997;28(6):513-517.

9. IMT B Scientific data. VisionCare Ophthalmic Technologies Ltd. http://www.visioncare.co.il/scientific.html. Accessed October 22, 2002.

10. Kaskaloglu M, Uretmen O, Yagci A. Medium-term results of implantable miniaturized telescopes in eyes with age-related macular degeneration. *J Cataract Refract Surg.* 2001; 27(11):1751-1755.

11. Werner L, Kaskaloglu M, Apple DJ, et al. Aqueous infiltration into an implantable miniaturized telescope. *Ophthalmic Surg Lasers.* 2002;33(4):343-348.

12. Klein R, Klein BE, Jensen SC, Cruickshanks KJ. The relationship of ocular factors to the incidence and progression of age-related maculopathy. *Arch Ophthalmol.* 1998;116(4):506-513.

13. Pollack A, Bukelman A, Zalish M, Leiba H, Oliver M. The course of age-related macular degeneration following bilateral cataract surgery. *Ophthalmic Surg Lasers.* 1998;29(4):286-294.

14. Pollack A, Marcovich A, Bukelman A, Zalish M, Oliver M. Development of exudative age-related macular degeneration after cataract surgery. *Eye.* 1997;11(Pt 4):523-530.

15. Pollack A, Marcovich A, Bukelman A, Oliver M. Age-related macular degeneration after extracapsular cataract extraction with intraocular lens implantation. *Ophthalmology.* 1996;103(10):1546-1554.

16. Van der Schaft TL, Mooy CM, de Bruijn WC, Mulder PG, Pameyer JH, de Jong PT. Increased prevalence of disciform macular degeneration after cataract extraction with implantation of an intraocular lens. *Br J Ophthalmol.* 1994;78(6):441-445.

17. Peli E. The optical functional advantages of an intraocular low-vision telescope. *Optom Vis Sci.* 2002;79(4):225-233.

# SECTION 2

## REFRACTIVE SURGERY

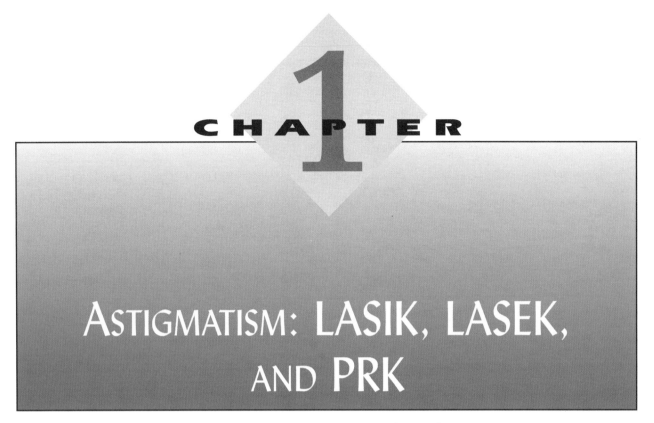

# CHAPTER 1

# ASTIGMATISM: LASIK, LASEK, AND PRK

*Noel A. Alpins, FRACO, FRCOphth, FACS and Carolyn M. Terry, BOptom*

Astigmatism occurs concomitantly with myopia and hyperopia in a high proportion of refractive corrections attempted with LASIK, LASEK, and PRK. Consequently, accurate measurement and analysis of preoperative astigmatism is an essential step in further understanding and determining appropriate corneal ablations for its surgical treatment.

## THE ASTIGMATISM PHENOMENON

The total amount of correction required to eliminate the astigmatism within an eye's optical system is gauged subjectively by a manifest refraction. This measurement is the sum of all astigmatic components, optical and perceptual, and is known as the refractive astigmatism.

The principal refractive surface of the eye, the cornea, can contribute an element of astigmatism, both from its anterior and posterior surfaces. The shape of the anterior corneal surface can be objectively quantified using manual keratometry or corneal topography methods and is described as corneal astigmatism.

Corneal astigmatism arising from the anterior corneal surface can be grouped into regular and irregular forms. Regular corneal astigmatism occurs when the principal meridians, flattest and steepest, of the anterior corneal surface are both orthogonal and symmetrical (Figures 1-1 through 1-3).[1]

Irregular corneal astigmatism describes the situation where there is a difference in the steepest corneal meridian across the hemi-division of the cornea—ie, where the astigmatism across the hemi-division is different in magnitude (asymmetry); not aligned across 180 degrees (non-orthogonal); or a combination of both of these factors.[2] The corneal irregularity itself can be idiopathic or occur secondary to:[3]

- Irregularity on the anterior corneal surface (eg, keratoconus [Figure 1-4], pellucid marginal degeneration, and keratoglobus)
- Trauma (eg, corneal incisions, excision or burns)
- Posttherapeutic healing or scarring
- Surgery (eg, keratoplasty, PRK, LASIK, LASEK, RK, or AK)

Residual astigmatism is a measure of the difference between the refractive and corneal astigmatism.[4] The amount of residual astigmatism can be measured directly from a spherical RGP contact lens overrefraction or mathematically calculated by vectorially subtracting the topographic from the refractive astigmatism at the corneal plane.[1] Both surfaces of the crystalline lens, any misalignment or tilt within the optical system, and an element of visual cortical perception[1,5] contribute to the amount of residual astigmatism present within an optical system.

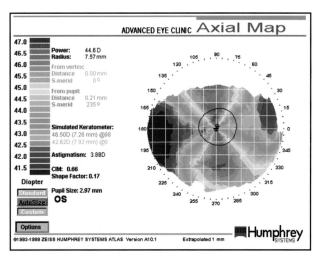

**Figure 1-1.** Regular with-the-rule astigmatism. The steepest axis of the anterior corneal surface is aligned along the vertical meridian.

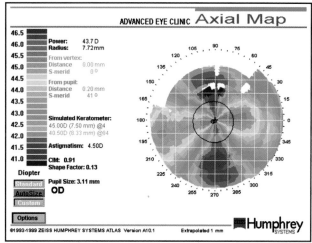

**Figure 1-2.** Regular against-the-rule astigmatism. The steepest axis of the anterior corneal surface is aligned along the horizontal meridian.

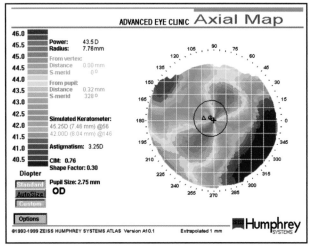

**Figure 1-3.** Regular oblique astigmatism. The steepest axis of the anterior corneal surface is aligned along an oblique orientation.

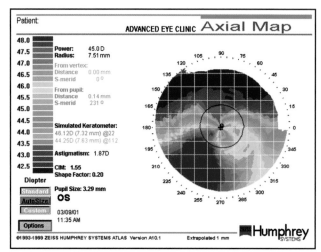

**Figure 1-4.** Irregular astigmatism. This anterior corneal display of keratoconus shows nonorthogonal and asymmetric astigmatism with steepening in the inferior hemidivision of the cornea.

# MEASUREMENT OF ASTIGMATISM

## Optical Astigmatism

### MANIFEST REFRACTION

The spherocylindrical result established from a manifest refraction determines how much optical correction is required to establish a single, clear focused image on the retina. The manifest refraction not only quantifies the amount of astigmatism due to the refracting surfaces of the eye, but also incorporates the component of astigmatism due to the perception of the retinal image by the visual cortex.[6]

This subjective mode of testing is largely dependent on observer response and testing conditions and subsequently can be prone to inconsistencies between individuals.

Variations in ergonomics due to differences in ambient lighting conditions and chart type, distance, illumination, and contrast can lead to unreliable comparison between data.[7]

### WAVEFRONT ABERROMETRY

Wavefront assessment devices are useful diagnostic tools that provide objective information regarding the optical aberrations within an ocular system. Small decentrations in all optical surfaces and shapes can produce optical aberrations even in "normal" eyes and cannot be corrected effectively by spectacles or contact lenses.[8] The wavefront devices available in clinical practice utilize the principle of outgoing reflection aberrometry (Shack-Hartmann, Adaptive Optics Associates, Cambridge, Mass), retinal imaging aberrometry (Tscherning) or ingoing adjustable refractometry (spatially resolved refractometer).[9] The Shack-Hartmann aberrometer is the most widely implemented technique.[9] In this technique, a beam of light is focused upon the retina from which a reflection passes backward through the media of the eye.[10] As the wavefront emerges from the entrance pupil, it is detected by a sensor and the resultant image is analyzed and compared to the uniform distribution produced by a perfect wavefront.[11]

The ensuing wavefront pattern provides a profile for the refractive error and expresses the ocular aberrations in terms of Zernike polynomials.[10] Second-order aberrations provide a measurement of defocus and astigmatism, not unlike the information derived from a manifest refraction. However, unlike a manifest refraction, a wavefront device is unable to provide effective information regarding cortical perception.[12] Third-order (trefoil, coma, and coma-like aberrations), fourth-order (spherical aberration and spherical-like aberrations), and higher order aberrations are also detected by these devices.[10]

## Corneal Shape

### KERATOMETRY

Keratometry provides a basic curvature measurement of the anterior cornea's 2 principal meridians. The resultant average corneal astigmatism value applies to a limited central area of the anterior cornea and cannot quantify any corneal irregularity that may be present on that surface.

### CORNEAL TOPOGRAPHY

Corneal topography mapping by computer-assisted videokeratography (CAVK) affords a more advanced technique of appraising corneal astigmatism by measuring values at multiple reference points over the anterior corneal surface. This objective measurement modality provides useful information regarding corneal irregularity and assists the quantitative and qualitative analysis of astigmatism.

The CAVK is also capable of producing an average curvature value for the whole cornea, not unlike a keratometry reading. However, these simulated keratometry values are a best-fit compromise. As the various commercially available CAVK devices establish these values using varied proprietary methods, variability between values can exist and render standardization difficult.

# SURGICAL TREATMENT OF ASTIGMATISM

Most excimer lasers in use today possess the ability to treat myopic, hyperopic and mixed astigmatism by LASIK, LASEK, and PRK up to a maximum ranging from 4.00 to 6.00 D.[13] The pattern of ablation application has varied widely with previous and current methods including scanning spots or slits, ablatable masks, expanding blades, rotating slits, and rotating masks.[13]

## Refraction and Wavefront Versus Topography and Keratometry

Situations where corneal and optical astigmatism precisely coincide are relatively uncomplicated to treat surgically by LASIK, LASEK, or PRK. In reality, individuals commonly display some variance between the refractive and corneal astigmatism parameters.

Upon first consideration, it seems feasible to achieve a plano spherical and astigmatism result by targeting either a spherical corneal shape or manifest refraction. However, when differences exist between these 2 parameters, either in their magnitude, orientation, or both, there will be some remaining astigmatism within the optical system of the eye following surgical treatment. This astigmatism will exist entirely on the cornea or the resultant manifest refraction depending on the initial emphasis for correction by the astigmatism treatment. Either way, there is the possibility that such a surgical approach at either extreme could create an inferior functioning optical system and lead to a poorer quality of vision.

For example, many think that if the aim of refractive surgery is to reduce or eliminate the requirement for spectacle correction, then the corneal ablation—for both the spherical and cylindrical components—should be solely defined by the manifest refraction. Disregarding the initial corneal shape means that there is the potential to leave excessive levels of corneal astigmatism remaining[5,6,7] and the chance of reduced quality of vision secondary to an increase in aberrations such as spherical aberration[14] or lower order astigmatism.

Conversely, an ablation guided entirely by topography, with the intention of generating a spherical anterior corneal surface, could potentially leave residual manifest refractive error from the other internal refracting surfaces of the eye.

The advent of wavefront analysis devices has added an additional dimension to consider when treating astigmatism. Much of today's research efforts have been placed on the development of customized corneal ablations to correct higher order aberrations. The majority of conventional ablations correct the lower order aberrations of blur and defocus by altering the natural prolate shape of the cornea. It is widely documented that the resulting postoperative oblate corneal shape may give rise to an increase in higher order monochromatic aberrations such as coma and spherical aberration, particularly under scotopic conditions.[15-18] This can subsequently lead to a decline in postoperative visual performance.

By evaluating these aberrations and applying individual customized treatments to the corneal surface, an increase in visual performance may result. In other words, all aberrations regardless of their origin—be they corneal, lenticular or retinal—would be compensated for on the anterior corneal surface. This theory, however, places little importance on the impact of any induced irregularity that could result from correcting all these aberrations on the corneal surface alone.[12]

There is some concern that the healing characteristics of the cornea, particularly the corneal epithelium, may negate the correction accomplished with wavefront ablations by reducing or masking its effectiveness.[19] Furthermore, the biomechanical and healing effects of the cornea following wavefront-guided treatments are yet to be determined or nomograms developed,[20] which could potentially improve visual results while reducing induced aberrations.[21] It is also likely that the aberrations within an optical system are not static[22] but may in fact be dynamically changing over time. These alterations can occur in the crystalline lens with age[12] and accommodation,[22] or via the nonoptical components of the visual system (ie, the cerebral integration of images).[12]

Consequently, in order to effectively treat astigmatism as part of the overall spherocylindrical correction, there is merit in considering both corneal and optical astigmatism components to formulate an integrated treatment strategy. Wavefront data adds another dimension to this treatment strategy and can be considered in conjunction with the parallel technology of corneal topography,[12,20] and integrated using vector planning for the ultimate determination of surgical astigmatic treatments.[12]

In an attempt to perform successful astigmatism surgery it is important to consider:
1. Optimizing surgical treatments according to prevailing corneal and optical parameters[6]
2. Targeting less overall corneal astigmatism by orientating the maximum ablation closer to the principal corneal meridian
3. Conducting valid analyses of astigmatic results using both corneal and refractive measurements. This is accomplished by predetermining the target values for the treatment of astigmatism[5-7]

## Vector Planning

The analytical approach of vector planning[5] provides a technique of implementing these objectives by incorporating each patient's unique corneal and refractive parameters in a customized treatment plan.

As astigmatism is described both by magnitude and direction, the mathematical approach of vectors can be used to assist the surgeon design astigmatic corrections with an associated spherical component. The basic principal of vector analysis assists the development of customized treatment plans by integrating corneal astigmatism and refractive astigmatism values. With the assistance of vectors, treatment parameters can be calculated and determined for the "maximal treatment" of astigmatism by complete elimination of refractive astigmatism (100% refraction), topographic astigmatism (100% topographic), or any combination of both

that totals 100% and leaves the minimum possible remaining.

## The Optimal Result

The optimal result of any given customized eye treatment can be determined by employing the following principles:[5,6]
1. Less astigmatism remaining is preferable to more
2. When remaining astigmatism is unavoidable after correction, then a WTR orientation for distance vision is more favorable to an ATR orientation

With the steepest meridian lying vertically, a WTR orientation places the clearest retinal image along this vertical orientation. This is likely to be associated with an increase in visual acuity with vertical strokes dominating the English alphabet.[23] It is probable that any oblique orientation would be least favorable.[6]

# VECTOR PLANNING PARADIGM: AN EXAMPLE

The ASSORT program treatment-planning module (ASSORT Pty Ltd, Australia) is used to illustrate the steps required in the calculation of surgical parameters for the symmetric and orthogonal treatment of astigmatism. This example shows small magnitude changes in conjunction with a minor astigmatism treatment but effectively represents the principles involved in vector planning (Figure 1-5).

## Ocular Residual Astigmatism

The vectorial value of ocular residual astigmatism (ORA) refers to the discrepancy that exists between the corneal and refractive astigmatism at the corneal plane. In other words, in cases where a discrepancy exists between corneal and refractive astigmatism, then the ORA represents the amount of astigmatism that cannot be eliminated from the optical system following the photorefractive treatment of astigmatism.[6] The best theoretical outcome or the maximal reduction in astigmatism possible following surgery occurs when the astigmatism remaining is equivalent to the ORA.[5] The astigmatism remaining can be refractive, topographic or any combination of both parameters. By using vector planning to determine the treatment, the surgeon has the ability to chose the proportion of any of the ORA remaining in the theoretical refraction, while reducing the targeted corneal astigmatism.[6]

## Planning the Treatment Using Surgical Vectors

The values of measured preoperative refractive and corneal astigmatism are used to generate the optimized treatment plan. Figure 1-6 shows the simulated keratometry val-

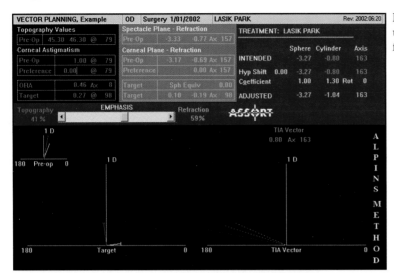

**Figure 1-5.** ASSORT treatment planning module. This example displays an optimized plan for the treatment of astigmatism.

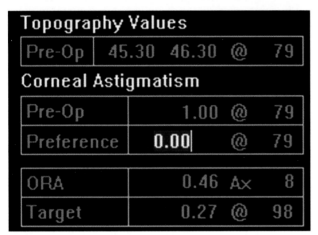

**Figure 1-6.** Topography: preoperative measurements and postoperative goals. As seen in Figure 1-5, the top left-hand side of the ASSORT screen shows the pre-operative corneal astigmatism extracted from the corneal topography, the preferred spherical outcome, the ORA, and the target corneal values.

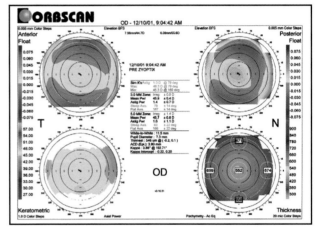

**Figure 1-7.** Vector-planning example: preoperative topography data. This Orbscan (Bausch & Lomb, Rochester, NY) indicates the preoperative corneal topography illustrated in the vector-planning example.

ues as determined by topography (Figure 1-7), the preference for remaining corneal astigmatism and target values. Figure 1-8 displays the refractive values, preferences, and targets as determined by manifest refraction or a wavefront analysis device (Figure 1-9). The preoperative refraction data is converted to the corneal plane for planning and analytical purposes. The facility also allows for a nonzero spherical equivalent to be targeted postoperatively.

A polar display of these preoperative measurements is displayed in Figure 1-10, the preoperative astigmatism for topography (dark blue line) of +1.00 D at a meridian of 79 degrees and refractive astigmatism of +0.69 D at 67 degrees being the power axis of the negative cylinder (light blue line).

## Determining Surgical Emphasis

The surgical emphasis bar defines the relative treatment preferences for a spherical cornea, spherical refraction, or any treatment at an intermediate point to these extremes. This adjustment apportions the ORA that is to be corrected in the corneal and refractive modalities.

### 100% CORRECTION OF REFRACTIVE ASTIGMATISM

Although, a spherical refraction will be achieved at this treatment emphasis, the topographic target will be at its maximum level and equivalent to the ORA but at 90 degrees to it in order to neutralize it. In this case, +0.46 D at a meridian of 98 degrees (Figure 1-11).

### 100% CORRECTION OF CORNEAL ASTIGMATISM

Despite a spherical equivalent of zero and a resultant spherical cornea, such treatment emphasis will result in a

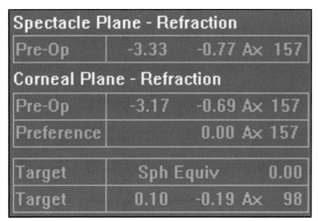

| Spectacle Plane - Refraction | | |
|---|---|---|
| Pre-Op | -3.33 | -0.77 Ax 157 |
| **Corneal Plane - Refraction** | | |
| Pre-Op | -3.17 | -0.69 Ax 157 |
| Preference | | 0.00 Ax 157 |
| Target | Sph Equiv | 0.00 |
| Target | 0.10 | -0.19 Ax 98 |

**Figure 1-8.** Refraction: preoperative measurements and postoperative goals. As displayed in Figure 1-5, the central top section of the ASSORT screen shows the preoperative refraction data converted from the spectacle to the corneal plane, as determined by the wavefront analysis device. It also displays the preferred refractive astigmatism outcome, the target spherical equivalent, and the calculated target refractive (spherical and cylindrical) values for the proposed treatment.

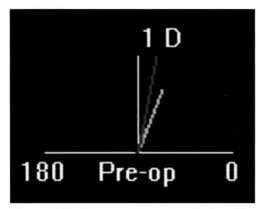

**Figure 1-10.** Preoperative polar display. The polar display of preoperative corneal astigmatism (dark blue line) and refractive astigmatism (light blue line) at the power axis of negative cylinder values

refractive target of sphere +0.23 D, cylinder -0.46 D, and axis 98 degrees (Figure 1-12).

THE OPTIMAL RESULT

A treatment emphasis of 41% corneal astigmatism and 59% refractive astigmatism provides a surgical balance of the 2 targeted zero-astigmatism goals. The resultant topographic target is +0.27 D at a meridian of 98 degrees and a refraction target of sphere +0.10 D, cylinder -0.19 D at an axis of 90 degrees (Figure 1-13).

*Target Induced Astigmatism Vector*

The target induced astigmatism vector (TIA) describes the amount and orientation of dioptric steepening force

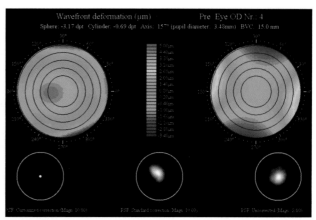

**Figure 1-9.** Vector planning example: preoperative refraction data. This figure exhibits the preoperative spherocylindrical error and point-spread function as determined by a wavefront analysis device.

required to achieve a desired astigmatic goal. Its axis coincides with the meridian of maximum ablation and relative steepening effect. Figure 1-14 shows the TIA necessary to achieve the astigmatic results targeted in Figure 1-13. To achieve a zero-refractive astigmatism target (light blue line) a TIA of 0.69 D Ax 157 would be required. Conversely, a TIA of 1.00 D Ax 169 is required to achieve a zero topographic target (dark blue line). The green line displays the TIA required to achieve the proposed astigmatic treatment that lies at an intermediate point between the corneal and refractive extremes. The magnitude of the astigmatic treatment is 0.80 D at a maximum ablation meridian of 163 degrees.

The maximum correction of astigmatism is achieved at all positions of treatment emphasis (0% to 100%) using this method of vector planning. Any remaining topographic or refractive astigmatism is at a minimum and orientated at 90 degrees to each other, when their sum is equivalent to the ORA.

Where possible, excessive corneal astigmatism (above 0.75 D) should be avoided by moving the emphasis left towards the full topography correction. Moving the maximum treatment closer to the principal flat corneal meridian can assist in minimizing lower order aberrations. In instances where the ORA is in excess of 1.50 D, due to larger differences between corneal and refractive values, it is advisable to share this load between the cornea and refraction by placing the emphasis at the midpoint (50%). A recent study showed that 33% of eyes have an ORA greater than 1.00 D, and 7% have an ORA greater than the preoperative astigmatism therefore resulting in an increase in corneal astigmatism postoperatively if refractive treatment parameters are used exclusively.[5]

*Determination of Treatment*

The treatment required to achieve the desired corneal and refraction targets is displayed by the ASSORT nomogram

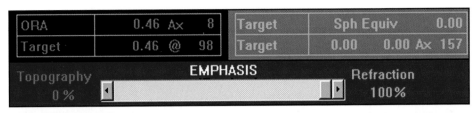

**Figure 1-11.** Surgical emphasis: 100% correction of refractive astigmatism.

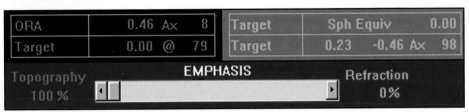

**Figure 1-12.** Surgical emphasis: 100% correction of topographic astigmatism.

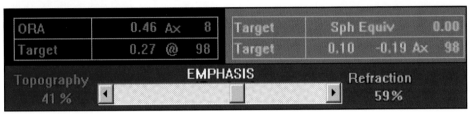

**Figure 1-13.** Surgical emphasis: optimal result with minimum astigmatism remaining.

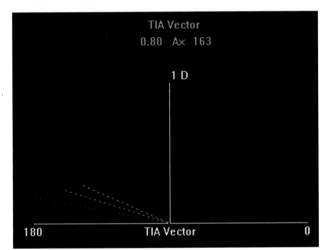

**Figure 1-14.** TIA polar diagram: optimal result. The treatment (TIA) vector (light green) applied to this eye lies between the treatment required to sphericize the refraction (light blue) or to sphericize the cornea (dark blue). In this example, the TIA lies closer to the refractive astigmatism correction line.

**TREATMENT: LASIK PARK**

|  |  | Sphere | Cylinder | Axis |
|---|---|---|---|---|
| INTENDED |  | -3.27 | -0.80 | 163 |
| Hyp Shift | 0.00 | -3.27 | -0.80 | 163 |
| Coefficient |  | 1.00 | 1.30 Rot | 0 |
| ADJUSTED |  | -3.27 | -1.04 | 163 |

**Figure 1-15.** Treatment. The intended treatment at the corneal plane comprises the spherical treatment required to achieve a zero spherical equivalent and the astigmatism treatment (TIA). The adjusted treatment, which will be applied to the cornea, has been modified for any spherical shifts or spherical and astigmatic nomogram adjustments.

adjustment table (Figure 1-15). The intended treatment should be mathematically adjusted according to the laser type used for the ablation, its manufacturers recommendations or the surgeon's previous experience and other prevailing conditions.

Following allowances for spherical shifts as a consequence of astigmatism changes, and nomogram adjustment for under- or overcorrection, an adjusted treatment appears detailing the corneal plane treatment plan. In this example, the nomogram adjustments, based on past experience, allow for a full correction of sphere and 30% of commonly found astigmatic undercorrection.

By using this approach of targeting less overall resultant corneal astigmatism, the optimization process can provide an advantageous surgical outcome without increasing the resultant refractive astigmatism present.

## ANALYSIS OF ASTIGMATIC OUTCOMES

Examination of surgical outcomes following treatments for astigmatism is an essential step in ascertaining the success of individual treatments and for the further development and refinement of treatment nomograms.[5] Fine adjustments in surgical nomograms may be necessary for under and overcorrections of sphere and cylinder and for the associated spherical shifts that accompany astigmatic treatments. Such surgical technique or systematic laser errors can be determined from the analysis of aggregate data.[7]

## Concepts and Terms of Analysis

The effectiveness of astigmatism surgery can be determined from the relationships between 3 fundamental vector quantities—the TIA, surgically induced astigmatism vector (SIA) and the difference vector (DV).[6,7]

The TIA, as mentioned previously, is the astigmatic change (magnitude and orientation) intended from surgery. The SIA, reflects the magnitude and orientation of corneal steepening that has been induced by surgery. When the SIA equals the TIA in both magnitude and orientation, the surgical astigmatic goal has been achieved. In cases where this has not been accomplished, the DV represents the astigmatic change that would be required to allow the initial surgery to achieve its target.[6,7]

The effectiveness of the astigmatic treatment can be gauged by comparing individual vector relationships to the TIA. The index of success (IOS) is a relative measurement of success that relates the magnitude of the difference vector to the magnitude of the TIA. Ideally, the IOS is zero. The correction index (CI) is the ratio of the SIA to the TIA. In situations where the CI is greater than 1.0, an overcorrection has occurred, whereas, a CI less than 1.0 indicates that an undercorrection has resulted. The inverse of the CI is the coefficient of adjustment (CA). When resolved from aggregate analysis, the CA can be used to gauge if any modifications to the surgical nomograms are required.[6,7]

Furthermore, arithmetic differences between the SIA and TIA can be calculated. The magnitude of error (ME) is the discrepancy between the magnitude of the SIA and the TIA. A positive ME indicates an overcorrection, while a negative ME an undercorrection. The angle of error (AE) quantifies the difference between the angle of the achieved correction compared to the angle of the intended correction. A positive AE implies that the achieved correction falls on an axis counterclockwise to the intended orientation while conversely, a negative AE denotes an achieved correction in clockwise orientation from that which was intended.

## Single Patient Analysis: An Example

It is valuable to perform parallel analysis of astigmatism outcomes, using all measurement methods. This assists the establishment of valid trends of relative success, error, and adjustment so the effectiveness of the astigmatic procedure can be analyzed in detail. This is particularly useful in comparing aggregate outcomes and in calculating retreatment parameters.

Postoperative results are shown by topography (Figure 1-16) and wavefront analysis (Figure 1-17). The corresponding corneal and refractive analyses for this individual data are calculated at the corneal plane using the ASSORT outcomes analysis program as displayed in Figures 1-18 and 1-19 respectively.

The treatment used in this example was determined with a surgical emphasis of 100% refraction, in order to achieve a plano refraction. That is, the astigmatic treatment TIA is 0.69 x 157 intending to induce 0.69-D steepening along the 157 degree corneal meridian to achieve a refractive astigmatic target of 0.00 D. The corneal target under these circumstances is 0.46 D at 98 degrees changed from a preoperative value of 1.00D at 79 degrees. From the resultant pre- and postoperative data the SIA can be determined. This vectorial change between these astigmatism values is 0.31 D (corneal) and 0.39 D (refractive).

The analysis display generated using the ASSORT program contains 3 graphical representations while the tabulated data within Figures 1-18 and 1-19 shows the AE, ME, CI, and IOS. Refractive and corneal analysis both show that there has been an undercorrection of astigmatism. This is evidenced in the CI values of 0.56 for refraction and 0.45 for topography. Although refractive data indicates that the treatment was 26 degrees off axis, the comparative topographic data shows a smaller 5-degree angle of error. The IOS for both data sets demonstrates that an improvement in astigmatism status was achieved.

# IRREGULAR ASTIGMATISM

The development of highly sophisticated diagnostic equipment, including CAVK and wavefront aberrometry analysis devices, has highlighted a higher prevalence of corneal irregularity existing within the population. Even individuals with otherwise "normal" eyes may exhibit some degree of irregularity.[3]

In addition to differences between refractive and corneal astigmatism, irregularity may exist across the corneal hemidivision either as a difference in dioptric magnitude (asymmetry) or orientation (nonorthogonal) or both.[2] The vectorial value of TD is a valuable tool for quantifying corneal irregularity. Topographic disparity represents the dioptric separation between the 2 corneal hemidivisions as displayed on a 720-degree double-angle vector diagram (DAVD). Significant irregularity is present cases where the TD is greater than 1.00 D and occurs in approximately 44% of eyes with treatable astigmatism.[2,3]

The theory behind vector planning can be applied with increased complexity to predetermine separate surgical plans and unique TIAs for each hemidivision. Despite the treatment options for irregular astigmatism having expanded with the advent of tailored corneal excimer laser ablations,

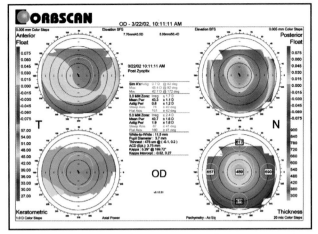

**Figure 1-16.** Vector planning example: postoperative topography data. This postoperative topography result is analyzed as part of the vector-planning example.

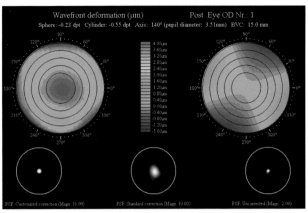

**Figure 1-17.** Vector planning example: postoperative refraction data. The refraction data for analysis has been determined from postoperative wavefront analysis.

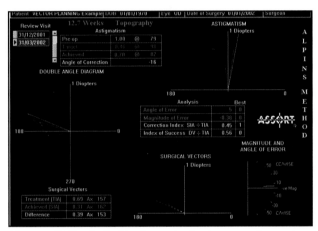

**Figure 1-18.** Individual analysis topography using ASSORT and the Alpins' method.

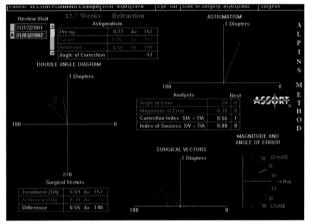

**Figure 1-19.** Individual analysis refraction using ASSORT and the Alpins method.

the patterns required for customized asymmetrical toric ablations are not yet readily available. The challenge exists to apply different treatments over 2 corneal hemidivisions while maintaining a smooth transitional zone over this ablated surface.[3]

Such asymmetrical treatments can be applied with the aim of[2,3]:

1. Reducing or rearranging the existing astigmatism

2. That is, the least favorable corneal meridian may be rotated toward the more favorable meridian to obtain alignment topographically. Alternatively this may be achieved by changing both in opposite cyclical directions without necessarily needing to alter the overall refractive state

3. Reducing the magnitude of remaining astigmatism and its meridian

4. Providing a combination of the above-listed objectives to obtain the minimum amount of regular astigmatism remaining

The ability to treat irregular astigmatism in such a way provides the potential to improve both best-corrected and unaided visual acuities while significantly enhancing overall visual performance.[2,3]

# CONCLUSION

It is important to consider and address differences between corneal shape and function to maximize the visual potential of the eye's optical system and improve visual results after photorefractive surgery. These differences in astigmatic status may occur between manifest refraction and keratometry or wavefront analysis and corneal topography or all of these. Therefore, addressing this conflict using vector planning may provide a method of developing improved customized treatment plans. Furthermore, the analysis of astigmatism results using vector analysis can help surgeons compare outcomes and develop more accurate nomograms for the effective treatment of astigmatism.

## ACKNOWLEDGMENTS

The authors wish to thank Drs. Peter Heiner and Darryl Gregor for permission to use their patient's Orbscan (Orbscan, Bausch & Lomb, Rochester, NY) and Wavefront data.

## REFERENCES

1. Alpins NA, Tabin GC, Taylor HR. Photoastigmatic refractive keratectomy (PARK). In: McGhee CNJ, Taylor HR, Gartry DS, Trokel SL, eds. *Excimer Lasers in Ophthalmology.* London: Martin Dunitz Ltd; 1997:243-259.

2. Alpins NA. Treatment of irregular astigmatism. *J Cataract Refract Surg.* 1998;24:634-646.

3. Goggin M, Alpins N, Schmid LM. Management of irregular astigmatism. *Curr Opin Ophthalmol.* 2000;11:260-266.

4. Duke-Elder S, ed. *System of Ophthalmology.* Vol 5. *Ophthalmic Optic and Refraction.* St Louis, Mo: Mosby; 1970;275-278.

5. Alpins NA. New method of targeting vectors to treat astigmatism. *J Cataract Refract Surg.* 1997;23:65-75.

6. Alpins NA. A new method of analyzing vectors for changes in astigmatism. *J Cataract Refract Surg.* 1993;19:524-533.

7. Alpins NA Astigmatism analysis by the Alpins method. *J Cataract Refract Surg.* 2001;27:31-49.

8. Seiler T, Mrochen M, Kaemmerer M. Operative correction of ocular aberrations to improve visual acuity. *J Refract Surg.* 2000;16:S619-S622.

9. Krueger, RR. Technology requirements for Summit-Autonomous CustomCornea. *J Refract Surg.* 2000;16:S592-S601.

10. Miller DT. Retinal imaging and vision at the frontiers of adaptive optics. *Physics Today.* 2000:31-36.

11. Harmam H. A quick method for analyzing Hartmann-Shack patterns: application to refractive surgery. *J Refract Surg.* 2000;16:S636-S642.

12. Alpins NA. Special article. Wavefront technology: a new advance that fails to answer old questions on corneal vs refractive astigmatism correction. *J Refract Surg.* 2002;18:737-739.

13. Wu H. Astigmatism and LASIK. *Curr Opin Ophthalmol.* 2002;3:250-255.

14. Seiler T, Reckman, Maloney R. Effective spherical aberration of the cornea as a quantitative descriptor in corneal topography. *J Cataract Refract Surg.* 1993;15:155-65.

15. Mrochen M, Kaemmerer M, Seiler T. Clinical results of wavefront-guided laser in situ keratomileusis 3 months after surgery. *J Cataract Refract Surg.* 2001;27:201-207.

16. Holladay J, Dudeja D, Chang J. Functional vision and corneal changes after laser in situ keratomileusis determined by contrast sensitivity, glare testing, and corneal topography. *J Cataract Refract Surg.* 1999;25:663-669.

17. Oshika T, Mijata K, Tokunaga T, et al. Higher order wavefront aberrations of cornea and magnitude of refractive correction in laser in situ keratomileusis. *Ophthalmology.* 2002;109:1154-1158.

18. Oshika T, Klyce SD, Applegate RA, Howland HC, El Danasaury MA. Comparision of corneal wavefront aberration after photorefractive keratectomy and laser in situ keratomileusis. *Am J Ophthalmol.* 1999;127:1-7.

19. Seiler T, Mrochen M, Kaemmerer M. Operative correction of ocular aberrations to improve visual acuity. *J Refract Surg.* 2000;16:S619-S622.

20. Schwiergerling J, Snyder R, Lee J. Wavefront and topography: keratome-induced corneal changes demonstrate that both are needed for custom ablations. *J Refract Surg.* 2002;18:S584-S588.

21. Roberts C. Biomechanics of the cornea and wavefront-guided laser refractive surgery. *J Refract Surg.* 2002;18:S589-S592.

22. Artal P, Fernandez EJ, Manzanera S. Are optical aberrations during accommodation a significant problem for refractive surgery? *J Refract Surg.* 2002;18:S563-S566.

23. Eggers H. Estimation of uncorrected visual acuity in malingerers. *Arch Ophthalmol.* 1945;33:23-27.

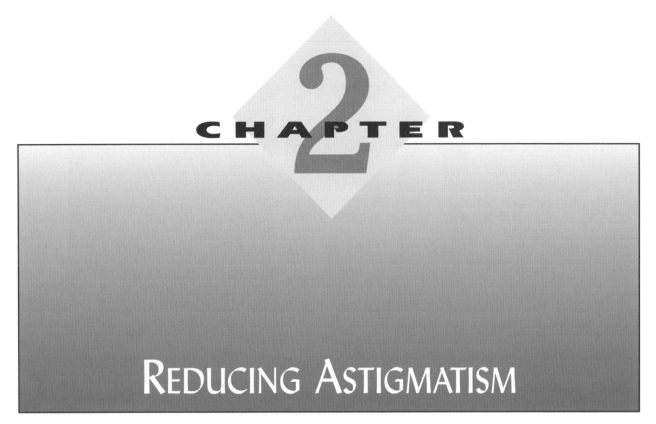

# CHAPTER 2

# REDUCING ASTIGMATISM

*R. Bruce Wallace III, MD, FACS*

## REDUCING ASTIGMATISM

To become less dependent on glasses after implanting an IOL, especially a multifocal lens, astigmatism must be reduced.[1] Fortunately, the surgical correction of corneal astigmatism has been improving and has been rapidly gaining popularity. Today, many patients become relatively astigmatism-free thanks to these new remedies.

## ASTIGMATISM IN THREE DIMENSIONS

In order to reduce unwanted astigmatism, the surgeon must lead the way in their practice to develop a systematic approach to surgical correction. Reducing astigmatism begins with effective preoperative assessment. Most cataract surgeons depend on trained technicians to perform preoperative astigmatism measurements, which include refraction, keratometry, and videokeratography, or corneal topography. Unfortunately, most technicians do not think about astigmatism in 3-D because these measurements only generate numbers or 2-D color maps. For technicians and surgeons to be effective in astigmatism control, it is helpful to understand and visualize astigmatism, especially corneal astigma-

tism, in 3-D. Such terms as the *flat axis*, the *steep axis*, and *coupling* become easier to grasp when thinking of corneal shapes rather than numbers or colors.

To determine if your office staff perceives astigmatism in 3-D, try this experiment. Ask your best-trained technicians to imagine that the oblong curvatures of an American football represent the astigmatic corneal surfaces of a patient's eye with the curvature in 1 axis steep, the other flat. Imagine that the football is lying flat on the ground. Would that resemble WTR or ATR astigmatism? If he or she answers WTR, he or she is correct and is probably thinking about astigmatism in 3-D (unless they are just good guessers). With this fundamental understanding of what the term "regular astigmatism" means, all members of the surgical team will find astigmatism correction easier to understand.

## SURGICAL PLANNING

The goal for astigmatism control should be the creation of a resultant cylinder of less than 1.00 D at any axis. Most patients enjoy good unaided visual acuity with this degree of astigmatism. Some studies suggest a benefit to leaving some amount of residual ATR cylinder so that uncorrected near vision after cataract surgery is improved. However, surgical practices utilizing multifocal IOLs and/or monovision will not find this to be an advantage because of the compromise of the loss of distance visual acuity with amounts over 1.00 D of cylinder.

One of the more challenging tasks that the surgeon faces is deciding which astigmatic preoperative measurements should be used when planning a surgical correction. Do we depend on the cylinder diopters and axis from the refraction, the keratometry or do we always need to perform corneal topography? One study showed the frequency of poor correlation of all 3 methods of measurement, especially with less than 2.00 D of astigmatism. Fortunately, unlike correction of spherical refractive errors, astigmatism correction is more forgiving, especially when treating moderate to low levels.

One way to plan surgical correction of astigmatism is to initially assess the refraction and the keratometry simultaneously. If good correlation exists as to the amount of cylinder and axis, the surgical planning for astigmatism correction during cataract surgery is fairly straightforward. If, however, there is poor correlation (even though keratometry should be more reliable) surgical correction can be less predictable, even with corneal topography. This is where the "art" of astigmatism correction applies. The surgeon needs to also judge the relative reliability of the astigmatic information. If after careful consideration, there is doubt as to a reasonable surgical plan, the astigmatism correction should be postponed until after cataract surgery and an adequate time for wound healing.

After years of placing phacoemulsification incisions on-axis, I have abandoned this use simply because temporal phacoemulsification incisions have so many advantages over incisions placed elsewhere on the cornea. LRIs have now become a mainstay of my practice, thanks to some of the early pioneers such as Dr. Stephen Hollis and Dr. James Gills. Induced astigmatism from my phaco incision is 0.50 D or less. If I did not perform corneal astigmatic surgery when using the multifocal lenses available today, I would encounter troublesome astigmatism in approximately one-third of these patients. My current nomogram leans heavily toward 1 LRI due to the relative safety and to what I have found to be long-term benefits of 1 incision. *Coupling* is a term that helps us to understand the aftereffects of these procedures and what it might do to the spherical equivalent postoperatively. A one-to-one steepening-flattening resulting from an LRI incision might not influence the K value and therefore the IOL calculation for most patients. However, longer incisions might induce an RK effect and the surgeon may need to increase the IOL power in order to achieve a good spherical result. Therefore, it is important to document the long-term effect on the spherical equivalent. Hoffer found a 0.175-D steepening of the cornea 1 year after 2.5 mm clear corneal oblique phaco incisions. Surgeons are encouraged to continue to assess the long-term astigmatic effects of their phacoemulsification incisions and astigmatic

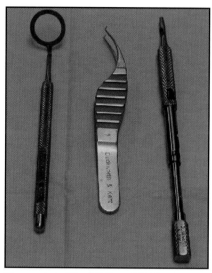

**Figure 2-1.** The Wallace LRI kit manufactured by Duckworth and Kent.

procedures and look for any need to adjust their future procedures to compensate for any unexpected late changes in the final refractive result.

## SURGICAL TECHNIQUE

I like the utilization of an LRI kit. This allows the surgeon to sterilize LRI instruments separately from their standard phaco instruments and call for this kit when LRIs are indicated. My preferred instrumentation at this time is the Wallace LRI Kit (Figure 2-1), manufactured by Duckworth and Kent (Hertfordhire, United Kingdom). This kit includes a preset 600-μm diamond knife with a tri-facet tip and titanium hand-piece. The value of the tri-facet tip is that it is less likely to dull after many uses. The diamond knife has a single footplate that, when placed posteriorly, allows the surgeon to visualize the diamond as it passes through corneal tissue. Also included is a Mendez axis marker or gauge. The value of this instrument is that it allows the surgeon to stay oriented because the ring has axis numbers and when the insertion of the handle into the ring is placed at the lateral canthus, these numbers are a helpful reference for axis location (Figure 2-2). The kit also includes a 0.12-mm forceps, which is used to mark the axis as well as the intended incision sites and is used to fixate the globe while the knife passes through corneal tissue (Figure 2-3). I pass the diamond knife 1.0 mm to 1.5 mm from the true limbus in clear corneal tissue so these procedures are really peripheral corneal incisions and not LRIs.

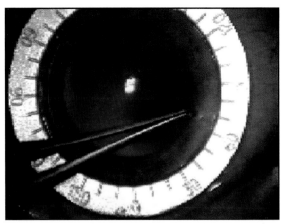

**Figure 2-2.** Mendez marker on eye with 0.12-mm forceps marking the axis.

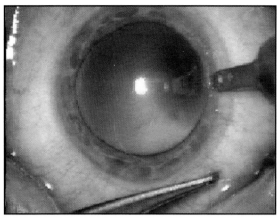

**Figure 2-3.** A preset 600-μm diamond knife used to cut the corneal arc.

## LRI Postoperation

We prescribe antibiotic and anti-inflammatory medications used for standard cataract surgery and typically add a topical NSAID such as Acular PF (Allergan, Irvine, Calif) or Voltaren (CIBA Vision, Duluth, Ga) QID for 3 days after these procedures. We also follow our astigmatic outcomes on a regular basis by measuring the actual amount of refractive cylinder at any axis. Our theory is that if a patient has less than 1.00 D at any axis, this will be considered a good refractive result. It also encourages us to keep score and continue to attempt to improve our results.

## Fine Tuning

Being able to fine tune our results after surgery is an important element in patient satisfaction. Not all patients will have the expected refractive outcome and may require additional astigmatic surgery, either in the surgery center or possibly in the office. Dr. Kurt Buzard now employs slit lamp astigmatic correction for those patients with troublesome residual astigmatism. Dry eye is a common problem after all lens surgery, but is particularly noticeable with multifocal intraocular lens implantation. Many studies are now emerging to show that benzochromium chloride, a common preservative in antibiotics and anti-inflammatory medications, is disruptive to corneal tear film, epithelium, and tear

function. Patients may require topical lubricants for months to years after surgery, especially if they have a previous history of dry eye syndrome. Many of their visual complaints after multifocal lens implantation may stem from an induced dry eye syndrome and not from optical aberrations from the implant.

## Summary

Reducing astigmatism requires a systematic approach, with the surgeon committed to correcting those patients who are expected to have over a diopter of residual astigmatism after surgery. LRIs are an important addition to our surgical approach to refractive cataract surgery and the effective use of multifocal intraocular lenses. If we follow our results, both short-term and long-term, we are likely to continually improve our refractive outcomes and the value we bring to the quality of life of our patients.

## References

1. Knorz M, Kock D, Marinez-Franco C, Lorger C. Effect of pupil size and astigmatism on contrast acuity with monofocal and bifocal intraocular lenses. *J Cataract Refract. Surg.* 1994; 20:26-33.

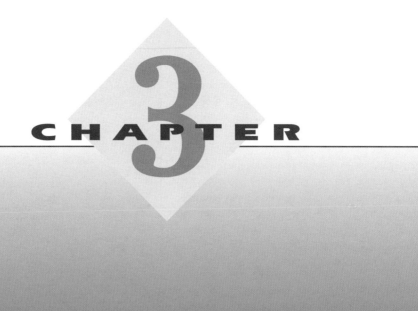

# CHAPTER 3

# TORIC INTRAOCULAR LENSES

*Stephen Bylsma, MD*

With the decree of "emmetropia" as the desired result from cataract surgery over the last decade, the necessity to correct preexisting astigmatism has become paramount. Astigmatic correction at the time of cataract surgery may be broadly categorized into tissue (structural) correction versus optical correction. Examples of structural correction involve changing the physical shape or tissues of the eye, and include the commonly performed procedures of LRIs, arcuate keratectomy, and LASIK. Some of these tissue-directed procedures are limited in the amount of astigmatism they may correct, and all share a dependence on the variable (patient-specific) healing response of the eye following treatment. In contrast, optical correction of astigmatism, as with glasses or contact lenses, is independent of an individual's tissue or healing response. The concept of a toric IOL incorporates both astigmatic and spherical powers directly onto an IOL to produce astigmatic correction that is highly predictable, reproducible, and more independent of the patient's healing response. In this chapter, we will examine how such a toric IOL may be used clinically to achieve the goal of emmetropia during cataract surgery.

Several attempts were made over the last decade at developing a toric IOL, including "custom" toric IOLs of PMMA[1,2] or adjustable silicone.[3] In 1998, a posterior chamber foldable silicone toric IOL (TIOL, Models AA4203-TF and AA4203-TL, STAAR Surgical, Monrovia, Calif) first became widely available following FDA approval of that lens.

The TIOL went on to receive "new technology" designation in the United States in recognition of the unique toric feature that promoted improved uncorrected visual acuity as a direct patient benefit associated with implantation of this IOL. As this model remains the predominant toric IOL available in the most of the world today, this chapter will focus primarily on the use of and results from this particular TIOL.

## TORIC IOL DESIGN

The TIOL is a single-piece plate-haptic IOL design for implantation into the lens capsule following successful phacoemulsification (Figure 3-1). The TIOL is made of first-generation silicone with a 6.0-mm optic and an overall length of either 10.8 mm (model AA4203TF, from 21.50 D to 30.50 D spherical equivalent power) or 11.2 mm (model AA4203TL, from 9.50-D to 23.50-D spherical equivalent power). Both models are available in 2 distinct toric powers: +2.00 D and +3.50 D. The recommended A-constant is for calculating the spherical equivalent power is 118.5 with an anterior chamber depth of 5.26. Two fenestration holes of 1.5 mm each are intended to promote early and long-term capsular adhesion and are found on the plate-haptic. The toric power resides on the anterior surface of the optic with the toric axis in line with the long axis of the plate-haptic of the TIOL. The TIOL is packaged with the toric surface facing up so that position of the toric surface is known. According to labeling that accompanies the TIOL, the anterior (toric) surface is intended for implantation facing the anterior capsule; as we will see, the TIOL may be intentionally reversed with the toric surface in contact with the posterior capsule. Regardless of anterior/posterior position, *the TIOL is a plus-cylinder lens* and is intended to be aligned along the steep keratometric axis, as would any plus-cylinder lens in spectacles. The TIOL is injected with a plunger and cartridge system that protects the lens from contacting extraocular tissue and fluids and enables reliable implantation through a 3.0-mm incision.

## PREOPERATIVE CONSIDERATIONS

Numerous issues are unique to the process of calculating the proper TIOL to use for each patient. The difference between TIOL models, toric powers, spherical equivalent (SE) powers, axis of alignment, and desired postoperative refraction must all be understood. Several steps specific to TIOL power calculation should be clarified.

The TIOL is available in SE powers from 9.50 to 30.50 D, and each SE power is available in 2 distinct toric powers (+2.00 and +3.50 D). It is critical to understand that calculating the TIOL SE power is no different from the usual IOL calculation used for nontoric (spherical) IOLs. Baseline data from axial length, keratometry, A-constant, and desired postoperative refraction are entered into the surgeon's preferred IOL calculation formula, and the result is a suggested IOL power. The process is the same for the TIOL calculation, and the result of the calculation suggests the specific TIOL SE power to use. So, for example, if the formula yields a suggested IOL power of 22.00 D to yield plano for a given eye, then the TIOL power to select would be 22.00 D. Although one must next select either the +2.00 D or the +3.50 D toric power for that 22.0 D TIOL, no specific change to the calculations are needed to arrive at the initial choice of the 22.00 D TIOL.

Having selected a 22.00 D TIOL for this hypothetical case, the next step is to select the toric power to use for that specific eye. For this, we turn to the keratometry. It is important to remember that following lens extraction, the only refractive element remaining is the cornea. Preexisting lenticular astigmatism will be gone. Therefore, it is the keratometry that determines which toric power to select as well as the proper axis of alignment of the TIOL.

It is also important to understand that the TIOL and the cornea are at different distances from the nodal point of the eye, so there is not a 1:1 correction between toric power and keratometry. When aligned in the proper meridian, the +2.00 D TIOL will correct 1.40 D of keratometric astigmatism (at the corneal plane), and the +3.50 D TIOL will correct 2.30 D of cylinder at the corneal plane. Initial recom-

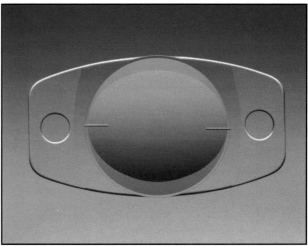

**Figure 3-1.** The toric IOL ( TIOL).

mendations are to use the +2.00 D toric power between 1.40 to 2.20 D of preoperative keratometric astigmatism, and use the +3.50 D toric power when the keratometry shows greater than 2.20 D of astigmatism. As we will see, these values change slightly if the optic is implanted in a reverse position.

If we return to the eye requiring the 22.00 D TIOL, and if we assume the keratometry showed 1.75 D of corneal asymmetry, then we would select the +2.00 toric power. As a result, our final IOL selection would be for the 22.00/+2.00 TIOL. If the 22.0/+3.50 D TIOL were chosen, an undesirable result would occur whereby the cylinder would be overcorrected and the refractive axis would be "flipped" at 90 degrees away from baseline.

Next, the TIOL model must be specified (model -TF vs. -TL), but only if the selected IOL is between 21.50 D and 23.50 D where these models overlap in power. Many surgeons prefer to use the longer -TL whenever possible, as it may be associated with less chance for off-axis rotation in the early postoperative period when compared to the shorter -TF model. For ranges above and below 21.50 to 23.50 D, only one TIOL model is available, and this step is omitted.

The final preoperative determination is to identify and record the intended axis in which to place the TIOL. The TIOL is a plus-cylinder lens, and should be aligned as would any plus cylinder lens to neutralize the keratometric cylinder. Topography is strongly encouraged to verify that the astigmatism is regular and to assist with determination of intended TIOL axis. While this approach may seem simplistic, it is essential to yield a TIOL implanted on the correct axis.

## CLINICAL RESULTS WITH TORIC INTRAOCULAR LENSES

A review of peer-reviewed publications demonstrates both the clinical importance and a potential drawback of using the

## Refractive Effect of Rotation

| Off-Axis Rotation (degrees) | Reduction of Toric Power (%) |
|---|---|
| 0 | 0 |
| 10 | 33 |
| 20 | 67 |
| 30 | 100 |
| >30 | Adds Cyl |

**Figure 3-2.** TIOL refractive power decreases as off-axis rotation increases.

TIOL. Numerous reports cite the efficacy of the TIOL in improving mean postoperative UCVA.[4-13]

Recently, Xiao-Yi and colleagues evaluated 175 eyes and found 84% of eyes in the TIOL group achieved 20/40 UCVA compared to 76% of eyes receiving limbal relaxing incisions with a spherical IOL.[4] In addition, the postoperative refractive cylinder (residual cylinder) was 31% less in the TIOL group than the limbal relaxing incision group. Also in that study, 25% of TIOLs were found to be rotated over 20 degrees off-axis, and 9% were repositioned to achieve improved UCVA.

Similarly, Ruhswurm found a mean reduction of refractive cylinder from 2.70 D preoperatively to 0.80 D postoperatively in 37 eyes, with 19% rotated off-axis up to 25 degrees and no TIOL rotation more than 30 degrees.[10] Likewise, Leyland's group found similar results but observed a greater than 30-degree rotation in 18% of 22 eyes implanted with the TIOL.[8] Numerous other studies are available that document clearly that the TIOL is associated with improved UCVA and reduction of residual cylinder for groups of eyes analyzed, yet individual eyes may undergo rotation of the TIOL with resultant diminution of UCVA that is improved by repositioning of the lens to the proper axis.[4-13]

Thus, the TIOL promotes excellent clinical results when it is aligned properly, but this lens has a consistent drawback that it may be found off-axis in the early postoperative period. While slight misalignment of the TIOL away from the intended corneal axis may mildly reduce the effective toric power, more substantial misalignments may create oblique astigmatism or worsening of preexisting refractive astigmatism.[7] As Figure 3-2 shows, when the TIOL axis is within 10 degrees of keratometric asymmetry, the full refractive power is realized. For off-axis rotations between 10 to 20 degrees, the refractive power of the TIOL is reduced by about one-third, for rotations of 20 to 30 degrees the effective power of the TIOL is reduced by two-thirds, and over 30 degrees the toric power is negated and may even add to preexisting

corneal astigmatism for significant malpositions. Thus, a major challenge to this technology is the stabilization of the TIOL within the capsular bag along the intended axis, as this alignment is critical for the predictable correction of astigmatism.

## STABILIZING THE TIOL AXIS

Very little data is available to identify specific reasons why the TIOL may rotate off axis. The primary reason for off-axis rotations is presumed to be a mismatch between the size of the capsular bag and the TIOL. Individual patients may have larger-than-normal capsular volume may allow the TIOL to rotate within the bag in the first 24 to 48 hours. Such "big bags" are thought to occur in harder, more advanced cataracts where the nucleus has grown significantly or in larger, myopic eyes. Recommendations have been made to avoid using the TIOL in eyes with a white-to-white of greater than 12.5 mm,[11] but the validity of this has not been confirmed in the literature.

A longer -TL model of the TIOL was manufactured in 2000 in the lower power ranges (9.50 to 23.50 D) for use in the larger myopic eyes. This new model measured 11.2 mm in overall length compared to the original -TF model that measures 10.8 mm and is still available in the power range of 21.50 to 30.50 D (spherical equivalent). To date, few reports are available to compare the rotation rate of these different-sized models. However, recent analysis of data from 1 center now suggests a method for stabilizing the TIOL, regardless of model.

## REVERSING THE OPTIC

Analysis of data from this author's center suggests that implanting the TIOL with the toric surface facing the posterior capsule significantly reduces the off-axis rotation rate.

When implanting the TIOL in eyes with "borderline" astigmatism, it is important to avoid overcorrecting the cylinder and "flipping the axis." In my early experience with the TIOL, eyes with 1.20 D to 1.30 D of keratometric cylinder were implanted with the +2.00 D TIOL optic "reversed," and eyes with 2.20 D to 2.30 D of keratometric cylinder were implanted with the +3.50 D TIOL optic reversed. Theoretically, this reversed position should decrease the toric power of the TIOL by about 8%, as the toric surface was then closer to the nodal point of the eye. The observation made upon implantation of the TIOL in "reversed" position was that the lens behaved differently intraoperatively; when rotating the reversed TIOL into final position, the surgeon appreciated significantly more resistance to rotation.

After 1-year experience with the TIOL, and after several off-axis (not reversed) implants required repositioning, all

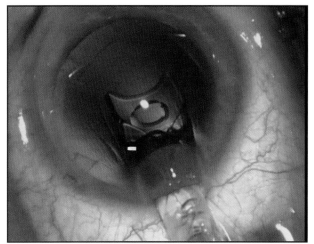

**Figure 3-3.** Implantation of TIOL through 3.0-mm incision.

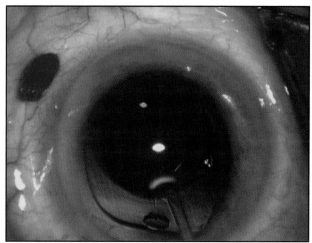

**Figure 3-4.** Placing trailing haptic of TIOL into capsular bag.

TIOLs were implanted in the reversed position (Figures 3-3 to 3-5). One year later, analysis of data was performed (submitted for publication). A retrospective analysis was performed on 171 eyes. Postoperative UCVA and residual refractive cylinder and compared between eyes implanted with the TIOL in the standard vs. reversed position. Surprisingly, a statistically significant increase in the percentage of eyes achieving 20/40 or better UCVA was found for the TIOL in the reversed versus standard position (83% vs. 58% respectively). Also, there was a significantly improved UCVA for the TIOL in the reversed versus standard position (0.60 + 0.18 versus 0.49 + 0.21). Finally, the reverse-TIOL position group showed a significant increase in the percentage of eyes achieving a residual refractive cylinder <0.50 D (56% vs 34%).

Thus, the TIOL in the reversed position was observed to promote improved UCVA and reduction of mean refractive cylinder despite the expectation that the toric power was 8% less in this position. The explanation for this finding was related to stabilization of the TIOL within the capsule: fewer off-axis rotations occurred in the reversed position group, so as a whole, the slight reduction of toric power was less important than the lack of off-axis rotation.

This data should not be misunderstood to suggest that any given TIOL provides more toric power when reversed. On the contrary, there is no doubt that a perfectly aligned TIOL with the toric surface facing the anterior capsule will produce greater astigmatic power than the same lens in the reversed position. The importance of the reversed position is that it stabilizes the TIOL against rotation. Therefore, for a large group of eyes, more standard-position lenses will be off axis, and the mean UCVA for that standard group will be worse than for the reversed group because the reversed group has many more on-axis IOLs. Thus, implantation in the reversed optic position appears to discourage postoperative off-axis rotation of the TIOL.

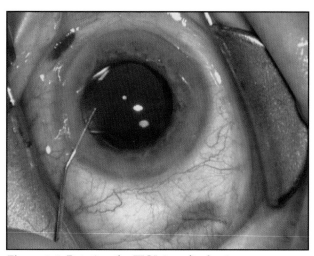

**Figure 3-5.** Rotating the TIOL into final axis.

# MORE SURGICAL PEARLS: ENHANCING RESULTS WITH TIOL

Clinical experience with the TIOL has lead to a greater understanding of how to achieve the best results with this lens. Just as with the observation that the reversed-optic position stabilizes the TIOL against rotation, many other issues have been elucidated over the last 5 years since FDA approval that may enhance consistency and predictability of the TIOL.

The first clinical pearl is to take the time to analyze the surgeon-specific change in keratometry that occurs when using a 3.0-mm CCI. To correct preoperative keratometric astigmatism, we need to accurately predict the postoperative magnitude and axis of corneal astigmatism. While most surgeons may believe their incisions are "astigmatically neutral,"

## Extended Range Nomogram

| K-asymmetry | Toric Power |
|:---:|:---:|
| ≤ 1.1 | 0 |
| 1.2 - 2.1 | +2.0 |
| ≥ 2.2 | +3.5 |

**Figure 3-6.** "Reversed optic" nomogram for selecting TIOL power.

when data is subjected to rigorous evaluation, few surgeons actually achieve such neutrality. One such rigorous program is the "vector plus" program that analyzes the astigmatic changes in vector format. The goal is to better predict how astigmatism will shift for a given patient, and use that knowledge to determine the intended axis of TIOL orientation.

Next, in selecting the TIOL, it is recommended to use the modified "reversed" nomogram (Figure 3-6). For keratometric cylinder, by topography, of less than 1.20 D, do not use the TIOL. For corneal astigmatism of 1.20 to 2.10 D, use the +2.00 D toric power in the reversed position, and for corneal astigmatism above 2.20 D, use the +3.50 D TIOL in the reversed position. Using this nomogram will insure the axis is not overcorrected and will yield the highest likelihood of keeping the TIOL on axis.

With a good understanding of the expected shape of the postoperative cornea and the proper lens chosen, the next issue is to identify the specific axis in which to align the TIOL. Topography is strongly preferred to keratometry in evaluating preoperative astigmatism and expected postoperative astigmatism. Topography will confirm the astigmatism as regular; using the TIOL in the presence of irregular astigmatism may not produce unpredictable results.

Once determined, the desired axis for TIOL alignment must be accurately recorded and conveyed for use in the operating room. While this may seem like a trivial step, mistakes in the recording of the TIOL axis for later use has been a clear source of sporadic errors at some centers. Transcription errors, plus-versus-minus cylinder conversions, misinterpretation of "steep" topographic axis, confusing the TIOL axis of orientation with the TIOL axis of power, and many other oversights may easily produce a TIOL unintentionally implanted on the improper axis. Also, there should be a strict protocol that 3 digits are always used for verbal communication by the staff in the operating room when referring to axis.

An alternate method for evaluating the proper axis does not require preoperative calculations. The use of qualitative keratometry intraoperatively projects uniform rings onto the cornea and allows the surgeon to view the "steep" axis by dis-

tortion of the reflected light. This method has the distinct advantage of simplicity and accuracy; however, if the Ks change postoperatively as the incision heals, there may be some "drift."

When qualitative keratometry is not used, the axis needs to be determined pre- or intraoperatively by some marking mechanism. Many surgeons prefer to mark the eye preoperatively while the patient is upright. This is thought to minimize torsional changes that may occur with the recumbent position or secondary to anesthesia. Other surgeons mark the eye after the patient is draped using a Mendez gauge to identify the proper axis. Regardless of the method used, when using methods other than qualitative keratometry, special attention must be made to the overall head and spine position of the patient.

Another important factor to prevent postoperative rotations is to implant the TIOL as slowly as possible. The author's observation is that if the TIOL is allowed to rapidly "shoot" out of the cartridge, then the TIOL will tend to drift back to that axis where the distal haptic first impacted into the distal capsule (data not shown). While evidence is not yet available to confirm this observation, is seems nonetheless important to allow the TIOL to unfold as slowly as possible.

Of further importance to prevent off-axis rotation is the removal of viscoelastic from the area between the the IOL and the posterior capsule. Such removal allows direct contact between the posterior capsule and the reversed toric surface. The TIOL may then be positioned into the desired axis. This final positioning is best done by alternately "dialing" the TIOL on both sides of the optic. If only 1 side is pushed, the posterior capsule may be distorted, which may tend to rotate the lens back. The best chance to prevent a postoperative rotation is to gently "nestle" the TIOL into final position with light pressure on alternate sides of the optic along the long axis. The final step is to verify the TIOL is still at the desired axis at the conclusion of the surgery.

In cases where the TIOL does rotate off-axis, the lens may be left as is or repositioned. Depending on the patient's tolerance of the malposition, BCVA, degree of anisometropia, amount of aberrations, and desire for the best possible UCVA, leaving the TIOL off axis may be the best course of action. When the off axis TIOL produces symptoms that warrant intervention, the TIOL is best repositioned between 1 to 3 weeks postoperatively. If repositioned earlier, fibrosis of the capsule may not be sufficient to prevent the lens from returning to its original orientation. After 3 weeks, the fibrosis of the capsule may be quite significant, making repositioning more difficult. At 2 weeks, the lens can be gently "rocked" free from capsular adhesions and moved to the desired axis. Rarely will the TIOL move again once repositioned in this fashion. If repositioning of a TIOL is attempted after 1 to 2 months, there may be excessive fibrosis, and the capsule may not allow the TIOL to assume a different axis; these cases are best handled by an IOL exchange for a spherical IOL, with toric correction by spectacles or other means.

Other clinical techniques have employed the TIOL in novel ways. Dr. Gills and others have used either LRIs with the TIOL or 2 TIOLs sutured together in piggyback fashion to correct excessively large amounts of astigmatism.[15-17] Others have combined the TIOL with a multifocal spherical IOL to allow simultaneous correction of astigmatism with near and distance refractive errors. Yet others have suggested using the TIOL to create "pseudoaccommodation," whereby low myopia and WTR astigmatism is combined to achieve good UCVA at distance and near. The common feature in all these newer applications is the predictability that the TIOL offers in correcting astigmatism.

As clinical experience is gained with the TIOL, surgeons become more confident and accurate in its use. The TIOL offers distinct advantages yet requires specific steps and particular care for optimum results. As we strive for the best for our cataract patients, the ability to correcting preexisting astigmatism optically rather than via tissue rearrangement increases the chances that we may reliably achieve emmetropia for all our patients who desire it.

# References

1. Frohn A, Dick HB, Thiel HJ. Implantation of a toric poly(methyl methacrylate) intraocular lens to correct high astigmatism. *J Cataract Refract Surg.* 1999;25(12):1675-8.

2. Shimizu K, Misawa A, Suzuki Y. Toric intraocular lenses. *J Cataract Refract Surg.* 1994;20:523-526.

3. Schwartz DM, Jethmalani JM, Sandstedt CA, Kornfield JA, Grubbs RH. Post implantation adjustable intraocular lenses. *Ophthalmol Clin North Am.* 2001;14(2):339-45.

4. Sun XY, Vicary D, Montgomery P, Griffiths M. Toric intraoxular lenses for correcting astigmatism in 130 eyes. *Ophthalmology.* 2000;107(9):1776-81.

5. Kershner RM. Toric intraoxular intraocular lenses for correcting astigmatism in 130 eyes (discussion). *Ophthalmology.* 2000;107(9):1781-2.

6. Sanders DR, Grabow HB, Shepherd J. The toric IOL. In: Grills JP, Martin RG, Sanders DR, eds. *Sutureless Cataract Surgery.* Thorofare, NJ: SLACK Incorporated; 1992:183-197.

7. Shimizu K, Misawa A, Suzuki Y. Toric intraocular lenses. *J Cataract Refract Surg.* 1994;20:523-526.

8. Leyland M, Zinicola E, Bloom P, Lee N. Prospective evaluation of a plate haptic toric intraocular lens. *Eye.* 2001;15(Pt 2):202-5.

9. Nguyen TM, Miller KM. Digital overlay technique for documenting toric intraocular lens axis orientation. *J Cataract Refract Surg.* 2000;26(10):1496-504.

10. Rushwurm I, Scholz U, Zehetmayer M, Hanselmeyer G, Vass C, Skorpik C. Astigmatism correction with a foldable toric intraocular lens in cataract patients. *J Cataract Refract Surg.* 2000;26(7):1022-7.

11. Novis C. Astigmatism and toric intraocular lenses. *Curr Opin Ophthalmol.* 2000;11(1):47-50.

12. Patel CK, Ormonde S, Rosen PH, Bron AJ. Postoperative intraocular lens rotation: a randomized comparison of plate and loop haptic implants. *Ophthalmology.* 1999;106(11):2190-5; discussion 2196.

13. Grabow HB. Toric IOL report. *Ann Ophthalmol.* 1997;(29):161-163.

14. Gills JP, Martin RG, Thornton SP, Sanders DR, eds. *Surgical Treatment of Astigmatism.* Thorofare, NJ: SLACK Incorporated; 1994:159-164.

15. Martin RG, Gills JP, Sanders DR, eds. *Foldable Intraocular Lenses.* Thorofare, NJ: SLACK Incorporated; 1993:237-250.

16. Gills J, Van der Karr M, Cherchio M. Combined toric intraocular lens implantation and relaxing incisions to reduce high preexisting astigmatism. *J Cataract Refract Surg.* 2002; 28(9):1585-8.

17. Till JS. Piggyback silicone intraocular lenses of opposite power. *J Cataract Refract Surg.* 2001;27(1):165-8.

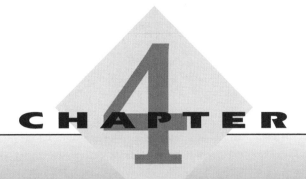

# CHAPTER 4

# HYPEROPIA AND MYOPIA TREATMENT AFTER RADIAL KERATOTOMY

*Joao Alberto Holanda de Freitas, MD and Paulo de Tarso da Silva Alvim, MD*

## INTRODUCTION

RK was developed to correct myopia and astigmatism through the use of a safe, well-accepted, and cost-effective incisional surgical procedure for patients who wish to decrease their dependence on spectacles or contact lenses. In the United States 250,000 cases usually were performed annually since its introduction in 1978 until 1994.

The Prospective Evaluation of Radial Keratotomy (PERK) study, and subsequent studies have shown that RK is a reasonably safe and effective surgical procedure for the correction of myopia up to 6.00 D.[1-8]

The PERK study also demonstrated that 43% of RK patients demonstrated a hyperopic shift in refraction in 1.00 or more diopters from 6 months to 10 years and concluded that this hyperopic shift continued through the 10-year follow-up.[1] Clearly this problem becomes magnified as the patient reaches a presbyopic age. Even though this refractive procedure is being performed less and less owing to the advent of the excimer laser, there are thousands of RK patients who seek further treatment of their residual myopia, astigmatism, overcorrection, or progression to hyperopia.

In addition to hyperopic shift, many RK patients experience fluctuations in vision on a daily basis. In RK patients, the fundamental problems of fluctuation of visual acuity and change in refractive error over time are most likely due to the fact that deep incisions destabilize the domed structure of the cornea. Eleven years after RK, 54% of eyes in the PERK study showed a diurnal fluctuation in refractive error of 0.50 D or more, most shifting in the myopic direction.[3] It has been postulated that this diurnal change may be the result of alterations in corneal topography caused by mechanic factors such as eyelid pressure; no correlation was found between changes in IOP or corneal thickness and refractive changes. It is this unpredictable destabilization of the cornea that can result in postoperative refractive errors many years after RK surgery. Diminishing the number and length of RK incisions has appeared to decrease the incidence of these problems, but only time will tell whether this adjustment will result in fewer undesirable long-term side effects.[5]

The biggest challenge in managing residual refractive error after RK is that whatever procedure one performs, the underlying destabilized corneas is in a dynamic state, so the effect of the enhancement may be lost or exaggerated over time. For example, hyperopic drifts continue to occur in many RK patients who undergo cataract surgery. In addition, diurnal fluctuations that are present are likely to persist. This becomes a very important point when one is counseling a patient about proposed enhancement. The purpose of this chapter is to describe some of the procedures used to manage over- and undercorrection post-RK.

# LASER-ASSISTED IN-SITU KERATOMILEUSIS

LASIK is gaining acceptance worldwide as the procedure of choice for retreatments of RK patients. LASIK is a predictable and safe refractive procedure for ametropia secondary to RK. Surface laser photoablation following RK is associated with a 5- to 10-fold increase in haze formation and at least a 20% reduction in refractive predictability. The 2 primary factors in producing regression following PRK enhancement following RK are haze formation and epithelial hyperplasia. The great advantage of LASIK over PRK for this group of patients is the elimination of both of these regression factors.

The main surgical issues with LASIK post-RK are the following:

1. Corrected application of suction to a destabilized and often irregular cornea
2. Care of the RK-treated flap
3. Perfect flap realignment

Before the operation, we must be certain that the RK incisions are well healed, so as to avoid separating them at the time of LASIK surgery. Enhancement of LASIK after RK is more difficult because there are risks of lifting the flap a second time and incisional dehiscence is possible. Ideally, the incisions should be narrow, with minimal scar tissue response and absolutely no deep epithelial facet formation.

Results of LASIK in undercorrected RK patients are very good and stable, and unlike with PRK, the patients are not at risk for developing haze. The visual improvement is faster when compared with PRK, and the patients have little if any discomfort.

It appears that the worst results post-RK enhancements results occur in patients with the greatest number of incisions and the smallest optical zones. Consequently, we must avoid to treat patients with greater than 8 radial incisions. The overriding concepts in these patients is the risk of corneal flap fragmentation. The risk of flap fragmentation is increased in RK patients with a high number of incisions, AK incisions that bisect a radial number of incisions, an optical zone smaller than 3.0 mm, or a history of peripheral redeepening or macroperforation. Epithelial inclusions within RK incisions increase the risk of epithelial ingrowth and possibly fragmentation. Furthermore, RK patients should wait at least 1 year before undergoing LASIK retreatment, and preferably 2 years if a lack of incision scarring is evident.[9]

LASIK after radial RK can be considered in the overcorrected RK patient as well. However, RK patients should be approached with more cautions as the results are less predictable and the hyperopic shift post-RK will continue. Results in cases with consecutive hyperopia post-RK are very good but less predictable, especially when associated with cylinder. In cases of post-RK hyperopia, there are 2 important considerations: first, whether the hyperopia represents a true overcorrection or hyperopic creep that has been progressive over time indicating corneal instability; and second, whether the hyperopia may simply be related to irregular astigmatism and not a true overcorrection amenable to hyperopic LASIK. Patients with spherical hyperopic overcorrections or with small degrees of hyperopic cylinder that have been documented as stable and have preserved best-corrected vision appear to do best.[9] Although patients should be told that starbursts phenomenon at night, the diurnal refractive fluctuations, and the gradual hyperopic shift in their vision with age cannot be corrected as the RK incisions will remain in the cornea.

We target the laser correction to slight myopia based on a morning cycloplegic refraction. Usually, post-RK patients should be treated 1 eye at a time with a high possibility of being treated on consecutive days. When performing the procedure, it is useful to use the deepest cut (200-μm depth cut with the ACS or a 180-μm plate with the Hansatome) possible as this will provide the most integrity for the flap and reduce the incidence of flap fragmentation and a central buttonhole caused by the corneal attenuation and the corneal flattening from the previous refractive procedure. The surgery is much more demanding than usual because the alignment of the corneal flap must be perfect.[10] If there is a need to retreat again, we prefer to recut the flap after several months trying to avoid flap fragmentation. However, some authors reported successful lifting the flap in RK patients within 1 week of the primary enhancement procedure when predictability was very poor.

# PHOTOREFRACTIVE KERATECTOMY

PRK enhancement after previous RK surgery is an alternative to standard RK enhancements (OZ reduction, additional incisions, and in-cut enhancements that be considered). Especially when one is concerned with an already small OZ or has maximized the number of safe radial incisions.[10] However, RK patients with smaller OZs and a greater number of incisions experience a higher incidence of confluent haze, regression, irregular astigmatism, and poor refractive predictability. Irregular astigmatism following RK is not amenable to surface excimer laser treatment.

Gimbel et al[11] have found that the use of a broad beam laser design is associated with a higher incidence of haze than occurs when enhancement is performed using a scanning slit-beam laser design. Of particular note is that if the patient has preoperative visual acuity fluctuations related to an unstable cornea, this symptom is not likely to abate following PRK enhancement. Furthermore, corneas that have undergone previous RK surgery have greater variability in healing and response to excimer laser ablation than do corneas that have had no previous surgery. We recommend targeting these patients for mild residual myopia because myopic enhancement is performed more easily than is hyperopic enhancement.

Intraoperatively, a transepithelial approach or gentle blunt debridement is acceptable. In many cases, epithelium is very thick centrally, as epithelial hyperplasia can occur following RK in response to corneal flattening. Because there may be a higher incidence of postoperative haze in eyes that have had the stromal keratocytes surgically disturbed by RK incisions, the authors recommend a less traumatic corneal epithelial removal system in place of standard manual debridement with a metal blade. A popular way to remove epithelium in these cases is by using PTK technique. Alternatively, manual removal assisted by 50% ethanol solution in a chemical "softening" may be helpful. The mechanical debridement must avoid opening healed RK incisions and the blunt spatula should be maintained parallel to the incisions. We prefer to start the debridement within the clear central optical zone and then extend the maneuver toward periphery between the RK incisions. Excimer laser ablation for residual spherical and astigmatic correction then can be performed in the usual technique. During the postoperative period, be very careful to avoid fast discontinuation of topical steroids because of the high risk of haze.[11]

# PHOTOTHERAPEUTIC KERATECTOMY

PTK is a useful adjunct to myopic and hyperopic PRK when one is enhancing an RK patient who has either some degree of irregular astigmatism or hypertrophic epithelial facet formation that causes elevated ridges over a healed RK incision. PTK can be performed using the patient's own epithelium as a "mask." Breakthrough patterns typically appear radially over the previous incisions. The pattern can be sketched and recorded for future reference. For analysis of results, the pattern can be drawn at progressively deeper levels and the micron level recorded for each drawing. Depending on what pattern is noted, PRK can be performed either immediately, or during subsequent enhancement if a significant refractive effect of the PTK surgery is anticipated. Some patients have reported improved quality of vision and less starburst around lights when this technique is used.

PTK techniques that remove haze while not produce increased hyperopia are possible by scanning limbus to limbus and ablating an equal amount of tissue from the entire surface.[11]

Majmudar et al[12] reported high efficacy of corneal epithelial debridement followed by a single topical application of Mitomycin-C 0.002% for 2 minutes followed by saline irrigation in preventing recurrence of subepithelial fibrosis in patients who have undergone corneal refractive surgery.

# LASER THERMOKERATOPLASTY

The treatment of the hyperopic overcorrected RK patient can also be done with the noncontact LTK technique trying to achieve more predictable outcomes.[13] Ismail et al reported good results without any complications in 38 cases operated. The corrections obtained had been more or less stable than in virgin hyperopic eyes. They reported superficial opening of an old RK incision in 3 cases that was safely managed by 24-hour eyepatching. These authors also recommend the application of the laser spots on the previous RK incision to avoid wound gape post-LTK.[14-16] In our opinion, the great challenge in this technique is the potential risk to produce irregular astigmatism secondary to the opening of the radial incisions.

# REFRACTIVE LENSECTOMY

Refractive lensectomy may be the preferred surgical procedure for significant refractive errors following RK if the patient is in the presbyopic age group and has developed early cataract. Significant myopia or significant hyperopia also would tip the scales toward lensectomy in this age group. Previous articles have demonstrated both the good results associated with clear lens extraction.[17,18] However, it poses a unique challenge with regard to IOL power calculation. It has become clear by the fact that previous corneal refractive surgery changes the architecture of the cornea so that standard formulas of measuring the corneal power cause it to be overestimated.[19-21] These difficulties in determining the true effective power of the cornea after RK is related to a relative proportional flattening of both the front and back surface of the cornea, which leaves the index of refraction relationship the same. The main cause of error is the fact that standard keratometry measures at the 3.2-mm zone of the central cornea, which often misses the central flatter zone of effective corneal power.

Four methods have been described in the literature to estimate corneal power following corneal power refractive surgery. These include: manual or automated keratometry, refractive history, trial contact lenses, and videokeratography.[19-21]

The clinical method history method[19-25] has stressed the importance of obtaining the precataract refractive records of eyes to eliminate cataract-induced added myopia. This method is based on the fact that the final change in refractive error that the eye obtains from surgery was due to a change in the effective corneal power. If this change (at the corneal plane) is added to the presurgical power, we will obtain the present effective corneal power.

The contact lenses method uses a hard contact of known power and base to calculate the effective corneal power. This can be done by noting the difference between manifest refractions with and without the contact lens.

Videokeratography theoretically may be more accurate than standard keratometry because of its ability to measure the corneal surface closer to the optical center; however, this has not been well documented.[19-20] The poor predictability of the IOL calculations must be considered and discussed fully with the patient. The effective refractive power of the cornea centrally can be difficult to measure with manual and automated keratometers, and even with corneal mapping devices. If one knows the refractive effect of the RK, the calculated effect of corneal power can be determined. One must keep in mind that continued hyperopia or induction of myopia by early cataract formation alters the true refractive effect of RK.

In addition to the difficulty associated with the accurate calculation of IOL power after RK, it is imperative that the surgeon be aware of the phenomenon of temporary hyperopic shift following lensectomy in these patients. This shift has been reported to cause as much as 6.00 D hyperopia, and the post-RK cornea can take up to 3 months to stabilize following lensectomy.[19] If the patient remains quite myopic, one might consider early IOL exchange; if the patient is more hyperopic than expected, it would be wise to wait for stabilization of the refraction before IOL exchange is considered.

Toric IOL implantation is an alternative to correct preoperative astigmatism. Astigmatic keratotomy may be combined with either lens implantation or phakic IOLs.

# PHAKIC INTRAOCULAR LENS IMPLANTATION

Phakic IOL implantation is another option for the correction of residual refractive errors following radial keratectomy. A major concern with phakic IOL implant is their effect on the corneal endothelium over time. Uncomplicated phacoemulsification and posterior chamber IOL implantation have been shown to cause 9% endothelial cell loss at 1 year and 15% at 5 years after surgery.[26] There is concern that phakic IOL implantation could cause a significantly higher rate of endothelial cell loss and may compromise corneal integrity over the life of the patient. The iris claw lens minimizes the risk. The ARTISAN (Ophtec, the Netherlands) PTIOL model can correct astigmatism from 2.00 to 7.00 D. Posterior chamber implantable contact lens introduces the risks of lens opacities and iris pigment epithelial chafing. These lenses are still undergoing clinical study and design modification, and additional time is needed to evaluate their safety and efficacy.

# LASSO TECHNIQUE

Several wound-tightening techniques have been described to correct hyperopia secondary to corneal overflattening following radial keratectomy.[27-35] These surgical procedures use suture material to steepen the central cornea. A "lasso" suture can be placed over and under existing RK incisions, then can be tied to result in a purse-string effect on the central cornea. These techniques all are done under topical anesthesia. All of these methods can reverse some of the hyperopia that is seen in overcorrected cases of RK; however they are somewhat imprecise. Furthermore, the effect can regress because the suture is cutting though incisions.

Alio et al reported a combination of a 10-0 nylon purse-string suture at 5.5 mm of the optical zone and 11-0 nylon suturing of 7.5 mm of the visual axis induced a wide range of central cornea steepness and eliminated previous wound gaping, respectively. The adjustment of the suture was done using a Placido ring under the operating microscope. Astigmatic overcorrection can also be reversed by suturing the astigmatic incision.[29,33-35]

# CONCLUSION

Although there are many options available to the refractive surgeon for the treatment of residual refractive errors following RK, each presents unique challenges. The unifying concept among each of these modalities in this setting is that post-RK cornea is dynamic. The possibility of short-term fluctuations and hyperopic shifts, as well as long-term drift toward hyperopia, in spite of additional refractive procedures, must be taken into account in the management and counseling of the undercorrected or overcorrected RK patient.

# REFERENCES

1. Waring GO III. Results of the prospective evaluation of radial keratotomy (PERK) study five years after surgery, *Ophthalmology.* 1991;98:1164.

2. Waring GO III. Results of the prospective evaluation of radial keratotomy (PERK) study ten years after surgery. *Arch Ophthalmol.* 1994;112:1298.

3. Deitz MR, Sanders DR, Raanan MG. A consecutive series (1982-1985) of radial keratotomies performed with the diamond blade. *Am J Ophthalmol.* 1987;103:417.

4. Salz JJ, Salz JM, Jones D. Ten years experience with a conservative approach to radial keratotomy. *Refract Corneal Surg.* 1991;7:12.

5. Werblin TP, Stafford M. The Casebeer system for predictable keratorefractive surgery. One-year evaluation of 205 consecutive eyes, *Ophthalmology.* 1993;100:1095.

6. Verity SM, et al. The combined (Genesis) technique of radial keratotomy: a prospective multicenter study, *Ophthalmology*. 1995;102:1908.

7. Waring GO III. One-year results of a prospective multicenter study of the Casebeer system of refractive keratotomy. *Ophthalmology*. 1996;103:1337.

8. Waring GO III, American Academy of Ophthalmology. Ophthalmic procedures assessment: radial keratotomy for myopia. *Ophthalmology*. 1993;100:1103.

9. Machat JJ, Slade SG, Probst LE. *The Art of LASIK*, 2nd ed. Thorofare, NJ: SLACK Incorporated. 1999;132-133.

10. Gimbel H. Experience during the learning curve of laser in situ keratomileusis. *J Cataract Refract Surg*. 1996; 22:542.

11. Gimbel H. Excimer laser photorefractive keratectomy for residual myopia after radial keratotomy, *Can J Ophthalmol*. 1997;32(1):25.

12. Majmudar. Topical Mitomycin-C for subepithelial fibrosis after refractive corneal surgery. *Ophthalmology*. 2000; 100(1):89-94.

13. Moreira H, Campus M, Sawuch MR, McDonnel JM, Sand B, McDonnel PJ. Holmium laser keratoplasty. *Ophthalmology*. 1992;5:752-761.

14. Ismail MM, Alio JL. Correction of hyperopia by holmium laser. ESCRS Congress; October 2-5, 1994; Lisbon, Portugal.

15. Ismail MM. Non-contact LTK for the correction of hyperopia. 15 months follow-up. ISRS Congress; July 28-30, 1995; Minneapolis, Minn.

16. Ismail MM, Alio JL, Artola A. Tratamiento de las hipercorreciones post-queratotomia astigmatica. *Archivos Sociedad Espanola de Oftalmologia*. 1994; 67:167-172.

17. Istafahani AH, Salz J. *Surgery for Hyperopia and Presbyopia*. Baltimore, Md: Williams & Wilkins; 1987.

18. Buzard KA, Fundingsland BR. Clear lens extraction for hyperopia. *Operative Techniques in Cataract and Refractive Surgery*. 1999;2;35-40.

19. Holladay JT. IOL calculations following radial keratotomy surgery. *Refract Corneal Surg*. 1989;5:36A.

20. Hoffer KJ. Intraocular lens power prediction for eyes after refractive keratotomy. *J Refract Surg*. 1995;11:490.

21. Lyle WA, Jin GJC. Intraocular lens power prediction in patients who undergo cataract surgery following previous radial keratotomy. *Arch Ophthalmol*. 1997;115:457.

22. Hoffer KJ. Calculation of intraocular lens power in post-radial keratotomy eyes. *Ophthalmic Practice (Canada)*. 1994;12(5):242-243.

23. Hoffer KJ. Ways to calculate IOL power in RK eyes. Refractive surgery update (Thornton). *Ocular Surg News*. 1995;13(10):86.

24. Hoffer KJ. How to do cataract surgery after RK. *Review of Ophthalmology*. 1996;20:117-120.

25. Hoffer KJ. Intraocular lens power calculation for eyes after refractive keratotomy. Consultation section. *Ann Ophthalmol*. 1996;28(2):67-68.

26. Werblin TP. Long-term endothelial cell loss following phacoemulsification: model for evaluating endothelial damage after intraocular surgery. *Refract Corneal Surg*. 1993;9(1):29.

27. Lindquist TD, Williams PA, Lindstrom RL. Surgical treatment of overcorrection following radial keratotomy: evaluation of clinical effectiveness. *Ophthalmic Surg*. 1991;22:12.

28. Starling JC, Hoffman RF. New surgical technique for the correction of hyperopia after radial keratotomy: an experimental model. *J Refract Surg*. 1986;3:119.

29. Alio JL, Ismail M. Management of radial keratotomy overcorrections by corneal sutures. *J Cataract Refract Surg*. 1993; 19:195-199.

30. Damiano RE, Forstot SL, Dukes DK. Surgical correction of hyperopia following radial keratotomy. *Refract Corneal Surg*. 1992;8:75.

31. Lyle MJ, Jin JC. Circular and interrupted suture technique for correction of hyperopia following radial keratotomy. *Refract Corneal Surg*. 1990;6:103.

32. Lu LW. Lasso technique refined to treat hyperopia following refractive surgery. *Ocular Surg News*. 1996;7(8):22.

33. Alio JL, Ismail MM. Management of astigmatic keratotomy overcorrections by corneal suturing. *J Cataract Refract Surg*. 1994;66:211-218.

34. Alio JL, Ismail MM, Artola A. Cirugia de la hipermotropia post-queratotomia radial mediante suturas corneales. *Archivos Sociedad Espanola de Oftalmologia*. 1994;66:211-218.

35. Ismail MM, Alio JL, Artola A. Tratamiento de la hipercorreciones post-queratotomia astigmatica. *Archivos Sociedad Espanola de Oftalmologia*. 1994;67:167-172.

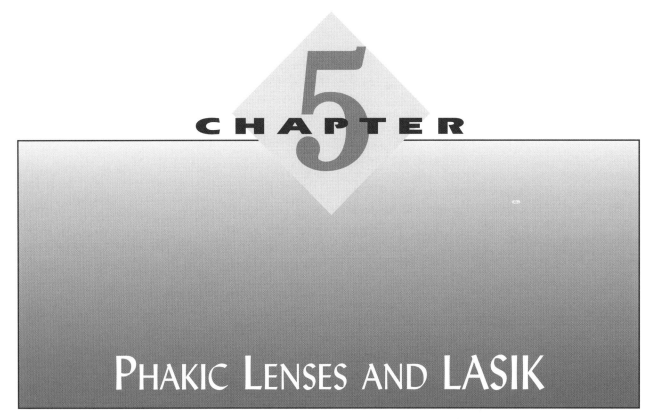

# CHAPTER 5

# PHAKIC LENSES AND LASIK

*Luis F. Restrepo, MD*

## INTRODUCTION

The term *bioptics* was originally coined by Roberto Zaldivar, MD, for the use of LASIK to refine the results of phakic lens implantation in high myopes.[1] They termed the 2-part phakic intraocular lens (PRL) LASIK procedure bioptics (2 optics) because the optical correction is split between 2 planes: the IOL plane and the anterior corneal plane. Nowadays, the meaning of bioptics has expanded to include all cases of using LASIK to enhance the results of implanting an IOL, phakic or aphakic, either having it planned in advance as a combined procedure or as a way to correct an unexpected refractive result. Bioptics comprises the following options: planned PRL plus LASIK, later use of LASIK for correct ammetropia after phakic lens implantation, LASIK for the correction of unexpected bad refractive result after cataract surgery, and planned LASIK after cataract surgery to obtain plano or almost plano in cases with preoperative astigmatism.

Bioptics considered as a single concept is a very difficult topic as it is constantly changing as advances are made in the fast-moving fields of phakic lenses, aphakic lenses, LASIK, and cataract surgery.

## PHAKIC INTRAOCULAR LENS PLUS LASIK

PRLs are becoming widely used for treating myopia and hyperopia, for those defects where LASIK is less predictable or desirable. There are many different types of PRL: anterior chamber angle or iris-supported, posterior chamber and floating lenses. Indications, surgical techniques, and difficulties vary for each type of lens and are beyond the scope of this chapter.

### Myopia

#### PHAKIC INTRAOCULAR LENSES FOR MYOPIA

In myopia, indications for implantation of PRLs vary among surgeons, some preferring phakic iols for myopic defects over as low as -3.00 D, other for defects over -9.00 D, or when the corneas are thin. The experience of each surgeon with LASIK and phakic implants plus the availability of the lenses decides the indication and the type of lens. In general, phakic IOLs seem to be very safe and reach predictable results for a wide range of myopic defects. Malecaze et al[2] reported an interesting comparison between LASIK and a PRLs in 25 patients with myopia. For each patient, 1 eye received LASIK and the other was implanted with the phakic lens. Myopia range was from -8.00 D to -12.00 D. Their conclusion was that both LASIK and the phakic lens seem to produce a similar predictability, but the BCVA and subjective evaluation of quality of vision were better for the lens. There are many other papers reporting the safety and predictability of phakic IOLs for the correction of spheric, or almost spheric, myopia for middle and high negative defects.[3-9] There are some others reporting complications and uneventful results.[10-12] An interesting fact is that phakic intraocular lens implantation seems to not induce significant astigmatism by itself. The main complication is cataract formation.

At the time of writing, toric phakic lenses are in development and trials, but not in general use. Leading manufacturers like Ophtec (the Netherlands) and STAAR Surgical (Monrovia, Calif) have torics lenses in clinical trials while others have announced their own developments. Georges Baikoff, MD, has designed and started implanting a phakic lens for the correction of presbyopia in emmetropic patients with no astigmatism.[13]

The surgeon who wants to correct high myopic defects faces many challenges. Clear lens extraction is more suited for presbyopic patients due to the loss of accommodation and also seems to increases the risk of retinal detachment. LASIK has the well-known limitations of the amount of tissue ablated and also the final keratometric readings becoming too flat. PRLs have demonstrated to be adequate for the correction of high myopia.[3-9]

### Myopic Bioptics

When Zaldivar and colleagues introduced the term bioptics, it was applied to the correction of high (extreme) myopia combining a posterior chamber PRL and LASIK in 67 eyes of 54 patients. The logic behind this approach is that bioptics offers 2 important theoretical advantages over PRL or LASIK surgery alone. First, the combination of the 2 procedures permits the maximizing the OZ size of each (ie, optics size of the lens is smaller at higher powers) and second, the final correction can be finely tuned as the excimer laser application is done after some time of the PRL implantation, when the refractive defect is stable and its measurement more reliable as a significant reduction of the defect has taken place.[1] The same logics apply to a wider range of myopic defects of lesser dioptric power in selected cases when the cornea is thin and a LASIK procedure to correct the complete defect would not be advisable. There is another great advantage of bioptics: the correction of astigmatism either preexistent or induced by the intraocular phakic lens surgery. However, toric PRLs are reaching the market and are being implanted.[14,15]

### Indications

In general, planned bioptics indications are myopic astigmatism of over -9.00 D of spherical equivalent and spherical defects greater than -15.00 D. Unplanned bioptics could be

also indicated for refining the results of implantation of a PRL with an undesirable refractive result, because of poor calculation or because of the rare cases of induced astigmatism.

## *Hyperopic*

### PRLs for Hyperopia

The results of different excimer laser systems determine the choice of PRL for the correction the hyperopia. It is known that over +3.00 LASIK results for hyperopia are less predictable and most refractive surgeons agree that either +5.00 of refractive defect or predicted keratometric readings over 49.00 D are the upper limit for hyperopic defect correction with excimer laser. PRLs are very safe and predictable up to +12.00 D[16] and have been used for higher corrections with good results. Nevertheless, the use of PRL for hyperopia faces more challenges than for myopia as the anatomical spaces used are usually more crowded, are of minor sizes, and have greater risk of complications.

### Hyperopic Bioptics

Hyperopic bioptics are much less common than myopic, and there are reasons for this. In the first place hyperopic phakic lenses have been available less time than myopic and secondly the anatomical considerations limit its use (the higher the power, the thicker the lens). A reasonably thorough search for published papers on the subject showed no results. Nevertheless there have been many presentations at congresses of selected cases showing good results in general.

### Indications

In the case of hyperopic bioptics, the only acceptable approach is as a planned combined surgery. The risks involved in doing a microkeratome pass after the PRL is in place surpass the possible benefits. Usually hyperopic astigmatism is very symptomatic. Bioptics are useful to correct the astigmatic part of the refractive defect and must be planned on a case-by-case basis. Bioptics could be considered when the astigmatic component of the defect is greater than 1.00 D. The final LASIK approach depends on the surgeon's experience with his own laser as the planned keratorefractive correction could be designed as hyperopic or mixed astigmatism by under or overcorrecting the spheric part with the PRL.

### Technique

By the time this technique was introduced and was gaining acceptance, LASIK was planned as a separate procedure done between 1 to 6 months after the implantation of the PRL. In spite of having been planned, the complete laser surgery was delayed including the creation of the corneal flap. Currently most surgeons pass the microkeratome as the first step of the bioptics procedure, creating the corneal flap but delaying the application of the excimer laser. This way avoids the risks derived of exerting the high pressure suction by the microkeratome when the PRL is in place. In summary those risks are: dislodging the lens for all models, and the possible contact between the endothelium and the PRL in the case of angle- or iris-fixated lenses. The management of the flap does not represent additional difficulty for the lens implantation and can easily be lifted any time after for the excimer laser application.

The anesthesia and other surgical conditions are determined by the technique used for the particular PRL to be used. The microkeratome pass could be done with topical, peribulbar, retrobulbar, or general anesthesia without major differences in the outcome. Let us say that in case of hyperopic bioptics, retrobulbar anesthesia could be advantageous as it "lifts" the globe from the orbit and could make the creation of the corneal flap in deep and small eyes easier.

The timing for the excimer laser ablation varies among surgeons. It is considered that the refraction is stable after 1 month of the PRL implantation in most cases so usually the laser is applied anytime after that.

# Pseudophakic Bioptics

Taking into account that nearly 6 million cataract surgeries are done each year worldwide and that cataract surgery is now considered a refractive procedure by itself, bioptics becomes a logic step in the search of plano or almost plano as a final result. According to Louis D. Nichamin, MD, standard cataract surgery represents a 50/50 chance for the patients to be free of glasses for most daily activities except reading, whereas with bioptics, the chance is over 95%.[17] Even the most experienced cataract surgeons have cases that end with undesirable refractive results. As with PRLs, pseudophakic bioptics could be planned and unplanned.

## *Planned Pseudophakic Biopics*

As a good refractive result becomes the expected outcome after cataract surgery, pseudophakic bioptics emerges as a way for ensuring such results. Among the advantages of bioptics is the fact that the learning curve is almost null for the average surgeon; there is no new technique to learn and even more important, the surgeon could be more tolerant about the incision placement and size in standard phacoemulsification surgery, as the astigmatic factor would be corrected by the excimer laser. The different available techniques to deal with preoperative astigmatism by means of incision placement or additional refractive incisions are not very precise and usually fail with astigmatisms over 3.00 D.[17]

## *Indications*

As a general guide, planned pseudophakic bioptics is indicated when the preoperative astigmatic factor exceeds 2.00 D.

## *Technique*

For planned pseudophakic bioptics, the corneal flap must be created before the lens surgery. Preference among surgeons varies, regarding the timing of the flap creation. The microkeratome can be passed the day before but there is not any good reason for this practice as the flap can be created as the first step of the cataract surgery and does not jeopardize the rest of the procedure even if epithelial defects are produced.

After the cataract surgery, the excimer laser application must be delayed at least 2 weeks. The refractive result of the implant surgery will be more reliable after 4 weeks and it could be more appropriate to wait this amount of time before proceeding to the ablation and even more so if a wavefront guided correction is going to be used. At the chosen time, the flap is just lifted and the excimer applied.

## *Unplanned Pseudophakic Bioptics*

As LASIK is becoming a widely practiced surgery among cataract surgeons, bioptics would become routinely used to refine the results of the intraocular lens implantation. LASIK usually has fewer risks and is easier than other options like IOL exchange or piggyback implants.

### Indications

Any uncomplicated cataract case that ends with an undesirable refractive result could be greatly improved with subsequent LASIK treatment for the residual refractive error. Pseudophakic bioptics has been used even with multifocal intraocular lenses as the Array (Advanced Medical Optics, Santa Ana, Calif).[17]

Jose Guell, MD, proposes another use of bioptics. He uses a bioptics approach in patients who want to try monovision along with the correction of high ammetropies. He adjusts the residual myopia with the excimer including the total correction in unsatisfied patients.[17]

Combined cataract surgery plus penetrating keratoplasty can be also complemented with late LASIK as a final step to reach a better refractive result.

Another interesting type of candidates are those patients requiring cataract surgery and who have previously had incisional corneal refractive surgery. Pseudophakic bioptics is particularly well suited to these patients as IOL calculation is difficult and less predictable and also because many of them have significant astigmatism.

Using a less strict definition, it could be said that CLE plus LASIK is another form of bioptics.

### Technique

The type of cataract surgery performed, the surgical incision, and the postoperative evolution are the major factors to be taken into account when unplanned pseudophakic bioptics is under consideration.

The stability of the incision used for the cataract surgery is by itself the main factor. For phacoemulsification patients with CCIs, it is considered that passing the microkeratome 1 month after the cataract surgery is safe. For limbal incisions, either phacoemulsification or other minimal incision techniques, opinion varies but 3 months must be the minimum lapse before constructing the flap being safer to wait up to the sixth month after the intraocular surgery.

In cases where penetrating keratoplasty has been practiced as a combined technique with IOL implantation, it is safer to wait more than 12 months to perform the LASIK procedure.

When the patient has had incisional corneal refractive surgery, it is very advisable to create the flap as an initial step and wait at least 4 weeks before proceeding to the laser applications as it is not unusual to find changes on the refractive error and axis shifting of the astigmatic portion.

### COMPLICATIONS

Obviously bioptics, either with PRL or pseudophakic, shares all the known complications of implanting IOLs and those of LASIK.

The most important complications of bioptics use are related to the effect of passing the microkeratome when the IOL (PRL or even pseudophakic) is in place. Other complications are the dislodging of the IOL and the causing contact between the optic of the lens and the endothelium with damage of the later.

Special attention must be given to the epithelium in older patients as it could become very loose because of the age, and also, this group of population has proclivity to dry eye so corneal abrasions are more common and heals slowly.

## SUMMARY

As a good refractive result has become of paramount importance for all types of IOL implantations (either PRLs or pseudophakic), bioptics as emerged as a very useful way to reach such results. Also, bioptics represents a safe method of correcting higher defects that are beyond the limits of LASIK alone.

Every refractive and cataract surgeon must consider bioptics among the options for treating his patients. Bioptics will become a routinely used approach as risks are low and custom ablation techniques will provide even more accurate results. Any innovation in LASIK, PRLs, and cataract surgery will improve bioptics consequently.

The beauty behind the concept of bioptics is that the surgeon can combine completely different methods of correcting the refractive defects (the keratorefractive and the intraocular), in such a way that the end result will be better than the one reached by either approach by itself.

## REFERENCES

1. Zaldivar R, Davidorf J, Oscherow S, Ricur G, Piezzi V. Combined posterior chamber phakic intraocular lens and laser in situ keratomileusis: bioptics for extreme myopia. *J Refract Surg.* 1999;15:299-308.

2. Malecaze FJ, Hunlin H, Bierer P. A randomized paired eye comparison of two techniques for treating moderately high myopia: LASIK and the artisan phakic lens. *Ophthalmology.* 2002;109(9):1622-30.

3. Maloney RK, Nguyen LH, John ME. Artisan phakic lens for myopia: short-term results of a prospective, multicenter study. *Ophthalmology.* 2002;109(9):1631-41.

4. Arne JL, Lesueur LC. Phakic posterior chamber lenses for high myopia: Functional and anatomical outcomes. *J Cataract Refract Surg.* 2000;26:369-374.

5. Uusilato RJ, Aine E, Sen NH, Laatikainen L. *J Cataract Refract Surg.* 2002;28(1):29-36

6. Landesz M, van Eij G, Luyten G. Iris-claw phakic intraocular lens for high myopia. *J Refract Surg.* 2001;17(6):634-640.

7. Zaldivar R, Davidorf JM, Oscherow S. Posterior chamber phakic intraocular lens for myopia of -8 to -19 diopters. *J Refract Surg.* 1998;14:294-305.

8. Sanders DR, Brown DC, Martin RG, Sheperd J, Deitz M, DeLuca M. Implantable contact lens for moderate to high myopia: phase 1 FDA clinical study with 6 months follow-up. *J Cataract Refract Surg.* 1998;24:607-611.

9. Pérez-Santoja JJ, Alió JL, Jiménez-Alfaro I, Zato M. Surgical correction of severe miopía with an angle-supported phakic intraocular lens. *J Cataract Refract Surg.* 2000;26:1288-1302.

10. Yoon H, Macaluso DC, Moshirfar M, Lundergan M. Traumatic dislocation of an Ophtec artisan phakic intraocular lens. *J Refract Surg.* 2002;18(4):481-483.

11. Sánchez-Galeana CA, Zadok D, Montes M, Cortés MA, Chalet AS. Refractory intraocular pressure increase after phakic posterior chamber intraocular lens implantation. *Am J Ophthalmol.* 2002;134(1):121-123.

12. Muzzi G, Cantú C. Vitreous hemorrhage following phakic anterior chamber intraocular lens implantation in severe myopia. *Eur J Ophthalmol.* 2002;12(1):69-72.

13. Henahan JF. A first look at the presbyopic phakic IOL. Available at: http://www.eyeworld.org/apr01/0401p76.html. Accessed October 15, 2003.

14. Gimbel HV, Ziemba SL. Management of myopic astigmatism with phakic intraocular lens implantation. *J Cataract Refract Surg.* 2002;28(5):883-886.

15. Cimberle M. Surgeon: toric artisan iol effective against astigmatism. Available at: www.osnsupersite.com. Accessed October 15, 2003.

16. Davidorf J, Zaldivar R, Oscherow S. Posterior chamber phakic intraocular lens for hyperopia of +4 to +11 diopters. *J Refract Surg.* 1998;14:306-311.

17. Lipner M. Bioptic vision: for 6 million like cataract results. Available at: http://www.eyeworld.org/nov01/1101p54.html. Accessed October 15, 2003.

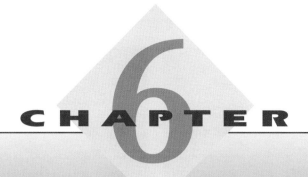

# CHAPTER 6

# HYPEROPIA AND CONDUCTIVE THERMOKERATOPLASTY

*José A.P. Gomes, MD and Daniela Endriss, MD*

## INTRODUCTION

Surgical correction of hyperopia has always been more challenging to ophthalmologists than the correction of myopia.[1-6] The results with lower amounts of baseline hyperopia are of particular interest, because 80% of adult hyperopes have refraction equal to or less than +3.00 D.[7] Different methods and techniques have been used to treat hyperopia. However, their results have been variable and not always satisfactory.

Nonincisional approaches to refractive surgery have been explored in the quest of finding a satisfactory solution to hyperopia.[1-6,8-19] Attempts to steepen the central cornea using thermal keratoplasty date back to the rabbit studies by Lans in the 19th century.[1-3,8,10-13] During the 1980s, hot wire thermokeratoplasty, a technique developed in the Soviet Union, was used to produce thermal burns (up to 600° C) that penetrated to 95% of corneal depth in hyperopic eyes. Studies showed that it resulted in substantial overcorrection followed by marked regression.[1,2,8,10]

*Conductive keratoplasty* (CK) is a new, nonablative method for the correction of mild to moderate hyperopia that consists of an electrical current-based technique for shrinking stromal collagen. The technique delivers low energy, high-frequency (radio frequency, 350 kHz) current directly into the corneal stroma by means of a Keratoplast tip

(Refractec Inc, Irvine, Calif) inserted at 8 to 32 treatment points in the midperipheral cornea (Figures 6-1 and 6-2).[8,9]

CK uses the electrical properties of corneal tissue to generate heat in the cornea. Collagen within the treatment zone is heated in a gentle, controlled fashion as a result of the natural resistance of stromal tissue to the flow of current.[1] Increasing dehydration of collagen increases resistance to the flow of the current, making the process self-limiting.[1,2,20,21] A thermal model predicts protein denaturation at each treated spot that results in a cylindrical footprint approximately 150 to 200 mm wide and 500 mm deep extending to approximately 80% of the midperipheral cornea. Striae form between the treated spots, creating a band of tightening that increases the curvature of the central cornea, thereby decreasing hyperopia. Unlike Fyodorov's original "hot needle keratoplasty" technique, the CK delivery needle stays cool as collagen is heated. This hyperopic correction is stable and has little regression through time.[1,2,8,9]

Histopathologic analysis of 6 human corneas that had radio-frequency current applied showed thermal injury to the epithelium, an intact Bowman membrane with discrete shrinkage of its fibers, and a shrunken and edematous stroma. No severe necrosis or inflammatory cells were present indicating that the technique gives more stable results.[8] A study reported to The American Society of Corneal and Refractive Surgery showed that the CK procedure did not

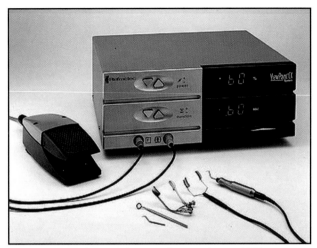

**Figure 6-1.** The conductive keratoplasty (CK) system (Viewpoint CK System; Courtesy of Refractec, Inc., Irvine, Calif).

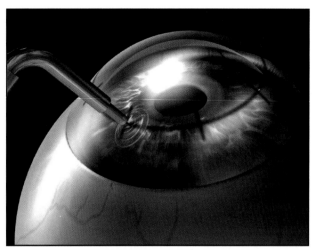

**Figure 6-2.** Conductive keratoplasty (CK) treatment with the keratoplast tip. (Courtesy of Refractec, Inc., Irvine, Calif.)

significantly change endothelial cell counts in the central or peripheral cornea despite penetration of treatment to approximately 80% of the corneal depth.[2]

# INDICATIONS AND CONTRAINDICATIONS

CK is designed to treat spherical, previously untreated hyperopia of +0.75 to +3.00 D. Treatment of presbyopia, astigmatism, and residual hyperopia following LASIK or other refractive procedures is another potential application. The best candidate is over 35 years of age, with pachymetry readings of no less than 560 mm at the 6-mm optical zone. Patients not eligible for CK treatment are those with active ocular disease, corneal abnormality, progressive or unstable hyperopia, or other significant ocular or physical history.[1,2,8,9]

# SURGICAL TECHNIQUE

A complete ophthalmologic exam is necessary before treating any patient. This includes visual acuity, manifest and cycloplegic refraction, slit lamp biomicroscopy, tonometry, fundoscopic examination, keratometry, pachymetry, and computerized corneal topography.

The procedure is explained to the patient preoperatively and it is very important to advise the patient that for the first few weeks, he or she will have a myopic effect. This is normal because at first the patient is overcorrected, allowing for the predetermined amount of regression to take effect. During this time, the patient may require visual aid with glasses for far vision.[1,2,8,9]

This procedure may be performed under topical anesthesia with 1 drop of 0.5% tetracaine, administered 3 times at 5-minute intervals. A lid speculum is placed in the eye to be

treated to obtain maximal exposure and to provide the electrical return path. It is important to ensure that the lid drape (if used) does not prevent direct contact of the lid speculum and eyelid, which would disrupt the electrical current return path. The fellow eye is taped closed. The operating microscope can be positioned over or in front of the eye to be treated. There is no need to fixate the globe. As the patient fixated on the microscope's light, the cornea is marked with a gentian-violet-dampened eight-intersection CK marker that creates a circle at the 7-mm optical zone and hatch marks at the 6-mm and 8-mm optical zones (Figure 6-3). The surface of the cornea is dried with a fiber-free sponge to avoid dissipation of the applied energy through a damp surface.

The Refractec corneal shaper system (Refractec Inc., Irvine, Calif) used to perform the CK procedure consists of a radio frequency energy-generating console. Attached to the probe is a single-use, sterile, penetrating tip, 90 mm in diameter and 450 mm long that delivers the current directly to the corneal stroma. At the very distal portion of the tip is an insulated stainless-steel stop (cuff) that assures correct depth of penetration (0.5 mm). The energy level default is 60% of 1 watt and the exposure time default is 0.6 seconds. These parameters are set on the console so that each foot pedal excursion delivers the same level and duration of energy to the keratoplast tip.[1,2,8,9]

The keratoplast tip is examined under the microscope to ensure that it is not damaged or bent prior to application. The appropriate treatment parameters are set on the console, and the eye is treated with the appropriate number of treatment spots, as specified in the nomogram. For example, to correct +1.00 D to +1.625 D of hyperopia, 16 treatment spots are placed: 8 at the 6-mm optical zone and another 8 at the 7-mm optical zone. When treating +0.75 D to +0.875 D, 8 treatment spots are applied only at the 7-mm optical zone. If astigmatism is present, greater amount of treatment will be needed in the flatter meridians to induce steepening in this area.[1,2]

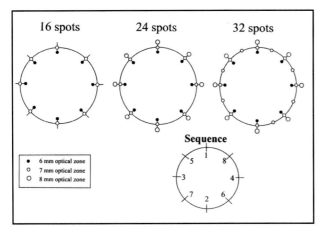

**Figure 6-3.** Number, location, and application sequence of the treatment spots. (Reprinted from *Ophthalmology,* 109, McDonald MB, Davidorf J, Maloney RK, Manche EE, Hersh P, Conductive keratoplasty for the correction of low to moderate hyperopia. 1-year results on the first 54 eyes, 637-49, Copyright [2002], with permission from the American Academy of Ophthalmology.)

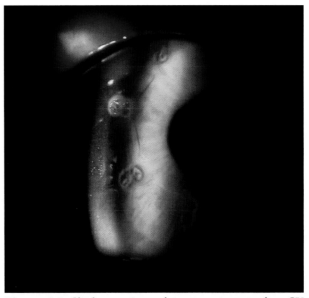

**Figure 6-4.** Slit-lamp view of treatment spot after CK showing bands of striae between spots. (Courtesy of Refractec Inc., Irvine, Calif).

The surgeons place the keratoplast tip on the cornea at the treatment markings, attempting to place it perpendicular to the corneal surface. The cuff around the probe, which settles perpendicular to the cornea, helps to achieve perpendicular placement. Light pressure is applied until the tip penetrates the stroma to its insulator stop. After each treatment spot, the tip is carefully cleaned with a fiber-free sponge, removing any tissue debris. Keratometry is performed after the full circle of treatments had been completed to check for any induced cylinder. Depending on the epithelium drying and edema, the patient may be able to have very good near vision immediately.[1,2,8,9]

After treatment, 1 drop of topical ophthalmic antibiotic solution and 1 drop of an ophthalmic nonsteroidal anti-inflammatory drug are administered and continued for 3 days. Topical corticosteroid is not used.

One hour after treatment, the opacities at each treatment spot are visible by slit lamp as small surface leukomas, with a band of striae connecting the treatment spots (Figure 6-4). Leukomas visible by slit lamp postoperatively are small because CK delivers energy deep into the stroma rather than on the surface. The striae between treatment zones remain visible at 3, 6, and 12 months, as reported by the United States CK clinical trial investigators, and suggest that the effect of treatment on the stroma is long lasting.[1,2]

## COMPLICATIONS

Some treatment-related adverse events include corneal edema between 1 week and 1 month postoperatively. After this period we can find peripheral corneal epithelial defect, recurrent corneal erosion, foreign body sensation, pain, or ghosting/double images.[1] Induced irregular astigmatism may be present when the application of the high frequency current is not done symmetrically on the entire treatment. Retreatment may be performed safely at the slit lamp.[8]

## OUTCOMES

McDonald et al[1] in a prospective multicenter study found encouraging results 1 year after CK (Figure 6-5). The predictability was good, but seemed to decrease with increased number of treatment spots. Regression after the CK procedure was low and decreased with time. The refraction appeared to stabilize at 6 months postoperatively. BSCVA was generally preserved after the procedure and incidence of induced cylinder is low.

Asbell et al,[2] also in a multicenter clinical trial, reported that efficacy results exceeded all FDA guidelines for performance of refractive surgery procedures. Mendez et al[8] reported an increased in postoperative visual acuity in all patients studied. The immediate postoperative refraction ranged from -1.50 D to -2.50 D, decreased to -1.00 D in 3 to 6 months, and reached plano at 1 year.

In an attempt to compare CK with laser techniques for the correction of hyperopia, we present a summary of the outcomes of well-known studies in Table 6-1. These preliminary results suggest that CK may be safer and more stable than PRK and as effective as LASIK for the treatment of low to moderate levels of hyperopia. The refractive correction after CK appears to be more stable for 1 year postoperatively than that after noncontact LTK. Conductive keratoplasty

**Figure 6-5.** Mean manifest refractive spherical equivalent (MRSE) refraction over time. D=diopters; SD=standard deviation. (Reprinted from *Ophthalmology*, 109, McDonald MB, Davidorf J, Maloney RK, Manche EE, Hersh P, Conductive keratoplasty for the correction of low to moderate hyperopia. 1-year results on the first 54 eyes, 637-49, Copyright [2002], with permission from the American Academy of Ophthalmology.)

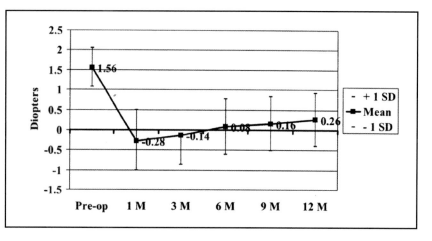

## Comparison of CK with LASIK, PK, and LTK Results for Treating Hyperopia

| | | CK[1]* | LASIK[6] | PRK[4]** | LTK[12] |
|---|---|---|---|---|---|
| Laser/instrument used | | Radio frequency (350 kHz) | Chiron-Technolas Keracor 117 | Aesculap-Meditec MEL 60 | Sunrise Holmium YAG |
| Follow-up | | 12 months | 12 months | 12 months | 12 months |
| Number of eyes | | 28 | 84 | 15 | 57 |
| Mean preoperative (SE±SD) | | +1.62 ± 0.53D | +4.50 ± 1.73 D | +4.20 ± 1.30 D | +3.80 ± 0.27 D |
| Range | | +1.00 to +3.00 D | +1.20 to +8.50 D | +1.50 to +6.00 D | +1.50 to +5.00 D |
| Mean postoperative (SE±SD) | | +0.26 ± 0.67 D | +0.88 ± 1.87 D | +1.43 ± NA | +1.73 ± 0.16 D |
| Efficacy | UCVA ≥ 20/20 | 57% | 35% | 6.3% | 47% |
| | UCVA ≥ 20/40 | 93% | 81% | 67% | 72% |
| Predictability | MRSE ± 0.50 D | 46% | 61% | 20% | 21% |
| | MRSE ± 1.00 D | 93% | 73% | 40% | 58% |
| Safety | 2 lines loss BSCVA | 0 | 6% | 6.6% | 0 |
| | BSCVA < 20/40 | 0 | 6% | NA | NA |
| Stability | | At 6 months | At 6 months | Most in 3 months | Total regression in 31% |

BSCVA=best spectacle-corrected visual acuity; CK=conductive keratoplasty; D=diopters; LASIK=laser in-situ keratomileusis; LTK=laser thermal keratoplasty; MRSE=manifest refractive spherical equivalent; NA=data not available; PRK=photorefractive keratectomy; SD=standard deviation; SE=spherical equivalent; UCVA=uncorrected visual acuity; YAG=yttrium-aluminum-garnet.
*Current nomogram; **Group 1 only

**TABLE 6-1**

may provide patients a full refractive correction that does not markedly regress.

As a nonexcimer laser technique for correcting hyperopia, CK preserves the central cornea, does not induce flap-related complications, and does not involve removal of any corneal tissue or cut corneal nerves. The decreased complexity of the procedure compared with LASIK results in the need for fewer staff members. The range of correction, however, is limited to low hyperopia, and the surgeon must turn to other procedures for patients outside of the treatment range of CK.

It is still too early to claim that this procedure results in a stable postoperative refractive error. Predictability needs to be improved, particularly in the ± 0.50 D range, and stability needs to be more firmly established. Research is still being done to make this procedure even more efficient. Many developments are underway which will enhance the intrastromal conductive keratoplasty procedure.[1,2,8]

# REFERENCES

1. McDonald MB, Davidorf J, Maloney RK, Manche EE, Hersh P. Conductive keratoplasty for the correction of low to moderate hyperopia. 1-year results on the first 54 eyes. *Ophthalmology.* 2002;109:637-49.

2. Asbell PA, Maloney RK, Davidorf J, Hersh P, McDonald M, Manche E. Conductive keratoplasty for the correction of hyperopia. *Tr Am Ophth Soc.* 2001;99:79-83.

3. Kohnen T. Advances in the surgical correction of hyperopia. *J Cataract Refract Surg.* 1998;24:1-2.

4. Pietilä J, Mäkinen P, Pajari S, Uusitalo H. Excimer laser photorefractive keratectomy for hyperopia. *J Cataract Refract Surg.* 1997;13:504-10.

5. Vinciguerra P, Epstein D, Radice P, Azzolini M. Long-term results of photorefractive keratectomy for hyperopia and hyperopic astigmatism. *J Refract Surg.* 1998;14:S183-5.

6. Esquenazi S, Mendoza A. Two-year follow-up of laser in situ keratomileusis for hyperopia. *J Refract Surg.* 1999;15:648-52.

7. Leibowitz M, Krueger DE, Maunder LR, et al. The Framingham eye study monograph. VIII: visual acuity. *Surv Ophthalmol.* 1980;24(suppl):472-9.

8. Mendez A, Mendez Noble A. Conductive keratoplasty for the correction of hyperopia. In: Sher NA, ed. *Surgery for Hyperopia and Presbyopia.* Philadelphia, Pa: Williams and Wilkins. 1997;163-71.

9. Mendez Noble A, Mendez A. Queratoplastia conductiva intraestromal para el manejo de la hipermetropia. In: Albertazzi R, Centurión V, eds. *La Moderna Cirurgia Refractiva.* Buenos Aires. 1997;243-5.

10. Souza L, Nosé W, Campos M, McDonnell PJ. Thermokeratoplasty for the treatment of hyperopia: a clinical follow-up. *Arq Bras Oftal.* 1997;60:136-45.

11. Eggink CA, Bardak Y, Cuypers MHM, Deutman AF. Treatment of hyperopia with contact Ho:YAG laser thermal keratoplasty. *J Refract Surg.* 1999;15:16-22.

12. Alió JL, Ismail MM, Sanchéz Pego JL. Correction of hyperopia with non-contact Ho:YAG laser thermal keratoplasty. *J Refract Surg.* 1997;13:17-22.

13. Koch DD, Abarca A, Villarreal R, et al. Hyperopia correction by noncontact holmium:YAG laser thermal keratoplasty. Clinical study with two-year follow-up. *Ophthalmology.* 1996;103:731-40.

14. Koch DD, Kohnen T, McDonnell PJ, et al. Hyperopia correction by noncontact holmium:YAG laser thermal keratoplasty. United States phase IIA clinical study with 2-year follow-up. *Ophthalmology.* 1997;104:1938-47.

15. Ismail MM, Alió JL, Pérez-Santonja JJ. Noncontact thermokeratoplasty to correct hyperopia induced by laser in situ keratomileusis. *J Cataract Refract Surg.* 1998;24:1191-4.

16. Daya SM, Tappouni FR, Habib NE. Photorefractive keratectomy for hyperopia. Six-month results in 45 eyes. *Ophthalmology.* 1997;104:1952-8.

17. Jackson WB, Mintsioulis G, Agapitos PJ, Casson EJ. Excimer laser photorefractive keratectomy for low hyperopia: safety and efficacy. *J Cataract Refract Surg.* 1997;23:480-7.

18. Argento CJ, Cosentino MJ. Laser in situ keratomileusis for hyperopia. *J Cataract Refract Surg.* 1998;24:1050-8.

19. Ditzen K, Huschka H, Pieger S. Laser in situ keratomileusis for hyperopia. *J Cataract Refract Surg.* 1998;24: 42-7.

20. Brinkmann R, Radt B, Flamm C, et al. Influence of temperature and time on thermally induced forces in corneal collagen and the effect on laser thermokeratoplasty. *J Cataract Refract Surg.* 2000;26:744-54.

21. Spörl E, Genth U, Schmalfuss K, Seiler T. Thermo-mechanical behavior of the cornea. *Ger J Ophthalmol.* 1997;5:322-7.

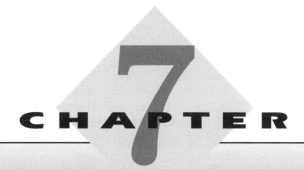

# CHAPTER 7

# HYPEROPIA: LASIK, LASEK, AND PRK

*Robin F. Beran, MD, FACS*

## INTRODUCTION

The surgical correction of hyperopia and hyperopic astigmatism by altering the shape of the cornea has always been a greater challenge than the correction for myopia and myopic astigmatism. Early attempts with incisional keratorefractive surgery, hexagonal keratotomy, found limited success. The hyperopic refractive error could be reduced, but at the expense of corneal instability and a high incidence of irregular astigmatism. The development of the excimer laser and hyperopic photorefractive keratectomy has achieved a more acceptable success rate with fewer complications. The range of correction, however, is still somewhat limited and postoperative recovery prolonged.

This chapter is intended to compare 3 photoablative techniques: LASIK, PRK, and LASEK. The expectation is to challenge the reader to critically analyze their utilization of these procedures and optimize their application. A common and popular misconception has been that there is 1 "best" procedure to be used in all situations. The refractive surgeon maintaining the philosophy of providing a diversification of techniques and selecting the most appropriate will most certainly better serve his or her patients.

## Corneal Anatomy and Physiology

There are numerous excellent references discussing corneal anatomy, physiology, and biomechanics.[1-4] The intention of this section is simply to expose the reader to aspects of those areas that are pertinent to the correction of hyperopia and hyperopic astigmatism by 1 of these 3 photorefractive procedures. Our understanding of many of these considerations remains limited; however, it is important to at least recognize these limitations so as to guide our surgical decisions. Patient expectations must be realistic. Failure to acknowledge the uncertainties surrounding wound healing and individual tissue variability can definitely lead to false expectations by both the patient and the surgeon.

The excellent precision with which corneal tissue can be ablated using the excimer laser tends to overshadow the factors that work to decrease the precision of these hyperopic corrective procedures. Epithelial healing, the laser ablation profile and characteristics, and variability in stromal hydration are just a few of these factors to be considered. The enthusiasm being generated about "supervision" associated with the development of wavefront technology and custom ablation must be tempered with the understanding that the limitations of the results of these procedures are related to the above factors, not only on the precision of the laser or its technology. We know that the changes made in the anterior curvature of the cornea do induce higher order optical aberrations. These ultimately limit the quality of postoperative vision. Our ability to be able to reduce or correct these should improve the level of visual functioning. Presently, poor control over individual tissue reactivity and wound healing has to raise concern over the claims of success being made for results obtained with wavefront refractions and custom ablations.

The cornea maintains 2 primary functions: to refract light rays onto the retina and to protect the intraocular contents. Excimer photorefractive procedures alter the anterior curvature of the cornea to change its ability to refract light. In accomplishing this, the transparency of the tissue as well as the strength and integrity must be maintained. The ability to alter the cornea's shape to correct hyperopia has proven to be a greater challenge than that to correct myopia. It is much easier to flatten the cornea by removing central tissue than to steepen it. The cornea's wound healing responses are much better at repairing the peripheral tissue removal, primarily through the epithelium's ability to thicken and fill in the defect. Fortunately, the hyperopic ablation is less likely to alter the structural integrity to the cornea since it is removing tissue in the midperiphery where the cornea is normally much thicker. However, one must not get careless and forget to calculate the residual posterior stroma especially in higher hyperopic treatments as well as retreatments. Dr. Steven Slade has presented a hyperopic PRK case in which multiple retreatments led to complete corneal perforation.

The corneal epithelium is integrally involved in the attempts made to steepen the anterior corneal curvature with either surface or lamellar photorefractive procedures. The epithelium functions as a barrier to both mechanical forces as well as diffusion of fluids and substances. In addition, its ability to provide a smooth optical surface is imperative to good visual function. It is composed of 5 to 7 cell layers normally 30 to 50 µm in thickness.[2] Each cell is approximately 7 µm in thickness, which can account for a half to three-quarters of a diopter of refractive effect. Thus the epithelial response seen to the peripheral tissue removal can significantly affect the refractive result just with a single extra cell layer. After LASIK and PRK the corneal epithelium will thicken as much as 75 µm.[1] It has been demonstrated that the epithelium thickens over areas of corneal thinning and especially over areas of irregularity in the LASIK flap.

The epithelium is composed of 3 types of cells: the surface squamous cells, middle polygonal wind cells, and regenerating basal cells. The glycoprotein layer in the plasma membrane of the squamous cell assists in protecting the cornea from infectious agents. Since LASIK does minimal damage to this layer, the risk of infection with lamellar procedures is significantly less than for surface ablative procedures. The polygonal cells have attachments to each other that are not destroyed by the 20% alcohol solution used in

LASEK and assist in permitting the epithelial flap to be detached in a single sheet. The basal cells are responsible for the regeneration of the epithelium. The accumulation of iron in these cells is the etiology for the iron lines seen after refractive surgery.

Not only does the structure of the epithelium participates in the results after photorefractive keratectomy, but its metabolism also plays an important role. Because the epithelium receives its oxygen supply from the tear film layer, during eyelid closure with sleep there is a reduction in the oxygen available. This results in anaerobic metabolism and increased lactic acid levels. The lactic acid will then lead to stromal swelling through increased osmolality and its toxic effects on the endothelium. Using a bandage soft contact lens in PRK and LASEK can increase the deleterious effect of this nocturnal hypoxia.

The basement membrane secreted by the epithelium assists in its attachment to the underlying stroma. It is postulated by Dr. Camellin that in LASEK, if the basement membrane is preserved, the re-epithelialization will be considerably faster.[5] Dr. Singh has work to suggest that the basement membrane is responsible for directing the nature of the differentiation of the underlying stroma.[6] Its presence may modify wound healing and eliminate the haze seen after surface ablative procedures.

The true function and value of Bowman's membrane has continued to evade identification. This uncertainty is an underlying factor in the controversy between surface (PRK and LASEK) and lamellar (LASIK) photorefractive procedures. Because Bowman's layer cannot regenerate, surface ablation greater than 1.00 D of correction will remove this layer exposing the underlying stroma. The interaction between the epithelium and this denuded stroma can lead to "haze" formation. This opacification is due to subepithelial and/or stromal wound repair.[7] As LASIK spares Bowman's and does not disturb its natural relationship to the epithelium and epithelial basement membrane, haze is rarely, if ever a consideration. One must not forget that LASIK does affect Bowman's layer as the incision does disrupt its integrity and biomechanical forces. If Bowman's layer has a role in maintaining the corneal shape, one would expect the LASIK flap to affect the surface topography. Indeed studies have shown that the simple construction of the lamellar flap can alter corneal topography.[8] More definite is the change in wavefront evaluation seen with flap construction.

It is not simply Bowman's layer that demonstrates this biomechanical weakening response. The underlying corneal lamellae are also under tension in the dome shape of the cornea. The LASIK flap relieves the strain in the anterior lamellae both peripheral to and central to the cut. The collagen fibers unwind and water moves into the tissue. This results in peripheral corneal thickening and central fiber uncoiling seen clinically as microstriae.[4]

The true effect of the laser ablation on the corneal endothelium is controversial. Whether or not the acoustic waves have a short-term or permanent deleterious effect on the corneal endothelium is not definite. It certainly does not appear clinically that there is any significant damage.[3] As mentioned previously, there is a transient effect on endothelial function when the cornea is under hypoxic stress. The question as to whether there is a different degree of acoustic effect on the endothelium based on the tissue thickness difference between surface and intrastromal ablation has been raised, but not answered.

A difference in the effect on corneal innervation is definitely present between surface and lamellar procedures. The LASIK flap deinnervates the ophthalmic branches of the trigeminal nerve corneal flap whereas surface ablation simply damages the endings. This is in part why one can see neurotropic keratitis as a complication of LASIK and not PRK. However, both types of ablation can be affected by the effect of deinnervation on the rate of epithelial healing.

# PREOPERATIVE EVALUATION

It can be argued that the most important part of the refractive surgery process is the preoperative evaluation. The preoperative evaluation includes more than just the physical ophthalmologic examination. The evaluation of a patient and his or her candidacy begins from the first communication or contact with any of the laser center's staff or physicians. Personality attributes, expectations, and demeanor all can assist in determining not only whether or not the individual is a good laser vision candidate, but also which procedure is most appropriate. The better trained and more astute the staff members, the more effective this process will be.

The initial patient contact is usually by phone. The phone receptionist and/or patient education coordinator should record any pertinent comments regarding their contact with the candidate. It is amazing the amount of information that can be gained through the first phone contact by an experienced staff member. The computer scheduling system should be utilized to record these observations. Obviously, scrutiny must be used as to how this information is recorded should it be observed by the candidate or other individuals. Many staff members have discrete codes they use to identify important characteristics such as impatience, attitude, or financial concerns.

A screening process for phone communications to make certain that appropriate candidates only are brought in for evaluation is essential. This is especially true if complimentary evaluations are performed. Time and effort spent on non-candidates is an added burden and expense. Although it is not always easy to be certain as to the candidates' true refractive error, in most cases one can determine if the candidate is hyperopic, myopic, or simply presbyopic.

Identifying the age, stability of refraction, expectations, and nature of visual problem further assist in advising the prospective patient. The history regarding past or present contact lens wear should be identified and the recommended instructions for removal prior to the examination provided. It is critical to maximize the efficiency of the preoperative assessment as the greater the amount of patient/staff/physician contact time the greater the chance of identifying potential problems. Every refractive surgeon can think of instances where their preoperative intuition was supported by the patient's postoperative behavior. With the rise of litigation one must not ignore any suspicious characteristics.

Personality characteristics include:

- ◇ Their understanding of laser vision correction
- ◇ Expectations based on this understanding as well as interaction with other laser vision correction patients
- ◇ Degree of education
- ◇ Visual/pain tolerance
- ◇ Level of anxiety, fears, concerns, and confidence
- ◇ Impatience
- ◇ Demanding, obsessive, compulsive
- ◇ Pleasant, friendly, considerate
- ◇ Abrupt, introverted

Lifestyle and occupational characteristics include:

- ◇ High-risk trauma
  1. Law enforcement
  2. Military
  3. Firefighters/paramedics
  4. Martial arts
- ◇ Low-risk trauma
  1. Golf
  2. Aerobic exercise
  3. Professional
- ◇ Infection risk
  1. Health care
  2. Agriculture
- ◇ Visual requirements
  1. Pilot
  2. Commercial driver
- ◇ Time demands
  1. Flexible
  2. Follow-up accessibility
  3. Recovery time
- ◇ The physical examination begins with a standard medical history. This includes previous medical problems, surgical procedures, medications, allergies, and pertinent family history. A thorough contact lens history is mandatory as well as the time of discontinued wear prior to testing

◆ Stability of the patient's refractive error must be established. Either records of past exams or checking old glasses' prescription is required. Uncorrected acuities at distance and near should be documented. Manifest and cycloplegic (1% cyclopentolate recommended) refractions along with best corrected acuities are measured

◆ Pupil size is measured in dark and light adapted states using the Colvard pupillometer (Oasis Medical, Glendora, Calif) or other similar standardized instrumentation. The pupillary reaction to light and the presence or absence of an afferent defect is checked.

◆ Ocular dominance is identified

◆ The Bausch & Lomb keratometer (Rochester, NY) is used to measure keratometry and qualitatively evaluate the mires. Orbscan (Bausch & Lomb) is used to record topography and pachymetry. If any question or concern about accuracy of corneal thickness, the manual pachymeter is used to confirm measurements

◆ IOP is checked using Goldmann applanation tonometry

◆ Slit lamp biomicroscopy evaluates the lids, cornea, anterior chamber, iris and lens. A qualitative evaluation of the tear film and tear meniscus is completed and then a zone quick screening test performed. Any low values are followed by a Schirmer's test. The reliability of recent tear analysis for lysosyme remains to be proven and is not cost effective at this time

◆ Gonioscopy should be performed on any hyperopic patient with suspiciously narrow angles on slit lamp biomicroscopy. Peripheral laser iridotomy should be performed if indicated prior to laser vision correction, since there may be a shift in the refractive error afterward

◆ Mydriatic and cycloplegic solution (1% cyclopentolate) is then instilled and the cycloplegic and fundus evaluation completed. The informed consent and patient education video is observed while the patient is dilating

# INDICATIONS AND CONTRAINDICATIONS

All refractive surgical procedures demand appropriate patient selection in order to achieve optimal results. Patient consent is paramount and one must remember that the patient may well have a preference as to the choice of surgical procedure. It is easiest and least confusing for the patient to consider first if they are a good laser candidate, then to determine which procedure is preferred.

## General Indications

◆ +1.00 to +6.00 D of spherical equivalent (DSE) at spectacle plane. For hyperopic astigmatism cylinder: cylinder not to exceed 4.00 D and SE not to exceed +6.00 DSE

◆ Patient consent

◆ At least 21 years of age

◆ <0.75 D difference between manifest and cyclopentolate refraction

◆ Refractive stability: patients whose hyperopia is progressing at a rate greater than 0.50 D per year should not be treated

## General Contraindications

Patients with systemic medical conditions—collagen vascular, autoimmune, or immunodeficiency disease. (Caution should be exercised with those diseases likely to affect to affect wound healing such as diabetes, atopy, and connective tissue disease.)

◆ Women: pregnant or nursing

◆ Patients with signs of keratoconus

◆ Patients taking medications: Isoretinoin (Accutane, Hoffman La Roche Inc, Switzerland), amiodarone hydrochloride (Cordarone, Wyeth, Madison, NJ), sumitripan (Imitrex, GlaxoSmithKline, Research Triangle Park, NC)

◆ Patients with history of keloid formation

◆ Not recommended at this time in patients with *herpes simplex* or *herpes zoster*

# OTHER SPECIFIC CONSIDERATIONS FOR PATIENT SELECTION

Remember it is extremely important to evaluate the specific characteristics with respect to each of the 3 laser vision correction procedures. The following to a large extent reflects my own personal approach to this task and will vary from surgeon to surgeon. However, I do believe that the principles are sound and demonstrate a true desire to maximize long-term safety and still achieve the desired visual result.

Patients need to be symptomatic with their hyperopia. Those patients, most likely younger than 35 years, who are not wearing corrective lenses, or do not have significant complaints are poor candidates.

The degree of hyperopia and astigmatism is important in determining the potential for improvement as well as being a factor in procedure selection. The majority of surgeons would agree that the visual results for hyperopia with or without astigmatism are optimal for between 1.00 and 4.00 D of correction. The results for 4.00 to 6.00 D are not as predictable. Above 6.00 D the patient is better served by a nonlaser keratorefractive procedure. Also, it can be very difficult to create a LASIK flap that is both large enough in diameter and is centered about an eccentric pupil to permit unrestricted ablation of the entire 9-mm treatment zone. With higher ablations, more treatment may be eliminated at the hinge, which can potentially affect the symmetry and completeness of the ablation increasing the chance for irregular astigmatism.

The degree and quality of the corneal curvature, anterior and posterior, significantly affect the choice of procedure. The Orbscan is 1 instrument that gives data for both these surfaces. The calculated postoperative anterior curvature should not be greater than 50.00 D for any procedure. Corneal curvatures in the 40.00 D or flatter range can lead to smaller flap diameters as well as greater incidence of flap construction complications. Therefore, a surface ablative procedure that eliminates the need for a flap and the inherent complications is preferred.

The quality of both anterior and posterior corneal surfaces must be considered. Keratoconus is the most common reason for preoperative irregular astigmatism. Certainly this is an uncommon finding when focusing on hyperopic eyes. The posterior curvature can assist in identifying keratoconic suspects that might get by with only anterior surface evaluation. One should never forget the value of a standard qualitative keratometer in looking for surface irregularities. Anterior basement membrane changes can also be detected, which should alert the surgeon to considering PRK as the preferred surgery. Extreme caution should be used in treating keratoconic suspects, but if surgery is chosen, it seems surface ablation is the least likely to alter the corneal integrity. LASIK should be contraindicated.

Controversy revolves around corneal thickness and what safety standards should be used. An overall corneal thickness of 500 µm is a reasonable minimum to permit safe flap construction without weakening the corneal structure. No matter the flap thickness (100 to 180 µm), this still seems to be an acceptable level. Leaving a residual posterior stromal thickness of 300 µm seems most prudent, although a number of LASIK surgeons use 250 µm as their minimum. For surface procedures there is even less agreement. Four hundred µm is a conservative amount, although 350 µm may be acceptable. The difficulty with basing surgery only on thickness without the input of tissue quality is that most probably each of these variables is equally important. To utilize only thickness means much more conservative levels must be used to compensate for any eyes with inherently weaker tissue.

The corneal diameter is much more important in hyperopic ablations than myopic ones. Since a larger flap diameter is necessary, the chances for a free cap and extension to

the limbus (eg, hemorrhaging) are higher. Surface ablation eliminates the potential for flap complications, but still increases the potential for hemorrhaging from limbal vessels or neovascularization with the larger ablation zone diameter.

The presence of a dry eye syndrome or tear dysfunction must be identified. Certainly all 3 procedures are affected by these problems and preoperative treatment must be implemented prior to surgery. It has been my experience that surface procedures are better suited to dry eyes, and LASIK with the potential for neurotropic keratitis is less desirable. The appropriate preoperative management is essential in achieving successful results. Patients must be educated as to the increased risk of postoperative problems and longer recovery.

Scotopic pupil size is another debated issue.[9] There does appear to be an increased incidence of low contrast and dark vision symptoms such as halos and glare with larger scotopic papillary diameters. Although a recent study by Dr. Shallhorn doesn't demonstrate this direct relationship,[9] this was performed in myopic eyes and I'm not aware that there is any prospective study on scotopic pupil size in hyperopia. Wavefront analysis should help to determine if preoperative higher aberrations may be a better indicator of scotopic visual side effects. Dr. Mia Pop's study revealed less subjective glare and halo effects with PRK than LASIK.[10] This is due to the fact that with LASIK there is a smaller effective optic zone than with surface ablation. Therefore, common sense dictates that in patients with larger scotopic papillary diameters and higher degrees of refractive error that the patient is informed of the potential increased risk, and that surface ablation be considered over LASIK.

Also, in hyperopic treatments it is important to identify an eccentric pupil. Failure to do so can result in a LASIK flap that does not permit a complete ablation profile. Surface ablation improves the ability to obtain a complete and large enough area of exposed Bowman's to insure a symmetrical ablation in many cases not suitable for LASIK.

Pupil considerations:

1. Scotopic pupil size >8 mm
2. Scotopic pupil size 7 to 8 mm/high hyperopia-hyperopic astigmatism
3. Eccentric pupil not permitting LASIK flap centration

The true effects of the significantly increased IOP that occurs with application of the fixation ring in LASIK have yet to be determined. There are ocular conditions that may be better served by avoiding this transient pressure elevation. Optic nerve disease is certainly a category that deserves consideration. In anyone predisposed to optic nerve or vascular problems such as central retinal vein occlusion, glaucomatous optic atrophy, or anterior ischemic optic neuropathy surface ablation may avoid the possible aggravation or development of these vision threatening problems. Again, it is important to emphasize that little if any proven information exists to prove these concerns; however, they do have merit based on our present knowledge and experience. Why take any unnecessary chances when safer and visually equivalent procedures exist?

Lattice degeneration and the overall increased risk of retinal detachment are obviously less applicable for the hyperopic eye than for the myopic eye. But application of the fixation ring with the abnormally abrupt and high elevation of intraocular pressure still may shift the vitreous. Consequently, it is reasonable to believe that this could increase the risk of retinal detachment in predisposed individuals. It is also appropriate to mention that eyes having had prior scleral buckling may be difficult to achieve adequate vacuum and fixation of the fixation ring. A surface ablation procedure can be helpful in these situations.

Any signs of cataractous lens changes are important in patient selection. It seems prudent to always factor in the degree of lenticular opacification, remaining accommodation, and degree of hyperopia to consider the possibility of lens extraction and intraocular lens implantation. In higher hyperopes, as mentioned earlier, the quality of postoperative vision for the IOL implant is superior to that achieved with laser ablation. Patients easily understand that it is preferable to perform cataract surgery earlier than to undergo laser vision correction only to need cataract surgery a year or so later.

And finally, once all these anatomical and specific ocular features have been identified, they should be considered in light of the personal and lifestyle characteristics of the individual patient to make appropriate recommendations as to the preferred options. The final decision or recommendation should have both short- and long-term safety as its foundation. The final decision is to be made by the patient. The choice of procedure should be based on honest and accurate information provided by the surgeon and staff. In some cases the surgeon's concern regarding safety may be overruled by the patient's desires. This is where it may be necessary for the surgeon to decide if he or she feels comfortable proceeding with the patient's choice. It is these situations that surgeons find most difficult.

# SURGICAL TECHNIQUES

## *Anesthesia*

The anesthesia technique used is the same for all 3 procedures. Topical anesthetic solution of proparacaine or tetracaine is sufficient. The administration of a mild oral sedative such as Valium (Roche, Nutley, NJ) can be beneficial, not only for the operation itself, but also for the comfort of the patient in the early postoperative period. Excessive sedation is undesirable as patient cooperation is mandatory to insure excellent patient fixation.

## *Procedure*

### PREOPERATIVE CONSIDERATIONS

Proper informed consent is obtained for the specific procedure LASIK, LASEK, or PRK.

A topical fluoroquinolone is routinely prescribed for qid usage the day prior to surgery. Thirty minutes prior to surgery a topical anesthetic, topical fluoroquinolone, and topical non-steroidal anti-inflammatory agent are instilled. Oral Valium is offered on an individual basis.

### OPERATIVE TECHNIQUES

1. LASIK
   - Microkeratome is assembled and proper functioning confirmed. The blade should always be examined under high magnification
   - The patient's hair is covered with a bonnet. Periocular areas are then prepped with Betadine solution and draped as a sterile field, making certain eyelashes are covered. A 4x4 gauze is placed on each side to absorb tears and solutions. The non operated eye is covered with an opaque shield
   - The patient is properly positioned under the operating microscope of the laser unit
   - Additional topical anesthetic and an adjustable wire lid speculum are placed
   - A cornea alignment marker with gentian violet is used to mark the corneal epithelium
   - Topical anesthetic is applied to the limbus in all four quadrants for 5 to 10 seconds each using a surgical spear
   - The fixation ring is then centered and vacuum applied
   - IOP is checked with an applanation tonometer, observation of papillary dilation, and patient's dimming of vision
   - BSS or preferred wetting solution is applied to the corneal surface
   - The microkeratome head is then inserted and the flap cut. The microkeratome and fixation ring are then carefully removed
   - A Chayet ring is placed about the limbus and the flap retracted. The stromal bed is carefully dried with a murocel spear or spatula
   - The patient fixates on the fixation light and the ablation performed being careful to protect the hinge from being ablation
   - The flap is then replaced and brief irrigation with BSS and one of several types of cannulas. The flap is allowed to settle into position. Several techniques ranging from wiping with a moist surgical spear to an applanation device or using air/oxygen to dry the edge of the flap are utilized

◆ Once the flap is determined to be stable, a viscous lubricant is placed and the speculum removed

2. LASEK

◆ The patient is properly positioned under the operating microscope of the laser unit

◆ A hair bonnet is placed and a 4x4 gauze pad is placed on each side to absorb tears and solutions. An opaque eye shield is taped over the nonoperated eye

◆ Additional topical anesthetic and an adjustable, bladed lid speculum are placed

◆ The appropriate diameter sharp, modified disposable trephine (a non-disposable trephine may be preferred) is placed and centered on the pupil, held between both right and left index fingers. Firm but gentle pressure is placed onto the cornea and the trephine slowly rotated 5 to 10 degrees in both clockwise and counterclockwise directions. A full thickness epithelial incision is desired. Even with a sharp edge this can be accomplished without significantly penetrating or damaging Bowman's layer

◆ The alcohol reservoir 0.5 mm larger than the trephine is placed very firmly onto the cornea. It is centered about the trephination incision. The patient should be reminded to keep both eyes open and directed to gaze straight ahead

◆ The 20% ETOH/BSS solution is injected into the reservoir with a metal cannula and glass syringe. The contact time is 30 seconds for routine cases. If the solution leaks out the eye should be immediately irrigated with BSS and the fornices dried with a surgical spear. The reservoir and ETOH/BSS solution are then reapplied for another 20 to 30 seconds

◆ An Intac's pocket hook is used to test and free the edge of the epithelial flap. If detachment does not occur easily, then one should reapply the EOTH/BSS solution. It is possible to get evaporation of the EOTH or a denatured vial, so always try a new vial of EOTH

◆ The microhoe is then used to slide back the epithelial flap. It is folded back on itself to the superior aspect of the hinge. It is not uncommon in the larger, hyperopic flaps to have a free flap

◆ The laser ablation is then performed. The nomogram adjustment is closer to that for LASIK than for PRK. It is recommended when starting out to use this adjustment and modify it according to the results

◆ The flap is then gently repositioned. The blunt tipped instrument is moistened in the tear film and the epithelium is then unfolded and pushed inferi-

orly. If a free cap occurs then traction superiorly at the edge permits it to be nicely repositioned. Since realignment of the flap is not important, epithelial markings are not necessary

◆ A drop or 2 of Muro 128 solution is then placed on the epithelial flap

◆ A Bausch & Lomb Purevision (Rochester, NY) (14.2-mm diameter and 8.6-mm base curve) or Biomedics 55 (14.2-mm diameter and 8.6-mm base curve) is placed

◆ The speculum is removed and gentle pressure with the 4x4 pad placed on the closed lid to stabilize the contact

3. PRK

◆ The patient is properly positioned under the operating microscope of the laser unit

◆ A hair bonnet is placed and a 4x4 gauze pad is placed on each side to absorb tears and solutions. An opaque eye shield is taped over the nonoperated eye

◆ Additional topical anesthetic and an adjustable, bladed lid speculum are placed

◆ The patient is briefly instructed on the fixation process and the sights, sounds, and smells of the procedure

◆ The epithelium is removed by preferred method
   a. Manual: debridement of a 9 mm to 10 mm with a spatula, 69 Beaver blade, or Amoil brush
   b. Alcohol: alcohol maybe applied to loosen the epithelium which is then easily removed with a surgical spear. A 9.5- to 10-mm reservoir is centered and then filled with 20% alcohol/BSS solution for 30 to 60 seconds. The solution removed with a surgical spear and the corneal surface irrigated with chilled BSS

◆ The desired hyperopic and astigmatic ablation is then performed

◆ A soft contact is then placed

◆ Lid speculum is removed

# MANAGEMENT

It is definitely true that the postoperative management of laser vision correction patients is critical to not only the surgical success but also patient satisfaction. Patient education is paramount and cannot be stressed enough. The general expectations of the nature of the visual recovery, potential discomfort, and realistic final visual result must be understood, especially with surface ablative procedures where there can be a significant amount of pain. These patients will interact with LASIK patients and it is essential that they are able to comprehend why their postoperative experience was different.

## Immediate Postoperative Period

### LASIK, LASEK, AND PRK

A drop each of the antibiotic, steroid, and NSAIDs are instilled. A less potent steroid such as fluoromethalone is used for surface ablation and more potent one such as prednisolone acetate for lamellar procedures. Clear shields or sunglasses are placed for protection. Oral pain medications are prescribed for surface ablation procedures. Patient instructions are to go home, take a nap, and instill the medication drops every 4 hours. PRK and LASEK are given a preservative-free nonsteroidal that is not used for LASIK. The patient is to use preservative-free artificial tears as necessary. An oral sleeping pill is given to take home at the patient's discretion.

## Postoperative Day 1

### COMFORT

1. LASIK: It is unusual to have any significant discomfort other than occasionally some dry eye symptoms
2. LASEK: The majority will be surprisingly comfortable. The first day is generally the best from a comfort standpoint for these patients
3. PRK: Most of the patients will experience only mild to moderate discomfort

### VISION

1. LASIK: The majority will be in the 20/20 to 20/50 range but not as common as in myopic LASIK. A degree of overcorrection is expected just as in surface ablation, however, usually not to the same extent
2. LASEK: Vision is similar to PRK in its range, but overall more see at the 20/25 to 20/40 level. Again, as with PRK, many or most will be myopic and functioning better at near
3. PRK: Vision will range from 20/25 to 20/400. Remember many if not most will be myopic with improved near vision

### EXAMINATION

1. External
   - LASIK: Almost all are normal lids unless patient has excessive blepharospasm, adverse reaction to topical medications, or rarely an infectious process
   - LASEK: Lids are normally quiet without significant edema. Lid edema if present is generally mild. It is due to excessive blepharospasm against the lid speculum, the presence of the soft contact lens, reaction to medication, or rarely an infectious process
   - PRK: Same as for LASEK

2. SLE: Conjunctiva
   - LASIK: Other than small subconjunctival hemorrhages generally normal. Injection might indicate inflammation, infection, or reaction to topical medications. Normal conjunctival appearance is the norm in eyes with diffuse lamellar keratitis and may help in differentiation from an infectious process
   - LASEK: As with PRK, the vast majority will be normal. Same reasons for injection are present
   - PRK: The majority are without injection. Injection may be related to the absence of the contact lens, a tight contact lens with hypoxia, adverse reaction to topical medication, inflammation or infection

3. Cornea
   - LASIK: Most cases the keratectomy should be almost invisible. Cornea is normally clear except for minute interface debris. Diffuse lamellar keratitis is almost always evident at this first visit. Superficial keratitis is not uncommon. Epithelium should normally be intact
   - LASEK: Stromal appearance similar to PRK. Epithelial flap in half the cases almost normal in appearance. Epithelial tissue over edge of limbal edge of defect will be edematous and easily identified
   - PRK: Contact lens should be well centered and minimal movement. A small percentage will demonstrate mild stromal edema with or without folds. There will be a large epithelial defect. Anterior surface should be clear. Careful attention should be paid to identify any early infiltrates

### MANAGEMENT

1. LASIK
   - If striae, lift flap and reposition
   - Continue topical antibiotic QID (fluoroquinolone)
   - Continue topical steroid QID (Pred Forte [Allergan, Irvine, Calif] or Lotemax [Bausch & Lomb, Rochester, NY]). If signs of DLK, increase to every 30 to 60 minutes. Consider flap irrigation if severe inflammation
   - Non-preserved artificial tears as necessary
   - Shields at bedtime
   - Activity as common sense dictates. Avoid swimming or hot tubs for 3 to 4 weeks. Caution against eye rubbing
   - Reassure that visual recovery is slower than with routine myopic LASIK

2. LASEK
   - Continue topical antibiotic QID (fluoroquinolone)

✦ Continue topical steroid QID (FML [Allergan] or Alrex [Bausch & Lomb, Rochester, NY]). If moderate to severe inflammation, then increase to 6 to 8 times a day

✦ Continue topical NSAID QID. Consider decreasing or stopping if no discomfort or inflammation. Recommend using Acular PF and only giving enough of the individual dispensers to last until the next visit. This will make it difficult to misuse and end up with sterile infiltrates

✦ Non-preserved artificial tears as needed

✦ Cool compresses as needed for pain

✦ Oral non-steroidal drug for mild discomfort, and darvocette N-100 or vicoprofen for moderate to severe pain. In most extreme cases use a narcotic such as Mepergan Fortis (Wyeth, Madison, NJ)

✦ Shields at bedtime

✦ Activity as common sense dictates. Avoid swimming or hot tubs for 3 to 4 weeks

✦ Reassure patient that not concerned about vision at this point. Normal to see better at near

✦ Change contact only if absolutely necessary. At this point even careful removal of the contact lens may loosen and likely remove the epithelial flap

3. PRK
   ✦ Same as for LASEK

FOLLOW-UP

1. LASIK
   ✦ 1 week if uncomplicated. If DLK or other concern see in 24 hours

2. LASEK
   ✦ Schedule for 2 days but see in 1 if any concerns or patient desires

3. PRK
   ✦ Same as LASEK

## Postoperative Days 2 Through 10

For all 3 procedures, patients need to understand the significant individual variability in the nature of the healing response. Although the majority of recoveries are similar for the procedures, the few extremely variable responses make it mandatory that patients be prepared. In doing so, it definitely helps in getting these exceptions through this difficult period. The patient expectations for refractive surgery are unquestionably unrealistic and must be tempered as much as possible with preoperative education. The better this education, the easier and more effective the postoperative management will be. Despite even the best education, it continually amazes me that patients will still ask during this early period, "Is this the best I'm going to see?" or "Is my vision going to improve?"

COMFORT

1. LASIK
   ✦ Other than foreign body sensation and dry eye symptoms there should be little if any discomfort unless there is some complication

2. LASEK
   ✦ Comfort generally continues to be good. Just as in PRK, hyperopic LASEK cases demonstrate less discomfort than myopic cases. The same factors responsible for pain with PRK are responsible for it in LASEK

3. PRK
   ✦ Comfort for hyperopic treatments tends to be better than for myopic treatments. At first this would seem to be the opposite that one would expect, as the epithelial defect and ablation is much larger than in a myopic ablation. However, my personal experience is that severe pain is unusual in the hyperopic cases. Patients who do experience discomfort need reassurance that this doesn't mean that there is a serious problem. A tight contact lens, hypoxia, poor tear function, adverse reaction to medication, and simply the natural wound healing response may all contribute to the discomfort

VISION

1. LASIK
   ✦ Vision is good. Not unusual to be myopic. One may need temporary spectacles to assist in driving

2. LASEK
   ✦ Vision will normally decrease as the epithelial flap is replaced by the new epithelium. Surprisingly, approximately 25% to 40% will maintain vision in the 20/25 to 20/50 range. As with PRK, vision normally improves 24 to 48 hours after the contact is removed and the epithelium is replaced

3. PRK
   ✦ Vision ranges from fair to poor. It is reasonable to tell the patient that the vision will tend to improve 24 to 48 hours after the contact lens is removed

EXAMINATION

1. External
   ✦ LASIK: Lids should be normal
   ✦ LASEK: Lids should be normal
   ✦ PRK: Lids should be normal

2. SLE: Conjunctiva
   ✦ LASIK: Should be normal other than resolving subconjunctival hemorrhages
   ✦ LASEK: Similar to PRK
   ✦ PRK: The conjunctiva is normally quiet. Injection is usually limbal when present. This is secondary to hypoxia due to a tight contact lens or reaction to the topical medication

3. Cornea
- ✦ LASIK: The flap should be clear without significant striae. Microstriae due to settling and that do not effect the vision are not as commonly seen as in those with high myopia. Interface inflammation may be detected after day 1, but it is usually due to a change in the person's vision as routine follow-up is 1 day and 1 week. SPK may still be present
- ✦ LASEK: The replacement of the epithelial flap can be followed by the changes in the mottled appearance of the edematous cells. As they slough and are replaced this mottled appearance disappears. The entire re-epithelialization may take from 4 to 8 days. The contact is generally removed at day four and the surface evaluated. A contact is replaced if not intact. As with PRK, stromal edema may be seen with contact wear and infiltrates need identified
- ✦ PRK: The epithelial defect will decrease covering the central cornea last. This usually takes 4 to 6 days in hyperopic corrections. Infiltrates need to be identified as sterile or infectious. Stromal edema may indicate a tight or dirty contact lens with resultant hypoxia

MANAGEMENT
1. LASIK
   - ✦ The development of any visually significant striae should be corrected by lifting and repositioning the flap. At this early stage, "ironing or stretching" of the flap with preferred method as well as careful hydration of the area of striae should correctly replace the flap. It is important to make certain that the epithelium over the striae is disrupted as it is the anterior folds in Bowman's layer that are the most recalcitrant
   - ✦ The topical antibiotic is continued QID for 1 week
   - ✦ The topical steroid is continued QID for 1 week. Its application in DLK is dependent on the level of inflammation. IOP must be monitored and the potential for fluid in the interface considered
   - ✦ Artificial tears prn
   - ✦ Shields at bedtime for 1 week
   - ✦ Activity as per day 1. If significantly myopic and trouble with distance functioning, then prescribe temporary spectacle correction
   - ✦ Reassurance that vision will fluctuate more than myopic cases
2. LASIK
   - ✦ Replace contact lens if tight or dirty. Contact lens should be removed when the corneal epithelium is completely intact and able to tolerate lid movement. If there is any question as to the integrity of the epithelium, it is always better to error on keeping the contact a day or 2 longer than to remove it and have the epithelium break down. On occasions in which there is a small defect or thickened area, it may be best to simply place a pressure patch for 6 to 12 hours. The defect may be slow to heal due to mechanical trauma or hypoxia from the contact
   - ✦ Continue topical antibiotic QID until the epithelium is intact and contact removed
   - ✦ Continue topical steroid QID. If epithelial healing delayed then decrease temporarily, and if increased inflammation then increase frequency
   - ✦ Discontinue topical nonsteroidal drug as soon as eye comfortable. Sterile infiltrates will develop occasionally despite the concomitant use of the topical steroid
   - ✦ Frequent use of artificial tears
   - ✦ Cool compresses as necessary
   - ✦ Continue oral nonsteroidal drug as well as analgesic prn
   - ✦ Shields at bedtime for 4 to 5 days
   - ✦ Activity as condition dictates. Vision will be primary reason for restricted activity
   - ✦ Reassurance as to slow visual recovery
   - ✦ When changing contact lens may need to gently debride loose tags of epithelial flap
3. PRK
   - ✦ Same as LASEK

FOLLOW-UP
1. LASIK
   - ✦ Patients are scheduled routinely at 1 month unless vision or other delays in recovery are present
2. LASEK
   - ✦ Patients are seen 1 to 2 weeks after the contact is removed and the epithelium intact
3. PRK
   - ✦ Same as LASEK

## *Postoperative Weeks 2 to 4*

COMFORT
1. LASIK
   - ✦ By this time most patients are comfortable. Dryness is not uncommon and should be aggressively treated with standard management
2. LASEK
   - ✦ Same as LASIK
3. PRK
   - ✦ Same as LASIK

VISION

1. LASIK
   + Vision should be improved with reduction in early myopic shift
2. LASEK
   + Vision for most should be considerably better. Myopia should be decreasing. May still be some irregular astigmatism due to epithelial reorganization
2. PRK
   + Same as for LASEK

EXAMINATION

1. External
   + LASIK: Normal
   + LASEK: Normal
   + PRK: Normal
2. SLE: Conjunctiva
   + LASIK: Normal
   + LASEK: Normal
   + LASIK: Normal
3. Cornea
   + LASIK: Normally clear. Interface opacities will be becoming less noticeable. If macrostriae develop, need to be treated. Epithelial ingrowth may be seen at this time
   + LASEK: Should be clear. As with PRK trace subepithelial haze (diffuse granular opacification) may be seen. Also one may identify anterior basement membrane changes
   + PRK: Should be clear. Trace subepithelial haze may be seen. Significant haze is rare

MANAGEMENT

1. LASIK
   + Late clinically significant striae need to be treated. Methods previously described are generally capable to correct these late defects. Rarely suturing is necessary as a last resort
   + Epithelial ingrowth that enlarges, threatens the visual axis, or does not decrease needs to be removed. The key is to remember that the etiology is poor wound apposition. The epithelium must be removed from the wound edges as well as the interface and then the wound edge repositioned and protected with a contact lens. Suturing may be needed in rare cases. Alcohol has been recommended by some, but seems unnecessary except in extremely rare instances
2. LASEK
   + Topical steroids should be administrated with respect to age, degree of correction, haze, and post-

operative refractive error. Hyperopic refractions dictate an increased frequency/potency of application and significant consecutive myopia with a reduction in the application. Some disagree with the effects of steroid administration, but there does appear to be significant clinical effects in many patients
   + Irregularity in epithelium may be added with hypertonic saline ointment or drops
3. PRK
   + Same as LASEK

FOLLOW-UP

1. LASIK
   + 2 to 3 months
2. LASEK
   + 2 to 3 months
3. PRK
   + 2 to 3 months

## Postoperative Months 2 Through 4

COMFORT

1. LASIK
   + Should be normal
2. LASEK
   + Should be normal
3. PRK
   + Should be normal

VISION

1. LASIK
   + Stabilization should be good by 1 month for the majority of cases
2. LASEK
   + There will still be some degree of fluctuation, but stabilization should be improving
3. PRK
   + Same as LASEK

EXAMINATION

1. LASIK
   + Clear with faint visible edge of flap not uncommonly detected
2. LASEK
   + Most will be clear. Occasional trace granular haze, but much less frequent than myopic cases. Check IOP if still on steroid
3. PRK
   + Similar to LASEK

MANAGEMENT
1. LASIK
   ✦ Taper steroids if treating DLK. Dry eye management as indicated
2. LASEK
   ✦ Continue to use topical steroid if concern regarding haze or regression.
   ✦ Dry eye management as indicated
3. PRK
   ✦ As per LASEK

FOLLOW-UP
1. LASIK
   ✦ 2 months to consider enhancement if necessary
2. LASEK
   ✦ 2 to 3 months if routine. Sooner if on steroid
3. PRK
   ✦ Same as LASEK

## Postoperative Months 6 Through 12

1. LASIK
   ✦ If regression or excessive myopia exists, retreatment should be performed
2. LASEK
   ✦ Watching for complete stabilization of refraction and visual acuity to determine if an enhancement is necessary
   ✦ Late haze should be managed with topical steroids and if severe, retreatment with mitomycin-C
3. PRK
   ✦ Same as LASEK

# COMPLICATIONS

## Preoperative

1. LASIK
   ✦ Error in preoperative measurements
   ✦ Poor patient selection
   ✦ Failure to diagnose keratoconus or other pertinent ocular problem
   ✦ Failure to have laser working properly
   ✦ Incorrect entry of ablation data into laser computer or calculation error of ablation parameters
2. LASEK
   ✦ Same as LASIK
3. PRK
   ✦ Same as LASEK

## Intraoperative

1. LASIK
   ✦ Inability to achieve adequate suction with the fixation ring. Unable to perform procedure with conversion to surface ablation
   ✦ Epithelial defect
   ✦ Flap abnormality-button-hole, thin flap, incomplete flap, and free cap
   ✦ Equipment malfunction
   ✦ Improper ablation due to poor focusing, excessive moisture, or excessive drying
   ✦ Inadequate repositioning of the flap
   ✦ Significant interface debris
2. LASEK
   ✦ Decentered ablation. Failure to maintain fixation during ablation
   ✦ Equipment malfunction
   ✦ Improper ablation depth due to poor focusing, excessive moisture, or excessive drying
   ✦ Excessive exposure of alcohol solution outside the reservoir
   ✦ Free epithelial flap or inability to construct epithelial flap, necessitating conversion to PRK
3. PRK
   ✦ Primarily the same as LASEK

## Postoperative

It is best to divide postoperative symptoms and problems into side effects (those that are usual and expected sequelae, and are normally self limited) and complications (those events that are unexpected and usually deleterious).

SIDE EFFECTS
1. Pain
   ✦ LASIK: Minimal
   ✦ LASEK: Intermediate in frequency and severity. Interestingly, unusual to have significant discomfort in first 12 to 24 hours like PRK. If discomfort occurs it is more likely at 48 to 72 hours
   ✦ PRK: Greatest in frequency and in potential severity. Usually lasts no more than 48 to 72 hours. Worst in first 12 to 24 hours. Bandage soft contact lens and topical nonsteroidal drug are most important in prevention. Dilute topical anesthetic judiciously used is very helpful
2. Foreign body sensation
   ✦ LASIK: Common during the first 24 to 48 hours until the epithelial incision heals completely. Also occurs if epithelial defects occur during the procedure

✦ LASEK: One of the most common symptoms related by patients in the postoperative period. Many patients blame this on the contact lens, but it is important to remind them of the benefits of the contact lens. This sensation is especially common after removal of the contact lens until the epithelium becomes smooth. The mainstay of management should be lubricants. Preferably preservative free and of increasing viscosity to control symptoms

✦ PRK: Same as PRK

3. Epiphora
   ✦ LASIK: Usually only the first 24 hours
   ✦ LASEK: Tends to be associated with the foreign body sensation. Very common during the first 3 to 4 days
   ✦ PRK: As with LASIK

4. Glare/Photophobia
   ✦ LASIK: Tends to be less photophobia than surface ablation since epithelium intact. Glare is similar. Halos tend to be subjectively more noticeable than with surface ablation due to the smaller effective optic zone
   ✦ LASEK: Is usually greatest 48 to 72 hours after surgery. Generally by 3 to 4 weeks it will have returned to its preoperative level. Halos are common and to be expected post-PRK and tend to decrease after 4 to 6 months
   ✦ PRK: Similar to LASEK

5. Vision
   ✦ LASIK: Vision normally improves to good acuity within the first 12 to 24 hours. All the visual side effects seen with surface ablation will be present, but usually to a much lesser degree. All of these secondary to the reepithelialization process should be avoided with LASIK. Stabilization is present in over 90% of eyes by 3 months
   ✦ LASEK: Very similar to PRK except that the vision in the first few days may be significantly better than that seen with PRK. If the epithelial flap maintains some viability and minimal edema, a number of LASEK patients are able to function relatively well during the first several days. On the other hand, if the flap is necrotic and edematous, the vision may be as bad or worse than with PRK
   ✦ PRK: Will undergo several common disturbances. Vision is routinely poor until the epithelium has regenerated over the area of ablation. As the surface quality improves and the epithelial structure normalizes, the vision will begin to stabilize. By 5 to 6 months most eyes have stabilized enough to con-

sider enhancement if necessary. A total regression of about 1.00 D is common. Ghost images (monocular diplopia) are frequently described by patients. They are due to irregular astigmatism related to the quality of the surface and ablation as well as any residual refractive error. Binocular diplopia may be related to anisometropia, unilateral surgery, or preoperative strabismus. Some fluctuation in vision both diurnally and day to day is common. Finally, almost all patients will notice a reduction of contrast sensitivity especially in low levels of illumination for the first 6 to 12 months

6. Residual or Induced Refractive Error
   ✦ LASIK: Similar to PRK (see below)
   ✦ LASEK: Similar to PRK (see below)
   ✦ PRK: The accuracy of the primary surgery depends on a number of factors including the degree of refractive error, the surgeon, and the surgeon's nomogram. The least controlled of these factors is the individual patient's tissue reaction and wound healing response to the procedure. Fortunately now most of the lasers are approved to treat any residual refractive error that remains

7. Keratitis
   ✦ LASIK: As with surface treatment, a superficial punctuate keratitis due to poor tear function, toxicity from topical medications or preservatives, and corneal deinnervation may be seen in the early postoperative period
   ✦ LASEK: Superficial punctate keratitis secondary to inadequate tear film or the effects of topical medication is the most common form seen
   ✦ PRK: Same as LASEK.

COMPLICATIONS
1. Irregular Astigmatism
   ✦ LASIK: Very much the same as for surface ablation procedures, although there is less contribution from the epithelium and more from the flap. Imperfections in the flap itself or in its repositioning are the primary reason for irregular astigmatism in LASIK. Microstriae that may form due to settling of the flap onto the ablation bed normally do not result in significant irregular astigmatism. Macrostriae do create irregular astigmatism and require repositioning of the flap. If left untreated, will result in an permanent loss of best corrected vision
   ✦ LASEK: This is most easily detected by the presence of a loss of BCVA. Retinoscopy, manual keratometry, and corneal topography can be used to further characterize the nature and degree of this problem. It is almost universally present in the early

postoperative period due to epithelial regeneration and modeling. Stromal edema also contributes to the problem. Permanent irregular astigmatism is due to decentration of the ablation, an asymmetrical ablation pattern, or an abnormal wound healing tissue response. Correction is difficult although the potential for custom ablations as well as the introduction of wavefront analysis gives us optimism for the future. Complete correction, however, may ultimately necessitate a deep lamellar or penetrating keratoplasty

◆ PRK: Similar to LASEK

An overlooked but important cause is the inability to deliver the entire hyperopic ablation under the flap. In small corneas, those flatter than 40.00 D, and with eccentric pupils not permitting a well centered flap, it is difficult if not impossible to deliver the complete diameter treatment. Asymmetry in the ablation will result in irregular astigmatism.

2. Subepithelial/stromal haze
   ◆ LASIK: Interface changes may infrequently occur, but subepithelial or anterior stromal haze should not
   ◆ LASEK: Basically similar to PRK, although in myopia the incidence for high myopia appears to be less. In the author's personal experience of 100 eyes >-9.00 D, only a 2% chance versus as high as 10% for PRK. The author has not experienced a single case of clinically significant haze in either hyperopic LASEK or PRK
   ◆ PRK: The development of haze with the resultant regression and loss of best corrected acuity is one of the major reasons for the decline in popularity of PRK and the increase of LASIK. The chance for the development of clinically significant haze depends primarily on the degree of refractive error (consequently the depth of the ablation), the quality of the ablation (smoothness), the diameter of the ablation and the transition of the edges, as well as the individuals wound healing response.[10] The incidence of haze in hyperopic ablations is significantly less than that for myopic, although it can occur. Time, steroids, retreatment, and the use of Mitomycin-C are all effective in clearing this complication

3. Infectious keratitis
   ◆ LASIK: The lowest incidence of infectious keratitis. However, bacteria, mycoplasma, and fungal organisms have all been identified as causes for early and late ulcers. Elevation of the flap and in some cases removal are required to adequately culture and treat these infections

◆ LASEK: Adequate documentation with respect to the incidence of infectious keratitis is not available. It would appear that the incidence should be either the same as PRK, or if the epithelial flap is viable and maintains some degree of functioning to protect the underlying stroma one would expect it to be lower

◆ PRK: Of the 3 procedures, PRK has the highest reported incidence of infectious keratitis (1 in 500 to 1000 cases). The occurrence is usually early in the postoperative period during the time the epithelial defect is healing and the bandage contact lens is in place. Later ulcers may develop and mycobacterial agents need be considered. Early diagnosis with cultures and sensitivity are imperative. Immediate medical management with fortified antibiotics should be instituted

4. Diffuse lamellar keratitis
   ◆ LASIK: Diffuse lamellar keratitis (DLK) is specific for LASIK. It is multifactorial, but in general is an immunologic inflammatory reaction occurring in the interface. Inciting agents include bacterial endotoxins, various chemicals and solutions, and contaminated microkeratome blades. Treatment consists of early detection, normally the first postoperative day, intensive topical prednisolone acetate (every 30 to 60 minutes), and in more severe cases elevation of the flap and irrigation of the interface
   ◆ LASEK: Not applicable
   ◆ PRK: Not applicable

5. Epithelial ingrowth
   ◆ LASIK: May occur in primary cases but is definitely more frequent after enhancements in which the flap has been lifted. Its incidence is unquestionably higher in hyperopic enhancements than in myopic ones. Isolated small areas of epithelium outside the visual axis will normally disappear spontaneously. Any suggestion of thinning or stromal melting of the flap warrants removal. Aggressive ingrowth is almost universally associated with a connection to the surface through an area of poor wound edge apposition. Removal of the ingrowth must address this defect or recurrence will be likely. Some have advocated the use of alcohol to destroy the epithelial ingrowth, but this is most probably not necessary if the wound defect is corrected
   ◆ LASEK: Not applicable
   ◆ PRK: Not applicable

6. Recurrent corneal erosions
   ◆ LASIK: Similar to PRK and LASEK (see below)

- ✦ LASEK: Similar to PRK. Does not appear to be any greater than PRK (see below)
- ✦ PRK: May be seen post PRK. Tend to be associated with preexisting anterior basement membrane dystrophy. Not uncommonly seen outside the area of ablation

7. Cataracts
   - ✦ LASIK: There has not been any evidence to implicate LASIK in the development of cataracts
   - ✦ LASEK: Exposure to the excimer's ultraviolet light does not appear to cause cataracts. Posterior subcapsular cataracts are associated with prolonged steroid administration in susceptible individuals
   - ✦ PRK: Same as LASEK

8. Ptosis
   - ✦ LASIK: Same as PRK (see below). Lid lacerations may occur with the use of some microkeratomes, especially the original Hansatome
   - ✦ LASEK: Same as PRK (see below)
   - ✦ PRK: Trauma to the levator muscle from blepharospasm against the lid speculum or related to lid inflammation/edema may result in ptosis

9. Secondary glaucoma
   - ✦ LASIK: May see with steroid administration. Need to watch for fluid in the interface which may give falsely low intraocular pressure readings
   - ✦ LASEK: Due to steroid response. Treat with topical anti-glaucoma medication and consider use of less potent steroid. This should be a transient condition and persist only until the steroid discontinued
   - ✦ PRK: Same as LASEK

10. Retinal detachment
   - ✦ LASIK: Still no conclusion for LASIK. More concern than with PRK because rapid increase and decrease in IOP related to fixation ring may result in shift of vitreous and traction on the retina
   - ✦ LASEK: Increased risk for retinal detachment has not been shown. Some concerned over potential shock waves to retina and vitreous. Less of a concern with hyperopic treatment than with predisposed myopic eyes
   - ✦ PRK: Same as LASEK

11. Anterior ischemic optic neuropathy
   - ✦ LASIK: Has been associated with LASIK procedures. Question if increased IOP due to fixation ring could affect microcirculation of the optic nerve and precipitate an attack. It should be more of a concern with hyperopic eyes since they are more likely to be predisposed to this with their optic nerve anatomy
   - ✦ LASEK: Not applicable

- ✦ PRK: Not applicable

12. Ectasia
   - ✦ LASIK: Controversy continues over both the total thickness of a cornea to be subjected to LASIK. Five hundred μm seems to be a comfortable overall thickness necessary to minimize the potential for ectasia even from simply the construction of the flap itself. For residual posterior stroma, somewhere between 250 to 300 μm appears to be acceptable, with the more conservative physicians choosing 300 μm. Again, it is imperative to take into account the possibility of keratoconic tendency especially on any suspicious appearing topography. In these cases, if laser vision correction is chosen, it seems wise to utilize surface ablation which should be much less likely to accelerate any ectatic process. The true flap thickness also plays into this discussion. How thin of flap can be safely and adequately constructed. Does the femtosecond laser permit a thinner more consistent flap to be made? All these can be debated and will factor into the discussion on the nature of iatrogenic ectasia after LASIK
   - ✦ LASEK: Parameters are the same as for PRK (see below)
   - ✦ PRK: Cases of ectasia have been reported; however, not with the frequency of that after LASIK. The absolute minimum corneal thickness necessary to avoid ectasia after PRK has not been established. Amounts varying from 400 to 300 μm have been proposed. The author's personal preference is to recommend leaving 400 μm, although I suspect 350 μm is acceptable. The factor that may be the most important is the quality of the corneal tissue. If the tissue is weaker or has a tendency toward ectasia (ie, keratoconus), then obviously more tissue would be necessary or it may not even matter if the cornea was destined to become spontaneously ectatic over time

## OUTCOMES

Caution must be exercised when interpreting and evaluating the results of these 3 refractive surgical procedures. The reported results must be taken in context and comparison with all variables considered. These variables range from the make and model of laser to the skill level of the surgeon. The rapid rates of procedural and technical modifications make it impossible in many instances to meaningfully compare results.

The majority of surgeons have their bias as to the procedure they prefer. Many times this is based on factors other than the proven or actual capability of the procedures to achieve satisfactory visual results. The technical difficulty, operative time, postoperative care, ability to comanage the postoperative care effectively—as well as simply what the patient wants—are just a few of the many reasons surgeons develop a choice of procedure.

The visual results of all 3 of these procedures are comparable. The choice of the procedure should be based on the factors discussed earlier in the chapter in order to achieve the best visual result with long term safety paramount. The reported outcomes described below support this belief.

## PRK

There has been far less information published regarding the correction of hyperopia and hyperopic astigmatism with PRK than for its use in the correction of myopia and myopic astigmatism. Also, most of the recent information has been concerning LASIK and not PRK, as LASIK has become the preferred technique because of its rapid and convenient postoperative recovery.

It is probably most appropriate to review the original study which resulted in the approval of hyperopic ablation for VISX by the FDA's Ophthalmic Device Advisory Panel in October, 1998.[11,12] The results are remarkably similar to those reported for other lasers and for LASEK and LASIK. This was a prospective, nonrandomized, unmasked, multicenter study performed a eight centers in the United States. One hundred and twenty-four eyes of 124 subjects with primary hyperopia were evaluated for 12 months after surgery. The mean preoperative sphere and cylinder were +2.28 SD 0.84 (range +0.38 to +4.00 D) and cylinder less than +1.00 D.

At 3 months, 55.9% and 80.8% of patients were within ±0.50 D and ±1.00 D respectively, of the intended correction. This became 74.1% and 90.5%, respectively at 6 months and 75.7% and 92.2% at 12 months. UCVA was 20/20 or better in 53.3% and 20/40 or better 96.0% at 6 months and 63.9% and 94.8%, respectively at 12 months. No eye had BCVA worse than 20/32.

Two years later in October, 2000, VISX received FDA approval for hyperopic astigmatism. The study included eyes up to a maximum spherical equivalent of +6.00 D with a range of spherical component of +0.50 to +5.00 D and a cylindrical component of +0.50 to +4.00 D. The visual and refractive results were similar to those for hyperopia alone. At 6 months 50.2% of eyes were 20/20 or better and 96.5% were 20/40 or better.

Dr. Keith Williams reported on 52 eyes with spherical equivalents of +1.00 to +6.00 D and cylindrical components of less than or equal to 1.50 D. Again, the outcomes were comparable to the original VISX study. At 6 months, 67% and 88% of the eyes, respectively were ±0.50 D and ±1.00 D. Improvement for the number of eyes within ±0.50 occurred by 12 months to 79%. At the 6-month evaluation 95.3% of the eyes were 20/40 or better. There was not any eye that lost BCVA and only mild transient corneal haze was identified.[13]

An early report by Dr. Bruce Jackson showed excellent results in 65 eyes of 38 patients. These were spherical hyperopic eyes from +1.00 to +4.00 D. At 1 year 80% were within ±0.50 D and 98% were within ±1.00 D. One eye developed clinically significant haze and some regression was noted from 1 to 6 months.[14]

Interestingly, the hyperopic results reported on a Technolas 116 laser from 1996 also appear favorable to these obtained on VISX units by the above authors. Thirty-six patients and 45 eyes were evaluated over the first 6 months after surgery. The mean SE was +3.33 SD 1.50 D (range +0.50 to +6.50 D) and mean cylindrical equivalent 1.51 SD 1.39 D (range +0.50 to +5.00 D). Overall 87% were within ±1.00 with a slight difference between HPRK (88%) and hyperopic astigmatic photorefractive keratectomy (HPARK) (85%). Visual results were 38% 20/20 or better and 93% were 20/40 or better—the former a little lower than above, but the latter certainly in line with those outcomes presented. A loss of 2 lines of best-corrected vision in 6.7% was higher than that from the other studies.[15]

A more recent study by Dr. Pacella using the Technolas 217 C showed not surprisingly somewhat better results than those with the 116. The mean SE was higher at 4.82 SD 2.11 D (range +1.00 to +7.75 D) and cylinder up to +0.50. At 18 months 46.4% of eyes were 20/20 or better and 100% better than or equal to 20/32. No eye lost 2 lines of best-corrected vision.[16]

Finally, a study by Dr. Carones with the Alcon LADARVision (Fort Worth, Tex) laser from 2000 evaluated 92 eyes of 57 patients. The mean spherical equivalent was +3.45 (range +0.50 to +6.00 D) and mean cylindrical equivalent 2.76 D. Eighty-two percent of the eyes were ±0.50 at 1 year with 53% 20/20 or better and 94% 20/40 or better. No eyes were reported to have lost BCVA.[7]

Obviously, this is an extremely simplified and gross comparison of studies and lasers. Overall, it seems fair to say that the results are comparable and 1 laser doesn't appear to be dramatically better for hyperopia and hyperopic astigmatism than the other.

## LASEK

For the past 2 years, LASEK has gained popularity and an increasing number of studies reporting results for the correction of myopia and myopic astigmatism. A paucity of data is available on the effectiveness of LASEK for hyperopia and hyperopic astigmatism. The best data I have is from my personal experience over the past 2 years.

Of the 1500 LASEK total procedures I have performed over the past 2 years, 37 have been for primary hyperopia and hyperopic astigmatism. These 37 eyes were of 24 patients. The VISX (Santa Clara, Calif) Star 3 excimer laser was used, as was a standard LASEK technique. All 37 eyes were prospectively evaluated. Data is reported for the 6 month evaluation and with 100% follow-up.

The average preoperative sphere and cylinder were +3.06 D (range +1.00 to +5.625 D) and 0.92 D (range 0 to 3.75 D), respectively. At 1 week, the mean UCVA was 20/40. At 3 months, 84% and 92% of patients were within ±0.50 D and ±1.00 D, respectively, of the intended correction. This became 80% and 94%, respectively at 6 months. By 6 months, 95% of the eyes were 20/40 or better. Surprisingly, for the 18 eyes in the high hyperopic group (SE greater than or equal to +3.00 D), 78% were better than or equal to 20/20 and 100% better than or equal to 20/40. No clinically significant haze or loss of best corrected vision was noted. The lower success rate for the lesser degrees of hyperopia was most likely due to using a less aggressive nomogram. There appears to be a need for a greater percentage of ablated tissue per diopter of correction than that used for the higher hyperopic eyes.

The main 2 advantages of LASEK over LASIK for hyperopia are definitely the elimination of the stromal flap complications inherent with LASIK and the ability to ensure the application of a complete ablation profile. It is simply impossible in all corneas to be able to achieve a flap of sufficient diameter and centration to guarantee that some of the ablation (especially in the area of the hinge) is blocked. Asymmetrical ablations may then lead to inconsistent results and possible irregular astigmatism with loss of best corrected vision. The low incidence of pain and absence of postoperative haze potentially make LASEK preferable to PRK.

## LASIK

Dr. Davidorf reported the results of hyperopic LASIK in 19 eyes in March 1999. One of these eyes had previously undergone radial keratotomy, but the other 18 were primary hyperopia. The mean spherical equivalent was +3.67 D and cylinder ranged from 0 to 2.00 D. The mean spherical equivalent at 3 months was 0.27 D. At 3 months, 63% of eyes were within ±0.50 D and 88% within ±1.00 D of the intended correction. While 100% saw 20/40 or better, 50% saw 20/20 or better. Loss of 1 line of best-corrected vision was seen in 5% of eyes.[17]

Results for the Technolas 117C laser are very similar for 2 separate studies from different surgeons. The first by Dr. Khaled Rashad from May 2001 included 85 eyes of 53 patients. The mean spherical equivalent was +3.31 ±0.69 D (range +1.25 to +5.00 D) and cylinder 0.91 ±1.06 D (range 0.00 to 3.00). At 1 year, 61.2% and 89.4% were within ±0.50 and ±1.00, respectively of the intended correction. While 92.9% achieved better than or equal to 20/40, only 24.7% recorded 20/20 or better. A loss of 2 lines of best-corrected vision occurred in 1.2%.[18]

The second study utilizing the Technolas 217C was by Dr. Lian in 2002. Fifty-four eyes of 35 patients were treated and the 1 year data reported. The mean spherical equivalent was +3.12 D (range +1 to +5.75 D) and the cylinder less than 1.50 D. Sixty-one percent were within ±0.50 D and 83.3% were within ±1.00 D. Visual acuity was 20/20 or better in 63% and 20/40 or better in 92.6%. The reported loss of 2 lines of best-corrected vision was 1.9%.[19]

In June 2000, Dr. Arturo Chayet reported on the results of hyperopic LASIK with the Nidek EC-5000 (Greensboro, NC) excimer laser. The outcomes for 2 groups, mild hyperopia <3.00 D (45 eyes) and moderate hyperopia +3.00 to +5.00 D (27 eyes), were evaluated at the 6-month period. In the low hyperopia group, 42.2% achieved 20/20 or better, and 95.6% 20/40 or better. The moderate hyperopia group was 25.9% and 77.8%, respectively. There retreatment rate was 25% overall, 20% in the mild eyes and 33.3% in the moderate eyes. Only 1 eye from the moderate hyperopia group lost 2 lines of best-corrected vision.[20]

A recent report by Dr. James Salz and the LADARVision LASIK Hyperopia Study Group included 360 hyperopic (152 eyes), hyperopic astigmatic (143 eyes), and mixed astigmatic (65 eyes) in a multicenter, prospective nonrandomized (self-controlled) comparative trial. Up to 6 D of hyperopia and 6.00 D of cylinder were treated. This excellent study contains a significant amount of important data, but to compare with the above data selected information will be extracted. For spherical hyperopia 20/20 or better was seen in 55.6% of low hyperopia group (+0.88 D to +2.90 D) and 47.8% of moderate group (+3.00 D to +6.00 D) at 12 months. Twenty/forty or better was reported in 95.9% and 88.5% respectively at the 1-year period. For hyperopic astigmatism, 64.1% in low group and 38.5% in moderate group were 20/20 or better. Ninety-five percent and 88.2% respectively were 20/40 or better. The loss of 2 lines of best-corrected acuity occurred in less than 5% for all groups.[21]

# CONCLUSION

Two studies that directly compare PRK and LASIK both demonstrate that the visual results for the 2 procedures are not significantly different. Dr. Jonathan M. Davidorf's study was a small sample of eyes and only 3 month follow up. Results appeared to slightly favor LASIK at this 3-month postoperative time, which is exactly what one would expect. Using the trend seen in the previous studies evaluating PRK for hyperopia, one would believe the PRK results would catch up to the LASIK results at 1 year. A comparison of the 2 procedures at only 3 months to demonstrate the end visual outcomes does not seem valid.

Dr. JP McCulley and colleagues at the University of Texas Southwestern Medical Center have reported their results comparing PRK and LASIK for the surgical correction of spherical hyperopia. The conclusion was that there was not any statistically significant difference in the uncorrected visual acuity at 1 year. However, postoperative pain and longer visual recovery were the clear disadvantages of the PRK group.[22]

Ugo Cimberle, MD, found the long-term visual and refractive results for LASIK and LASEK comparable in hyperopic treatment. His conclusion was that the advantage of LASIK's early refractive stability is balanced by the greater ability of larger optical zones with LASEK.[23]

As mentioned previously, it is extremely difficult to review the information available and identify 1 procedure that is unquestionably the best. There are simply too many factors involved and different individuals assign varying importance to each. If one's primary concern is speed of visual recovery, then LASIK is unquestionably the choice. If a cornea is too thin to permit safely creating a flap and maintaining its structural integrity, then a surface ablation procedure is indicated. The decision as to performing LASEK or PRK once a surface ablative procedure is needed is more controversial. Only further investigation and experience will assist in this concern. The greatest obstacle at this time is that patient acceptance is much better with LASEK than PRK. The predominance of LASIK and its promotion over PRK by surgeons has created a situation in which it is hard to overcome the patient's perception. This is extremely unfortunate as surface ablation does without a doubt have a place in refractive surgery, especially for the correction of hyperopia and hyperopic astigmatism. Once again, we see greed and the self promotion of some our colleagues has created a hole for us to climb out of in order to best serve our patients.

# REFERENCES

1. Fagerholm P. Wound healing after photorefractive keratectomy. *J Cataract Refract Surg.* 2000;26:432-447.

2. Dohlman CH. Physiology of the cornea. In: Smolin G, Thoft RA. *The Cornea: Scientific Foundations and Clinical Practice.* Boston, Mass: Little, Brown, and Company; 1983:3-16.

3. Friend J. Physiology of the cornea. In: Smolin G, Thoft RA. *The Cornea: Scientific Foundations and Clinical Practice.* Boston, Mass: Little, Brown, and Company; 1983:17-42.

4. Waring GO. Corneal anatomy and physiology as applied to refractive keratotomy. In: Waring GO. *Refractive Keratotomy for Myopia and Astigmatism.* St. Louis, Mo: Mosby; 1992:17-35.

5. Grendahl MJ. *LASIK/PRK Biomechanics, Molecularbiology, and Physiology. Aspen Ophthalmic Surgery Symposium:* Aspen, Colo; March, 2001.

6. Camellin M. LASEK. *Ocular Surgery News.* July 2000:14-17.

7. O'hEineachain R. Flying spot laser PRK provides accurate treatment of hyperopia. *Eurotimes.* 2000 Sept:8.

8. Guell JL, Velasco F, Roberts C. Topographic changes induced by flap creation. *Ocular Surgery News.* 2002 Sept:12.

9. Shallhorn S. Pupil size irrelevant to post-LASIK complaints. *Ocular Surgery News.* 2002 March:24.

10. Singh D. Mechanism of corneal haze after photorefractive keratectomy. *LASEK Symposium.* May, 2002, Houston, Texas.

11. VISX. Photorefractive keratectomy. In: *VISX Star S2 Excimer Laser System. professional use information.* Santa Clara, Calif: VISX Incorporated; 2000.

12. Smith SE. VISX hyperopic PRK results are good at 1 year. *Ocular Surgery News.* 1999 Jan:32.

13. Williams DK. One-year results of laser vision correction for low to moderate hyperopia. *Ophthalmology.* 2000;107(1):72-76.

14. Jackson WB, Casson E, Hodge WG, Mintsioulis G, Agapitos PJ. Laser vision correction for low hyperopia. *Ophthalmology.* 1998;105(9):1727-1738.

15. Daya SM, Tappouni FR, Habib NE. Photorefractive keratectomy for hyperopia. *Ophthalmology.* 1997;104(11):1952-1958.

16. Pacella E, Abdolrahimzadeh S, Gabrieli CB. Excimer laser photorefractive keratectomy for hyperopia. *Ophthal Surg Lasers.* 2001;32(1):30-34.

17. Davidorf JM, Eghbali F, Onclinx T, Maloney RK. Effect of varying the optical zone diameter on the results of hyperopic laser in situ keratomileusis. *Ophthalmology.* 2001;108(7):1261-1268.

18. Rashad KM. LASIK for correction of hyperopia from +1.25 to +5.00 diopters with the Technolas Keracor 117C laser. *J Refract Surg.* 2001;17(2):113-122..

19. Lian J, Ye W, Zhou D, Wang K. Laser in situ keratomileusis for correction of hyperopia and hyperopic astigmatism with the Technolas 117C. *J Refract Surg.* 2002;18(4):435-438.

20. Zadok D, Maskaleris G, Montes M, Shah S, Garcia V, Chayet A. Hyperopic laser in situ keratomileusis with the Nidek EC-5000 excimer laser. *Ophthalmology.* 2000;107(6):1132-1136.

21. Salz JJ, Stevens CA. LASIK correction of spherical hyperopia, hyperopic astigmatism, and mixed astigmatism with the LADARVision excimer laser system. *Ophthalmology.* 2002;109(9):1647-1658.

22. el-Agha, Johnston EW, Bowman RW, Cavanagh HD, McCulley JP. Excimer laser treatment of spherical hyperopia: PRK or LASIK? *Trans Am Ophthalmol Soc.* 2000;98:59-66; discussion 66-9.

23. Cimberle U, Cimberle M. LASIK, LASEK comparable in hyperopic treatment. *Ocular Surgery News.* 2002 Sept:16.

# BIBLIOGRAPHY

Argento CJ, Cosentino MJ. Comparison of optical zones in hyperopic laser in situ keratomileusis: 5.9 mm versus smaller optical zones. *J Cataract Refract Surg.* 2000;26:1137-1146.

Bethke WC. Laser treatment of hyperopia: tips and techniques. *Review of Refractive Surgery.* 2000 September:44-48.

Bethke W. How to handle the hyperope. *Review of Ophthalmology.* 1999 February:52-58.

Charters L, Brint SF. Early results good in LASIK hyperopic astigmatism trial. *Ophthalmology Times*. 1999 June:23.

Ditzen K, Fiedler J, Pieger S. Laser in situ keratomileusis for hyperopia and hyperopic astigmatism using the Meditec MEL spot scanner. *J Refract Surg*. 2002;18(4):430-434.

Guttman C. LASIK, PRK procedures hold promise for hyperopia. *Ophthalmology Times*. 1999 March:36.

Lee JB, Ryu CH, Kim, JH, Kim EK, Kim HB. Comparison of tear secretion and tear film instability after photorefractive keratectomy and laser in situ keratomileusis. *J Cataract Refract Surg*. 2000;26:1326-1331.

Lindstrom RL, Linebarger EJ, Hardten DR, Houtman DM, Samuelson TW. Early results of hyperopic and astigmatic laser in situ keratomileusis in eyes with secondary hyperopia. *Ophthalmology*. 2000;107(10):1858-1861.

Moller-Pedersen T, Cavanagh HD, Petroll WM, Jester JV. Stromal wound healing explains refractive instability and haze development after photorefractive keratectomy. *Ophthalmology*. 2000;107(7):1235-1245.

Pineda-Fernandez A, Rueda L, Huang D, Nur J, Jaramillo J. Laser in situ keratomileusis for hyperopia and hyperopic astigmatism with the Nidek EC-5000 excimer laser. *J Refract Surg*. 2001;17(6):670-675.

Pop M, Payette Y. Photorefractive keratectomy versus laser in situ keratomileusis: a controlled study. *Ophthalmology*. 2000; 107(1):251-257.

Schultz MC. Recurrent regression after hyperopic LASIK. *J Cataract Refract Surg*. 2002 June:45-46.

Singer HW. LASIK is the clear choice for treating hyperopia. *Ocular Surgery News*. 1999 May:18.

Stein RM. Ten pearls for treating hyperopic astigmatism. *Refractive Eyecare*. 2000;4(12):1,29-30.

Van Gelder RN, Steger-May K, Yang SH, Rattanatam T, Pepose JS. Comparison of photorefractive keratectomy, astigmatic PRK, laser in situ keratomileusis, and astigmatic LASIK in the treatment of myopia. *J Cataract Refract Surg*. 2002;28:462-476.

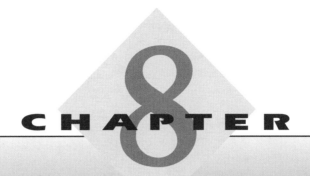

# CHAPTER 8

# HYPEROPIA: TREATMENT WITH ACCOMMODATIVE ESOTROPIA AND/OR NYSTAGMUS

*Hugo Daniel Nano Jr, MD*

## INTRODUCTION

Refractive accommodative esotropia (AET) is a common type of strabismus. Uncorrected hyperopia leads to an increased accommodative effort, which may lead to an accommodative convergence. The treatment of accommodative esotropia has traditionally consisted in full optical correction of hyperopia using glasses or contact lenses. Now, with all the technological advances involved in this subject, we have developed new techniques that offer the patients a much more gratified solution.[1-4]

We live in a "LASIK happy society," and glasses have become less acceptable and comfortable. Therefore, refractive surgery is the best option for those patients who want to replace their glasses for a permanent and much more untroubled solution, or even for those who do not tolerate the contact lenses.

The controversy generated by pediatric ophthalmologists is based on the fact that they believe it is inconvenient to perform this treatment in children because they are not capable to do it by themselves and they are forced to transfer their patients to other capable ophthalmologists. Despite this debate, this technique is still the most modern and adequate option for the majority of the cases.

Theoretically, any means able to reduce hyperopia should relax the accommodation process and would therefore decrease accommodative convergence and accommodative strabismus.

In the following sections, I will develop the pros and cons of the treatment proposed, which will lead us to a useful conclusion. Hopefully, it will help us all decide what is the best treatment to chose for each of our patients so that they will always feel gratified with the results obtained.

## EVALUATION

All patients must carry out a complete eye examination, including the measurements of visual acuity (uncorrected and best-corrected), as well as manifest refraction and cycloplegic refraction, corneal topography, and pachymetry. A sensorimotor examination (primary position alignment with and without glasses) should also be done.

If the patient presents amblyopia, the visual result will depend in the degree of the latter. The patient must be aware of this detail.

The response to glasses would be predictive of the response to LASIK or LASEK.

# INDICATIONS

1. Age: Between 20 to 60 years old. It has been demonstrated that hyperopia increases every year for the first 7 years of life. It rapidly decreases when the patient reaches the age of 13, and decreases in a slower manner at the age of 20, and it remains relatively constant after the age of 20. The presbyopic patients with previously controlled AET may experience an increase in esotropia late in life; requiring additional hyperopic correction.
2. Hyperopia between 1.00 to 6.00 D; associated or not with astigmatism of 1.00 to 6.00 D, presenting an spherical equivalent not over 6.00 D.
3. Cases of accommodative esotropia.
4. Aneisometropia.
5. Intolerance to contact lenses or glasses.

# CONTRAINDICATIONS

1. Dry eye.
2. Glaucoma.
3. Collagen pathologies.

# SURGICAL TECHNIQUES

## *For LASIK*

### PRESURGERY
1. Topical anaesthesia (lidocaine chlorhidrate 0.4%).
2. Suction ring slightly discentred nasally.
3. Perform the cut with microkeratome (diameter 8 to 9 mm).
4. Evert the flap and place it on the conjunctiva.
5. Centre the excimer laser with patient fixation.
6. PRK procedure under the laser, protecting the flap.
7. Astigmatism will be treated following the topography axis and subjective refraction.
8. If lint or debris is found under the flap, it has to be irrigated out with a cannula with BSS.
9. Finally the flap is repositioned and the adherence is assessed.

### POSTSURGERY
1. Use a protector patch for 24 hours.
2. Medications:
   - Tobramycin 0.3% drops; Fluorometholone 0.1% drops: 3 times a day the first week, 2 times a day for the second week; and once a day for the third week.
   - Artificial tears are needed during the first 3 months.

Preservative free drops are preferred.

## *For LASEK*

### PRESURGERY
1. Topical anaesthesia (lidocaine chlorhidrate 0.4%).
2. Use of diluted alcohol 20% for about 40 to 60 seconds.
3. Lift the epithelial flap with spatula, leaving adherence in the hinch zone.
4. PRK procedure.
5. Astigmatism is treated following the topography axis and subjective refraction.
6. The epithelial flap is repositioned.

### POSTSURGERY
1. Use contact lens for 24 to 72 hours.
2. Medications:
   - Tobramycin 0.3% drops: Artificial tears every 3 hours until the re-epithelialization has been completed.
   - Tobramycin 0.3% drops: Fluorometalone 0.1% drops: 3 times a day for the first week, 2 times a day for the second; and once day for the third.
   - Artificial tears as needed for the first 3 months.

# COMPLICATIONS

1. Low esotropic persistence.
2. Decentration.
3. Epithelial defects.
4. Small or irregular flap (in LASIK).
5. Epithelial cysts (in LASIK).
6. Haze (in LASEK).

# OUTCOMES

1. Mean spherical equivalent evolution.
2. 40 eyes studied.
3. My own experience.

# CONCLUSION

After all the information previously presented, we can say that the LASIK/LASEK technique is relatively safe and adequate to be applied in many cases. It is also effective when it comes to reducing the esodeviation in most of our patients. Further study is indicated to determine whether additional factors, such as reduction in contrast sensitivity after refractive surgery, may adversely affect fusional potential.

The dominant limitation seen after using this treatment was that, although all patients were less hyperopic after LASIK, they were not emmetropic. Moreover, some accommodative stimulus persisted after the procedure.

The presence of nystagmus must not be taken as a limitation when it comes to performing refractive surgery. With the aid of technological advances, such as eye trackers and the use of forceps (Bores or Kramer) to hold the eye allows us to overcome this problem and perform the surgery.

LASEK must be considered like a treatment option for those patients that present any sort of impediment to do a flap.

Refractive surgery must be taken into consideration as one more tool available even for pediatric as well as adult cases.

## REFERENCES

1. Nemet P, Levinger S. Refractive surgery for refractive errors which cause strabismus:. a report of eight cases. *Binocular Vision and Strabismus Quarterly*. 2002;17(3):187-190.

2. Kushner JB, Ronano PE, Molteno AC. BJ Correspondence. *Binocular Vision and Strabismus Quarterly*. 2000;5(4):315-318.

3. Stidham DB, Borrissova O, Borrison V. Effect of hyperopic laser in situ keratomileusis on ocular alignment and stereopsis in patients with accommodative esotropia. *Am J Ophthalmol*. 2002;109(6):1148-1153.

4. Nano HD Jr, Muzzin S. Excimer laser photorefractive keratectomy in pediatric patients. *J Cataract Refract Surg*. 1997; 23:736-739.

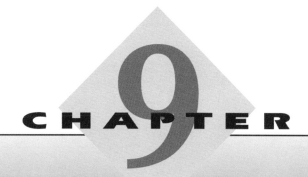

# CHAPTER 9

# PHAKIC LENS IMPLANTATION IN MYOPIA AND HYPEROPIA

*Daljit Singh, MS, DSc*

## EVALUATION

A phakic lens implantation is intraocularly invasive. If an aphakic lens could be sequestrated as we do with an in the bag IOL, it could be classed a safe procedure on a long-term basis. However, that is not the case.[1-5]

Every phakic lens touches, presses, or erodes a uveal tissue. It occupies an ever-shrinking space. Phakic lens surgery may or may not introduce an astigmatic error, but it usually leaves the preexisting one untouched.[6] With a phakic IOL, it is difficult indeed to fine tune refraction to emmetropia. Every phakic lens patient needs a lifelong regular, thorough follow-up including endothelial count. The need for a regular follow-up increases with the passage of time. If and when a cataract develops, a phakic lens shall need explantation before cataract surgery.[12] Whether an implanted phakic lens will lead to an earlier onset of cataract or accelerated depletion of endothelial cells in a certain percentage of cases is not known, though entirely possible.

The great advantage of a phakic IOL is that a good cataract surgeon can safely do the procedure without buying costly additional equipment. A phakic lens procedure is reversible (explantation) if a situation so demands.[7,8] A phakic lens implant procedure therefore has the potential of getting adopted far and wide. In some countries, the lens implantation is reimbursable, while a laser refractive procedure is not.

A moderate blunt trauma to the eyeball may produce cataract years after the incident. A disturbance in the anterior chamber during the performance of phakic lens implantation, may induce a biophysical or biochemical trauma that may manifest years later as cataract.[12] Phakic lenses are yet in their infancy. Even the materials and designs of the lenses are changing. Only recently foldable Artisan and angle-supported lenses have been introduced. It is too early for a competent answer to the most important issues of long-term tissue tolerance and their possible role in the initiation of inflammation, glaucoma, and cataract in implanted eyes. Their possible unmonitored widespread use in less than most competent hands is fraught with a grave danger (Figure 9-1). The world might experience an unprecedented epidemic of phakic lens related ocular morbidity in the coming years and decades.

Phakic IOLs appeared in mid-80s as attractive alternatives to RK for myopia and RK with deep cautery for hyperopia. The early phakic lens studies soon got nearly drowned in the flood/dawn of excimer laser corneal surgery. Excimer laser PRK was abandoned very early in favor of the more corneoinvasive LASIK. In spite of serious operative and postoperative complications connected with the use of a keratome, LASIK has thrived.

Besides other simmering safety issues, there has recently been an increasing concern about the upper refractive limits for LASIK. Thus restrained, many refractive surgeons are

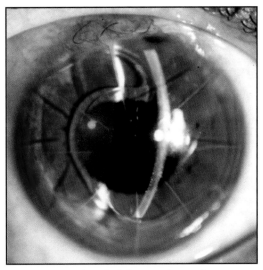

**Figure 9-1.** A dreaded future. An angle-supported phakic lens implanted to correct hyperopia resulting from RK, in a child 12 years old. The endothelial cell count is 1200 cells. The quality of the surgery appears to be poor.

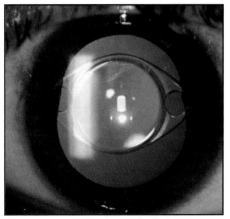

**Figure 9-2.** Well-tolerated phakic Artisan lens for myopia, 14 years postoperative, in a 34-year-old patient. The endothelial cell count is 2300. The pupil can be fully dilated for fundus examination.

turning to a phakic IOL solution all alone or as a combination of phakic lens with LASIK to achieve higher refractive corrections. A new approach for hyperopia is to overcorrect hyperopia with a phakic plus lens followed by laser refractive surgery for the resultant myopia and astigmatism. For high myopia, the approach is to somewhat undercorrect with a phakic minus lens and follow it with laser refractive surgery for the remaining myopia and astigmatism if any. Myopia laser surgery approach is preferred for final correction, since it is more accurate than hyperopia correction.

Three types of phakic IOLs exist:

1. Precrystalline lens (implantable contact lens)

2. Angle supported lens

3. Iris-fixated lens (Artisan lens)

Implantation of any kind of a phakic lens needs to be learned from a master. Early postoperative problems are related to the lens design and the meticulous details of the surgery and postoperative management. The late complications result from a prolonged interaction of the IOL with the adjacent tissues. Lifelong regular follow-up is therefore necessary.

To implant a phakic lens to correct hyperopia or myopia, a momentous decision has to be made after detailed examination and consultation with the patient. The pros and cons of the options of contact lens, extracapsular cataract extraction (ECCE) with monofocal or multifocal IOL, phakic IOL, and excimer laser procedure for the individual patient are considered. The surgeon has to convince himself and the patient why a phakic lens is the right procedure for the latter. The surgeon's own experience and the type of facilities available with him or her create a bias in favor of a particular technique. If a phakic IOL is decided upon, then a choice with a bias is made between a phakic posterior chamber, an angle-supported and an iris-supported lens. The phakic lenses are available from powers of ±1.00 D upward. What is the most sensible lowest limit of a phakic lens implant is debatable. Phakic lenses are also available to treat pure plus or minus cylindrical errors.

I have been using phakic iris claw (Artisan, Ophtec, the Netherlands) lens implantation for high myopia and high hyperopia since 1987 (Figure 9-2), PRK for myopia (1991) and hyperopia (1994) with a scanning slit beam excimer laser, and PRK with flying spot laser cum wavefront analyzed assisted corneal ablation (WASCA) since August, 2001. The results of PRK for all grades of myopia were satisfactory from the beginning and they improved steadily. Results with WASCA are certainly better than with unassisted PRK. Eight years back, over a dozen patients received a phakic lens in 1 eye and PRK procedure in the other. In spite of initial slow recovery with PRK, most of the patients thought both the procedures as equally good. In my practice phakic lens for any degree of myopia, was gradually discontinued in 1996. For very high myopes, an planned residual myopia after PRK is helpful in coping with the near vision problems created by the present or the future central retinochoroidal changes. Hyperopia phakic lens in my practice, however, continues to be a good choice in suitable high error cases.[11]

Laser refractive surgery scores over a phakic lens in that beyond a few months to a year, regular lifetime attention is not required. It also reduces or removes existing astigmatism, which a phakic lens normally does not. Our choice of a phakic iris-claw lens/Artisan lens is based on its long track record (Figure 9-3). The only place this lens touches the tissues is where it holds the iris. Our own 23 years of experience with aphakic and 15 years of phakic implants shows that the lens

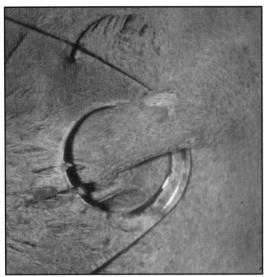

**Figure 9-3.** The iris tissue in the claw of an Artisan lens shows limited loss of pigment, which was shed by manipulations at the time of implantation. The surrounding iris looks healthy. One year postoperative hyperopia patient.

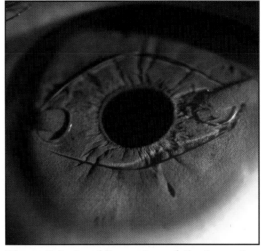

**Figure 9-4.** An oblique view of the lens edge showing the floating vaulted Artisan lens, which is fixed at the claws.

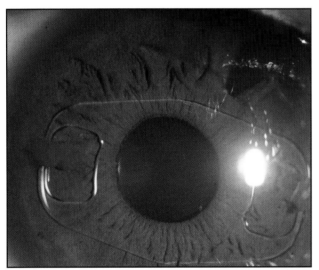

**Figure 9-5.** A 7.25 mm wide, with 4.25-mm optic, Artisan plus lens with claws 180 degrees apart. There is slight downward decentration 1 year after surgery.

is well tolerated. It does not produce angle-related, posterior pigment epithelium and crystalline lens-related problems. However, forceful rubbing of the eye can cause endothelial touch in case of Artisan as also angle-supported lenses.

## ANATOMY

The availability of space for lens implantation, its lifetime tolerance by the related tissues, and age-related dimensional changes in the tissues and spaces are important.

The posterior chamber has a volume of 65 μm, base-out apex in, with zero depth at pupillary margin. The narrowest part of this space gets occupied by the thickest part (optic) of a posterior chamber lens. A phakic posterior chamber lens shall also touch, press, or rub the ciliary epithelium (that overlies highly permeable large caliber capillaries), the anterior surface of the crystalline lens and the posterior pigment epithelium of the iris, somewhere or the other. The increasing volume of the crystalline lens with age, from 150 μm to 240 μm in a matter of 60 years, encroaches on this already cramped space. Some increase in resistance to the free flow of aqueous is therefore possible.

The average anterior chamber depth is 3.15 mm. The volume of the anterior chamber is 250 μm, which decreases by 7.5% per decade, an important issue of concern for angle supported and iris supported lenses. The iris is about 0.5 mm thick at the root and 0.6 mm at the collarette. It is thicker in brown and black eyes. An Artisan lens gets fixed through its claws that hold the midperiphery of the iris. The concave back curvature of phakic Artisan lens keeps it not only away from the crystalline lens, but also away from the iris surface. A correctly fixed lens optic and its 0.17 mm thick haptic are far away from the angle and the corneal endothelium. The maximum width of Artisan lens is 8.5 mm with an optic of 5 mm or 6 mm. However, I prefer to use lenses that are 7.25 mm wide and have an optic of 4.25 mm. The reason is that in the scotopic conditions, the pupil in my black-eye population is smaller than in blue-eye patients (Figures 9-4 through 9-7).

The blood vessels in the anterior border layer of the iris have thick adventitia that helps the claw of the Artisan lens grip better. The capillary endothelium in the human iris is nonfenestrated, therefore less prone to blood-aqueous barri-

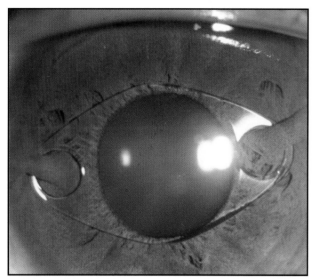

**Figure 9-6.** A 7.25 mm wide, with 4.25-mm optic iris claw lens. With eccentric claws in a dark eyed patient, 1 month after surgery.

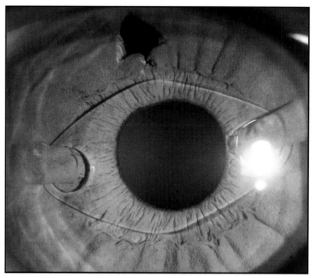

**Figure 9-7.** A 4.25 mm optic, 7.25-mm wide, well-centered hyperopia Artisan lens, 1 year postoperative.

er breakdown, as compared to ciliary capillary endothelium that is fenestrated as if designed to leak.

There is minimum touch/friction between the edge of the vaulted optic and the anterior surface of the iris. It is as if the Artisan lens floats in the aqueous, while it is anchored to 2 points on the iris. The main cause of an early dislocation is a poor fixation. The iris tissue that is actually caught inside the claws gets compressed from day 1 onwards. A breakdown of blood-aqueous barrier in the early postoperative period is possible. If the compressed iris tissue in the claw gets atrophied as it often does, usually it does not affect the fixation. This state can be likened to the passage of an earring through the lobule. However if the tissue bite had been small, the lens get dislocated. The inclusion of excessive iris tissue in the claws during surgery can push the implanted lens against the iris and the natural lens. This can interfere with the free circulation of the aqueous through the pupil, sometimes resulting in the formation of posterior synechia.

A well-designed angle-supported lens is said to rest against the scleral spur. Actually it presses against the corneoscleral trabeculae, Schlemm canal, the ciliary body in the angle recess and sometimes the blood vessels and nerves in the vicinity. Sizing of an angle-supported lens is difficult. There is nothing like a correct size. A lens has to be somewhat over-sized (press the tissues too) to stay in place. Even a slight undersize will make the lens move around, if not fixed by tissue reaction. Over a period of time, a haptic may press on the segmental blood supply of the iris, causing ischemia and iris atrophy that manifests as progressive ovalization of the pupil. A haptic can also erode the angle tissues and lodge in the ciliary body. Uveitis-glaucoma-hyphema

(UGH) syndrome and its reflection in the retina as CME are fearful possibilities.

In every kind of phakic lens implantation, the role of lifelong microtrauma and macrotrauma in causing implant tissue friction, pressure, or erosion should be kept in mind. All of the iris claw lens and most of the angle-supported lens can be observed under the slit lamp microscope. Gonioscopy can reveal the uveal-haptic relationship. The most crucial periphery of a posterior chamber phakic lens and its relationship/interaction with the uveal tissues cannot be examined. If the pupil fails to dilate due to any reason, only ultrasound-biomicroscopy can provide an indirect partial information about the tissue-implant status.

# PHAKIC LENS POWER CALCULATION

The lens power calculation is based on corneal curvature (K), the anterior chamber depth (ACD) and the spectacle correction (at 12-mm vertex). The following tables provided by Ophtec are useful in selecting a myopia or a hyperopia lens (Tables 9-1 and 9-2).

# INDICATIONS AND CONTRAINDICATIONS

Indications are obvious. A patient who is averse to use a pair of glasses or contact lens, who does not wish to be treated with PRK, LASEK, or LASIK for his refractive error, but

# Myopic Refractive Correction: IOL Power Needed to Make the Eye Emmetropic in Relation to Spectacle Correction

| ACD | 2.5 mm | | | 3.0 mm | | | 3.5 mm | | | 4.0 mm | | |
|---|---|---|---|---|---|---|---|---|---|---|---|---|
| K | 38 | 43 | 48 | 38 | 43 | 48 | 38 | 43 | 48 | 38 | 43 | 48 |
| -1 | -1.2 | -1.2 | -1.3 | -1.3 | -1.3 | -1.3 | -1.3 | -1.3 | -1.4 | -1.3 | -1.4 | -1.4 |
| -2 | -2.3 | -2.4 | -2.4 | -2.4 | -2.5 | -2.5 | -2.5 | -2.5 | -2.6 | -2.5 | -2.6 | -2.7 |
| -3 | -3.4 | -3.5 | -3.5 | -3.5 | -3.6 | -3.7 | -3.6 | -3.7 | -3.8 | -3.7 | -3.9 | -4.0 |
| -4 | -4.5 | -4.6 | -4.6 | -4.6 | -4.7 | -4.8 | -4.7 | -4.9 | -5.0 | -4.9 | -5.0 | -5.2 |
| -5 | -5.5 | -5.6 | -5.7 | -5.7 | -5.8 | -5.9 | -5.8 | -6.0 | -6.2 | -6.0 | -6.2 | -6.4 |
| -6 | -6.5 | -6.6 | -6.8 | -6.7 | -6.8 | -7.0 | -6.9 | -7.1 | -7.3 | -7.1 | -7.3 | -7.6 |
| -7 | -7.5 | -7.6 | -7.8 | -7.7 | -7.9 | -8.1 | -7.9 | -8.1 | -8.4 | -8.1 | -8.4 | -8.7 |
| -8 | -8.4 | -8.6 | -8.8 | -8.7 | -8.9 | -9.1 | -8.9 | -9.2 | -9.4 | -9.2 | -9.5 | -9.8 |
| -9 | -9.3 | -9.5 | -9.7 | -9.6 | -9.8 | -10.1 | -9.9 | -10.2 | -10.5 | -10.1 | -10.5 | -10.9 |
| -10 | -10.2 | -10.5 | -10.7 | -10.5 | -10.8 | -11.1 | -10.8 | -11.1 | -11.5 | -11.1 | -11.5 | -11.9 |
| -11 | -11.1 | -11.4 | -11.6 | -11.4 | -11.7 | -12.0 | -11.7 | -12.1 | -17.4 | -12.1 | -12.5 | -12.9 |
| -12 | -12.0 | -12.2 | -12.5 | -12.3 | -12.6 | -12.9 | -12.6 | -13.0 | -13.4 | -13.0 | -13.4 | -13.9 |
| -13 | -12.8 | -13.1 | -13.4 | -13.2 | -13.5 | -13.8 | -13.5 | -13.9 | -14.3 | -13.9 | -14.4 | -14.9 |
| -14 | -13.6 | -13.9 | -14.2 | -14.0 | -14.4 | -14.7 | -14.4 | -14.8 | -15.2 | -14.8 | -15.3 | -15.8 |
| -15 | -14.4 | -14.7 | -15.0 | -14.8 | -15.2 | -15.6 | -15.2 | -15.7 | -16.1 | -15.6 | -16.1 | -16.7 |
| -16 | -15.2 | -15.5 | -15.9 | -15.6 | -16.0 | -16.4 | -16.0 | -16.5 | -17.0 | -16.4 | -17.0 | -17.6 |
| -17 | -16.0 | -16.3 | -16.7 | -16.4 | -16.8 | -17.2 | -16.8 | -17.3 | -17.8 | -17.2 | -17.8 | -18.5 |
| -18 | -16.7 | -17.1 | -17.4 | -17.2 | -17.6 | -18.0 | -17.6 | -18.1 | -18.6 | -18.0 | -18.7 | -19.3 |
| -19 | -17.5 | -17.8 | -18.2 | -17.9 | -18.3 | -18.8 | -18.3 | -18.9 | -19.4 | -18.8 | -19.5 | -20.1 |
| -20 | -18.2 | -18.6 | -18.9 | -18.6 | -19.1 | -19.6 | -19.1 | -19.6 | -20.2 | -19.6 | -20.2 | -20.9 |
| -21 | -19.9 | -19.3 | -19.7 | -19.3 | -19.8 | -20.3 | -19.8 | -20.4 | -21.0 | -20.3 | -21.0 | -21.7 |
| -22 | -19.6 | -20.0 | -20.4 | -20.0 | -20.5 | -21.0 | -20.5 | -21.1 | -21.7 | -21.0 | -21.7 | -22.5 |
| -23 | -20.2 | -20.7 | -21.1 | -20.7 | -21.2 | -21.8 | -21.2 | -21.8 | -22.5 | -21.7 | -22.5 | -23.2 |
| -24 | -20.9 | -21.3 | -21.8 | -21.4 | -21.9 | -22.5 | -21.9 | -22.5 | -23.2 | -22.4 | -23.2 | -24.0 |
| -25 | -21.5 | -22.0 | -22.4 | -22.0 | -22.6 | -23.1 | -22.5 | -23.2 | -23.9 | -23.1 | -23.9 | -24.7 |

The corneal curvature (K), the anterior chamber depth (ACD), and the spectacle (at 12-mm vertex) correction are the parameters from which the desired lens power can be derived.

Note 1: The Artisan Myopia IOL 5/8.5 (and 6/8.5) is situated at a distance of 0.8 mm from the natural lens. Therefore 0.8 mm should be deducted from the measured anterior chamber depth to find the ACD-value.

Note 2: Preexisting astigmatism higher than -2.00 D cannot be corrected with a phakic IOL model 204 and model 206 because of their spherical optic. High astigmatism cannot be corrected with these lenses. By making the incision in relation to the cylinder, the surgeon may alter the curvature of the cornea to correct some of the remaining astigmatism. The result, however, is not predictable. High preexisting astigmatism may be corrected with custom-made toric PIOLs.

Table courtesy of Ophtec BV.

**TABLE 9-1**

likes the idea of a phakic refractive IOL, after understanding the pros and cons of various modalities, is a candidate for this surgery. The other group of patients has high refractive errors, for which usually the surgeon suggests a phakic lens or a dual operation of phakic lens implant, followed after some interval, by a laser refractive technique so that a most accurate refractive correction is achieved.

A myopic patient should not be younger than 18 years. Some suggest minimum age to be 30 years. There is no hard line for hyperopia, because in them the eye does not continue to grow. Phakic IOL is contraindicated in myopia other than axial, in the presence of lens sclerosis or early cataract, history of uveitis, presence of posterior synechia, history of glaucoma or IOP more than 20 mm, personal or family history of retinal detachment, diabetes mellitus, arthritis, and when the depth of the anterior chamber is less than 3 mm. Some of the above contraindications are relative to the discretion of the surgeon and on the needs of the patients.

## Hyperopic Refractive Correction: IOL Power Needed to Make the Eye Emmetropic in Relation to Spectacle Correction

| ACD | 2.0 mm | | | 2.5 mm | | | 3.0 mm | | |
|-----|------|------|------|------|------|------|------|------|------|
| K | 38 | 43 | 48 | 38 | 43 | 48 | 38 | 43 | 48 |
| 1 | 1.1 | 1.1 | 1.1 | 1.1 | 1.1 | 1.2 | 1.2 | 1.2 | 1.2 |
| 2 | 2.2 | 2.3 | 2.3 | 2.3 | 2.4 | 2.4 | 2.4 | 2.5 | 2.5 |
| 3 | 3.5 | 3.5 | 3.6 | 3.6 | 3.6 | 3.7 | 3.7 | 3.8 | 3.9 |
| 4 | 4.7 | 4.8 | 4.9 | 4.9 | 5.0 | 5.1 | 5.0 | 5.1 | 5.3 |
| 5 | 6.0 | 6.1 | 6.2 | 6.2 | 6.3 | 6.4 | 6.4 | 6.6 | 6.7 |
| 6 | 7.3 | 7.4 | 7.5 | 7.5 | 7.7 | 7.9 | 7.8 | 8.0 | 8.2 |
| 7 | 8.6 | 8.8 | 8.9 | 8.9 | 9.1 | 9.3 | 9.3 | 9.5 | 9.8 |
| 8 | 10.0 | 10.2 | 10.4 | 10.4 | 10.6 | 10.8 | 10.8 | 11.0 | 11.3 |
| 9 | 11.5 | 11.7 | 11.9 | 11.9 | 12.1 | 12.4 | 12.3 | 12.6 | 13.0 |
| **Refraction** | | | | | | | | | |
| 10 | 13.0 | 13.2 | 13.4 | 13.4 | 13.7 | 14.0 | 13.9 | 14.3 | 14.7 |

The corneal curvature (K), the anterior chamber depth (ACD), and the spectacle correction (at 12-mm vertex) are the parameters from which the desired lens power can be derived. Artisan Hyperopia IOLs are not available in dioptric powers above +12 D.

*Note 1*: The Artisan Hyperopia IOL 5/8.5 (6/8.5) is situated at a distance of 0.6 mm from the natural lens. Therefore 0.6 mm should be deducted from the measured anterior chamber depth to find the ACD value.

Table courtesy of Ophtec BV.

**TABLE 9-2**

There are relative contraindications like the age and the intelligence of the patient, when the patient cannot be prevented from habitual rubbing the eye. Some lens designs are not available for phakic eye implantation, if the corneal diameter is smaller than normal. The presence of amblyopia is not a contraindication.

## ANESTHESIA

While it is possible to implant a phakic lens after surface-cum intracameral, subconjunctival, peribulbar or retrobulbar anesthesia, my preference is general anesthesia. With general anesthesia, the surgeon's only concern is a good operation under ideal surgical conditions. The operation takes about 5 to 7 minutes in all.

## PREPARATION FOR OPERATION

1. Calculation of phakic IOL power from the results of refraction, the depth of the anterior chamber and the keratometric readings, with the help of the tables for different types of intraocular lens. The myopia and hyperopia tables for Artisan lens are given above

2. Conjunctival swab for culture and sensitivity

3. Instillation of ofloxacin or ciprofloxacin eye drops 6 to 8 times on the preceding day and 4 to 6 times on the morning of the operation

4. Pilocarpine 2% drops to contract the pupil, for Artisan or angle-supported lenses. The pupil is dilated for posterior chamber phakic lens implant

In the operation theater:

1. Painting the skin around the eye with povidine-iodine 10%

2. Washing the conjunctival sac with povidine-iodine 5%

3. Passing a superior rectus suture and a suture through the lower lid

4. Plastic adhesive drape and an eye speculum. I use none of these, because they seem to put pressure on the eye ball. The cilia are cut if they are likely to touch the operating instruments or the IOL. The lid margin and the conjunctival sac are thoroughly washed with povidine-iodine 5%

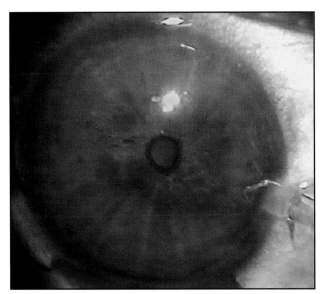

**Figure 9-8.** Making a side pocket incision with a trifacet diamond knife.

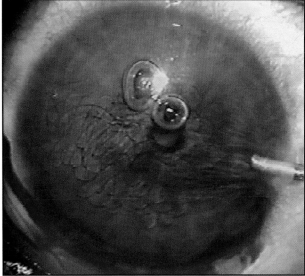

**Figure 9-9.** Making the eye firm by injecting HPMC from the side port. A firm eye helps in making a good pocket incision at the upper limbus.

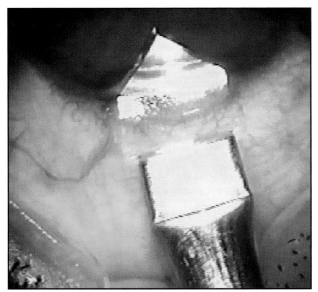

**Figure 9-10.** A 4.25 mm wide pocket incision with a diamond knife. The pocket should be 1.5 mm deep. This sharp-tipped knife should never point towards the iris or lens.

# STEPS OF PHAKIC LENS IMPLANTATION

## *Artisan Lens*

For incisions, a trifacet adjustable depth diamond knife is used to make 0.3 mm deep grooves on the limbus, 1 mm wide on the sides and 4.25 mm to 6 mm (according to lens size) at the upper limbus. The side ports are opened in to the anterior chamber as 1 mm deep pockets in the clear cornea (Figure 9-8).

A sharp, pointed diamond knife is not used, for fear of an accidental injury to the iris or the lens. The anterior chamber is filled firmly with viscoelastic material. I use 2% hydroxypropyl methylcellulose (HPMC). It is available in a syringe pack of 2 mL. HPMC should be injected, after taking the cannula clearly in to the anterior chamber (Figure 9-9). Injecting merely inside the pocket can sometimes cause a disastrous separation of the Descemet membrane. The top incision is made with a 4.25-mm diamond knife and a 1.5-mm pocket is fashioned. A diamond knife makes the cleanest cut. While making pocket incisions, it is important to watch the tip of the diamond knife, lest it strikes the iris or the lens. The knife should be moved in the plane of the iris and never toward it (Figure 9-10).

### PERIPHERAL IRIDECTOMY/IRIDOTOMY

If so desired, a peripheral iridectomy or iridotomy is performed close to the internal opening of the upper pocket incision. A peripheral iridectomy somewhat reduces the tendency of the iris to prolapse during phakic lens implantation. In the postoperative period, it is a safety valve, if for any reason the pupil gets blocked. To do an iridotomy or iridectomy, a utility forceps lifts the iris just inside the incision. The iris is snipped by a scissors inside the anterior chamber. The iris is never pulled out of the incision line, as this can tear the iris root and cause bleeding. The other option is to proceed, the iridectomy being done later (Figures 9-11A and B).

### LENS IMPLANTATION

Make sure the pupil is contracted. If not, an intracameral preparation of carbachol, acetylcholine, or pilocarpine is used to effect the same. The Artisan lens is vaulted and has a

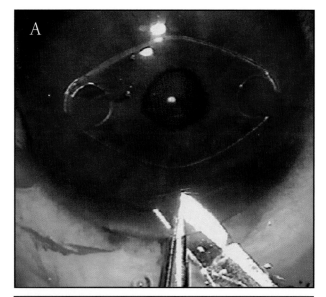

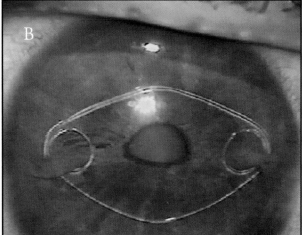

**Figure 9-11A and B.** Peripheral iridectomy/iridotomy is performed by taking the forceps and the scissors inside the anterior chamber.

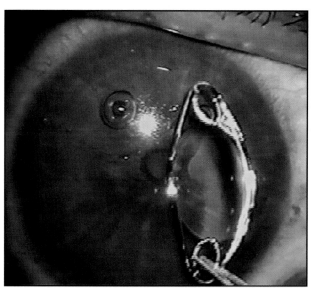

**Figure 9-12.** Convexo-concave vaulted construction of the phakic Artisan lens. The eccentric claws are clearly visible.

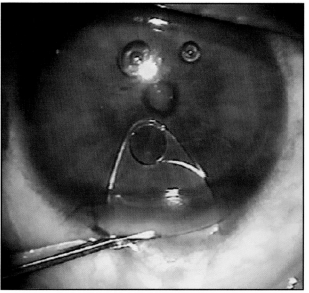

**Figure 9-13.** The phakic Artisan lens is introduced parallel to the iris surface. Note the pocket of the incision.

convexo-concave optic (Figure 9-12). The lens is introduced inside the anterior chamber, taking care of the position of the claws (Figure 9-13). I commonly use a lens with eccentric claws, which need to face superiorly for proper fixation. When a lens with claws 180 degrees apart is used, no such precaution is necessary (see Figures 9-5 and 9-14). The IOL is slipped in so that it crosses the pupil without touching the iris or the crystalline lens. Keeping the anterior chamber well supplied with HPMC, the IOL is rotated to make it horizontal (Figure 9-15). The rotation can be effected by an irrigating cannula, either physically or by the push of viscoelastic material. Any fine lens hook can do the same. I like to see the lens floating in the anterior chamber, so that when the lens holding forceps enters the anterior chamber, the upper edge of the IOL floats in to the open jaws of the lens-holding forceps.

The lens-holding forceps is designed to hold an IOL with a concave posterior surface (Figure 9-16). It is shaped like the tail of a dolphin. The grip on the lens is excellent.

The basic philosophy of Artisan lens implantation is to hold the centrally positioned lens steady, with the lens holder, while a second instrument introduced through the side port passes a fold of the iris through the claw of the lens (Figure 9-17).

Passing a fold of iris through the claw needs to be understood clearly. Each haptic of the Artisan lens has a springy flexible claw. The claw can be opened by anything stiff—a thin forceps, a hook, or a cannula. The iris can be introduced into the claw either by:

1. Carrying it along with the stiff instrument that opens the claw.

2. By gently pressing the claw on the iris, while an instrument opens the claw in a fluid motion; the moment

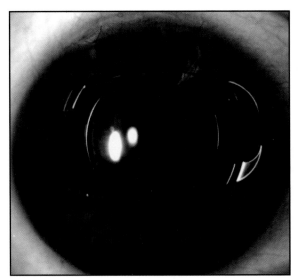

**Figure 9-14.** An Artisan lens with a 5-mm optic and a 8.5-mm width in a myopic eye. Six-mm optic lenses are also available, which considerably reduce the glare problem in lightly pigmented eyes. This lens is decentered upward. The claws are 180 degrees apart.

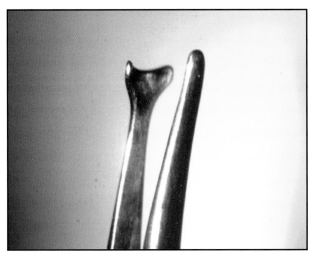

**Figure 9-16.** Dolphin tail like lens-holding forceps especially designed to hold convexo-concave optic.

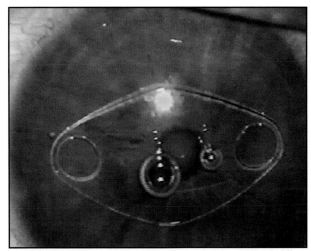

**Figure 9-15.** The lens is rotated inside the HPMC filled anterior chamber so that the eccentric claws are superior in position.

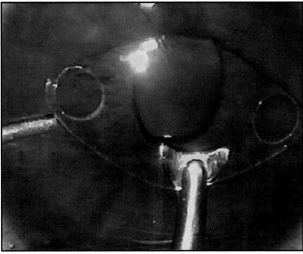

**Figure 9-17.** The phakic lens is held by the dolphin tail forceps, while the 25-gauge HPMC connected cannula is in place to raise a fold of the iris that can be pushed into the claw. At this moment the claw is right over the cannula, but is not clearly visible. The reason is that the claw is only a cut in the haptic.

the 2 sides of the claw fall back, they immediately pinch the iris immediately underneath. The amount of the iris in the claw can be increased or decreased by feeding more iris as before or by opening the claw backward and letting the desired amount of the iris out of the claw respectively.

During the time of claw fixation, it is important that the anterior chamber should not collapse, lest the lens-holding forceps rub against the corneal endothelium or the crystalline lens (Figures 9-18 and 9-19). Because the incision line is fairly large, during manipulations in the anterior chamber, the HPMC moves out fast. If Healon has been used, it may come out as a big blob.

Lack of control on the depth of the anterior chamber upsets the surgeon. If the iris also follows the viscoelastic material, the situation becomes nightmarish. To overcome these problems I have 2 simple solutions.

The maintenance of the anterior chamber and the passage of the iris through the claw is done with a simple device (Figure 9-20). A small stiff 25-gauge cannula is attached to an irrigating handle, which in turn is connected through 6 inches long silicone tubing, to a 2-ml syringe containing HPMC. The instrument is handled by the surgeon, while HPMC is pushed by the assistant on command. The pushing job can be done by a mechanical device controlled by a foot switch.

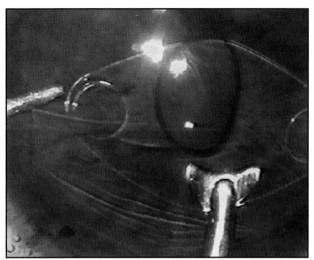

**Figure 9-18.** The iris fixation is completed on 1 side. Notice slight inadvertent drag on the iris produced by the lens holding forceps. Clumsy handling can injure the crystalline lens, which may or may not manifest for years.

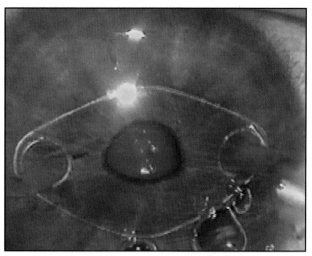

**Figure 9-19.** Both the claws of Artisan lens are in place. The HPMC irrigating/claw fixating cannula ensures that at no time the anterior chamber becomes flat.

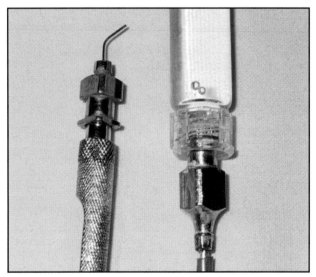

**Figure 9-20.** Irrigating cannula HPMC filled syringe assembly is joined by the silicone tubing. HPMC is pushed by the assistant on command, who also keeps observing the depth of the anterior chamber and the process of iris enclavation.

However, by entrusting 1 function of pushing in HPMC to the assistant, the surgeon can concentrate better on the job at hand.

HPMC should be injected into the anterior chamber in small amounts, with the sole aim of simply keeping the instruments and the Artisan lens separated from the tissues.

Overfilling the anterior chamber makes the claw fixation and the tendency of the iris to prolapse more difficult to control. When the Artisan lens is steadied in front of the pupil, the claw is fixated with an instrument through the side port.

A shift in the position of the lens-holding forceps, will lead to a misplaced fixation. Fixation close to the angle of the anterior chamber and excessive iris enclavation can cause a tear in the iris root and bleeding. There is no need to panic. Just wait for the bleeding to stop, fill the anterior chamber with HPMC, open the claw, and refix the lens at the proper site.

A simple way for a beginner is to make a small iris fixation on 1 side, take out all instruments, fill the anterior chamber with HPMC, reassess the optic centration and the fixation of the first claw, make the fixation of the second claw at the proper place, then go back to the first claw and complete the fixation or release it and refix properly. The point to understand is that the centration and fixation of the Artisan lens has to be done by the surgeon himself and the implanted lens will remain at the same position, for the rest of the patient's life. A misplaced lens not only creates optical problems, but is also a threat to the integrity of the adjacent tissues.

Another way to fix the implant is to use any horizontally or vertically acting plain lens holding forceps, to hold the lens haptic close to the claw, while another device (forceps or cannula or a hook) is used to pass the iris through the claw. Yet another way is to hold the lens with dolphin tail forceps while the iris is passed through the claw with the help of a hook passed through the same upper incision. How much iris is to be enclavated in the claw? Too little iris tissue in the claw of the lens can be responsible for dislocation months or years later. Too much iris tissue inside the claws, makes the lens optic press against the iris tissue, thereby reducing the freedom of the aqueous to move freely under the lens edges. It also encourages synechia formation between the iris and crystalline lens. Dr. Kiranjit Singh, looking at one of my

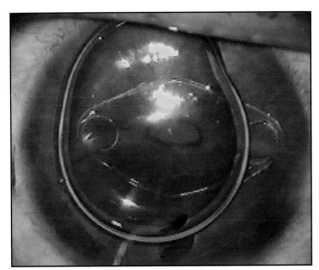

**Figure 9-21.** A moderate sized air bubble inside the saline filled anterior chamber ensures good closure of the pocket incisions.

cases used the term "suffocation" to describe the situation. The final answer to the question is neither too little, nor too much iris should go in to the claws.

### CLEARING THE ANTERIOR CHAMBER OF HPMC

The anterior chamber is cleared of HPMC by patient irrigation with a wide bore cannula. I irrigate with an 18-gauge cannula under low pressure. This helps remove HPMC without much turbulence. The existence of the HPMC in the anterior chamber is appreciated by its syrupy appearance, which gets diluted and eradicated by continued irrigation.

### CLOSING THE INCISION LINE

Since the corneal pocket has a width of nearly 1.5 mm, the 2 walls of the pocket can be brought together effectively with the help of a medium-sized air bubble. When the patient sits up and the air bubble moves upward, the apposition becomes even better. If the pocket incision is of an uncertain quality, it better to apply 1 or 2 superficial sutures, which may or may not be removed later, depending upon their contribution to the resulting astigmatism. The side pockets do not need a suture.

Having no suture and no air bubble in the anterior chamber runs a risk of leakage or aspiration. A medium-sized air bubble is a great help (Figure 9-21). When the patient sits up, the air bubble helps to bring the 2 sides of the pocket incision together and gives further safety to the incision.

If a patient with a large air bubble sits up, the bubble blocks the peripheral iridectomy as well as presses the lens optic against the iris, initiating a pupil block glaucoma. Such a patient is made to lie supine looking straight. The air bubble moves towards the center of the anterior chamber, and the peripheral iridectomy becomes functional.

### SUBCONJUNCTIVAL INJECTION

A subconjunctival injection of 20 mg of gentamycin and 2 mg of dexamethasone is given, under the superior conjunctiva.

## Angle-Supported Lens

Steps of operation for the insertion of a Baikoff angle-supported lens:

1. A 6-mm corneoscleral incision is made in the steepest meridian, attempting to correct the preoperative astigmatism
2. The pupil is contracted with acetylcholine
3. The anterior chamber is filled with HPMC
4. A 5-mm silicone Sheets glide is introduced in to the anterior chamber. More HPMC is injected over the glide
5. The phakic IOL is held with a utility forceps and the inferior haptic is slipped into the anterior chamber
6. The IOL is slid over the glide, until both ends of the inferior haptics are in contact with the angle. The glide is then pulled out gently
7. The upper haptic is pushed in to the anterior chamber and under the posterior lip of the incision, using a double-tip nucleus manipulator
8. The phakic IOL is rotated with Sinskey hook, to the horizontal meridian, where white-to-white distance is measured
9. A small peripheral iridectomy is performed
10. If the pupil is not round, the Sinskey hook is used to pull the haptic away from the angle; then, it is released.
11. Verify that the optic is centered, the pupil is round and there is no iris traction by the footplate
12. Apply 2 to 3 bite running 10 zero nylon. Before the knot is tied, HPMC is carefully washed out. Nylon is used to close any conjunctival flap made
13. After the incision is closed, gonioscopy is performed to make sure about the position of haptic ends and that there is no iris tuck. Many surgeons omit this important step

## Posterior Chamber Lens

A few days before lens implantation, a peripheral iridectomy is performed with Nd:YAG laser. Before the surgery the pupil is fully dilated. The surgical steps are as follows:

1. One 0.6-mm side port is made. It is needed to inject viscoelastic material in the anterior chamber
2. For a precrystalline lens, a 3.2-mm CCI is made on the steep meridian
3. The lens is introduced with angled-suture forceps, then it is positioned behind the iris on a horizontal axis with a cyclodialysis spatula
4. The lens is manipulated to center the optic on the pupil
5. The viscoelastic material is removed from the anterior and posterior chambers with an aspiration syringe (23-gauge cannula) or by copious irrigation with saline

6. The pupil is contracted with intraocular acetylcholine 1%, or pilocarpine 0.5% solution

7. The incision is closed by hydrating the corneal incisions. A suture is rarely needed

It is obvious from the 3 descriptions of lens implantation given above, that the implantation of every phakic lens needs thorough knowledge of a procedure and an average degree of surgical skill. The skill gets fine tuned with increasing experience.

## ALTERNATIVES AND PITFALLS

Laser refractive surgery especially by PRK cum WASCA should not be lost sight of especially in cases of myopia. PRK is a great procedure that needs to be rediscovered after shedding all prejudices, that were generated with the advent of LASIK. Cooling of the cornea with chilled saline immediately prior to and after PRK and application of a bandage contact has tremendously reduced the incidence of post-PRK pain. Nobody today talks about the possible adverse effect of loss of Bowman membrane with PRK, as was a fashion earlier.

Being an invasive procedure, a phakic lens implantation is not to be taken lightly. Phakic lens implantation is not a single event as an act of insertion, but is the beginning of a life long possible intraocular process that requires regular monitoring for inflammation, synechia, pigment shedding, glaucoma, and cataract formation. Besides, a regular watch is needed on endothelial cell counts. It is a pity that not many clinics, even in advanced countries, have such an important instrument as a specular endothelial microscope. Accurate endothelial cell count, at regular intervals gives an assurance to the patient and the surgeon as well.

Endothelial cells can be lost in every kind of phakic IOL, due to a variety of known (clinical and subclinical inflammation, glaucoma, and endothelial touch) and unknown reasons. Subclinical inflammation can be monitored by a laser flare meter only.

## MANAGEMENT AND COMPLICATIONS

### Postoperative Management

Because the surgery is performed on a healthy phakic eye, usually of a young patient, it is imperative that there is minimal or nil postoperative reaction.

#### ANTI-INFLAMMATORY

Prednisolone 40 mg daily for the first 3 days, 20 mg for the next 7 days, 10 mg for the next 15 days, and 5 mg daily for the next 15 days. This is followed by indomethacin slow release 250 mg capsule once daily for the next 30 days.

Next, fluoromethalone 0.25 % drops are given 6 times a day for 2 weeks, 5 times a day for next 2 weeks, reducing by 1 time every 2 weeks. Non-steroidal agent ketorolac tromethamine 0.5 % is added 6 weeks after the surgery. It is instilled 3 times a day and it is continued for 4 to 6 months. The anti-inflammatory regime might appear excessive, but the stakes are too high to take any chance with the operated healthy eye. A watch is kept on the IOP.

#### DILATATION OF THE PUPIL

The pupil is kept moving by the instillation of homatropine 2% and phenylepherine 5% once a day at bed time. If need be, phenylepherine is instilled during day time also. At the slightest sign of posterior synechia, the treatment is intensified.

#### REFRACTION

The first postoperative refraction may be done after 1 or 2 days.

#### FOLLOW-UP

The patient is examined daily for 3 days (Figure 9-22). The next examinations are performed after 15 days, 1 month, 2 months, 3 months, 6 months, and then twice a year. At every visit, UCVA and BCVA is recorded. The eye is examined under the slit lamp microscope, with pupil fully dilated. IOP is measured. Six months postoperative and then twice a year thereafter gonioscopy is done in angle support and posterior chamber lens cases. Endothelial cell count is done in every case.

#### WARNING TO THE PATIENT

The patient to advised to report immediately if there is pain, redness, or a fall in the sharpness of vision.

### Complications

#### EARLY COMPLICATIONS

1. Pigment disturbance. Pigment and cells are evident on the very next day of surgery. Many of them are deposited on the posterior surface of the lens optic. This helps to visualize the relationship of the crystalline lens to the posterior surface of the phakic lens. It takes a few weeks for the cells to disappear. They have no effect on the visual acuity (Figures 9-23 and 9-24)

2. Uveitis as manifested by the presence of multitude of cells on the artificial lens and aqueous flare. It occurs within 6 weeks of surgery and is generally due to non-compliance with the prophylactic anti-inflammatory postoperative regimen (Figure 9-25). This inflammation is readily controlled by a short course of steroids, followed by local steroids and oral long acting indomethacin for a month. Such a case is followed very carefully, lest there is a recurrence. A more severe form of blood-aqueous barrier breakdown may manifest as an inflammatory membrane on the anterior and the posterior surface of an Artisan (Figure 9-26) or an anterior chamber lens. Pupil dilatation and anti-

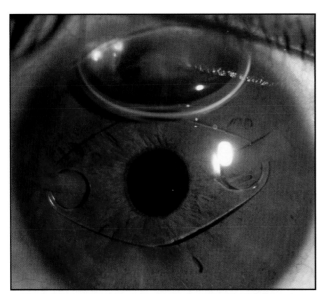

**Figure 9-22.** One day postoperative, the air bubble supports the pocket incision and blocks the peripheral iridectomy also. However, it does not affect fluid circulation, since the aqueous can escape under the edges and sides holes of the vaulted Artisan lens.

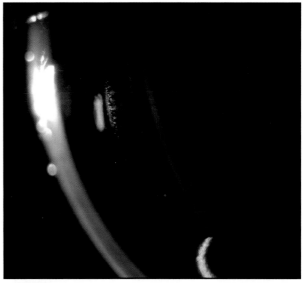

**Figure 9-23.** In the first postoperative week, some of the pigment liberated by surgical trauma can be seen deposited on the optic, especially the posterior. This helps to visualize the distance between the optic and the anterior surface of the crystalline lens. A phakic Artisan lens or an angle-supported lens never touches the crystalline lens.

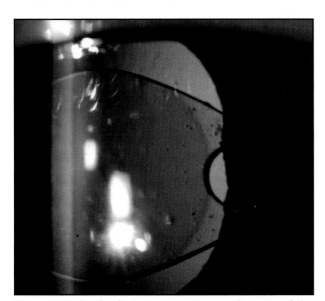

**Figure 9-24.** In the first postoperative week, some of the pigment liberated by surgical trauma can be seen deposited on the optic, especially the posterior. This helps to visualize the distance between the optic and the anterior surface of the crystalline lens. A phakic Artisan lens or an angle-supported lens never touches the crystalline lens.

inflammatory treatment is started. No attempt should be made to clear the IOL with Nd:YAG shots that may injure the natural lens. The condition resolves fast under treatment. However, if such a reaction occurs in a posterior chamber implanted lens case, the wisest course will be prompt explantation of the lens, plus medical treatment

3. Glaucoma. In the early postoperative period, it is due to pupil block. In an Artisan lens case it is due to a large air bubble. In a posterior chamber phakic lens, it is due to the closure of the pre-implant laser peripheral iridectomy with viscoelastic or pigment or the haptic of the implanted lens. The iridectomy may be reopened or a new one made to clear the block. If nothing helps then explantation may be considered

4. Hyphema. Manipulations made to implant an Artisan or an angle-supported lens can cause hyphema, which is usually minor and clears spontaneously

5. Cataract formation and fast visual deterioration days or weeks after phakic lens implantation is most probably traumatic in origin. The right course is an explantation with ECCE and suitable power IOL, as and when an opportune time is chosen for surgery

LATE COMPLICATIONS

1. Pupil ovalization is fairly common problem with angle-supported lenses. It raises the nagging question whether the lens should be explanted immediately or later and if later, when?

2. Glaucoma may be a coincidence or due to the crowding of the angle by a lens in the posterior chamber, or due to the damage to the angle of the anterior chamber by the haptics of anterior chamber lens. There is a risk of pigment shedding from the posterior pigment

**Figure 9-25.** Cell deposition 1 month after phakic lens implantation. The vision was somewhat reduced. Such cases clear up fast with anti-inflammatory medication. Close attention is required for many months to prevent any recurrence.

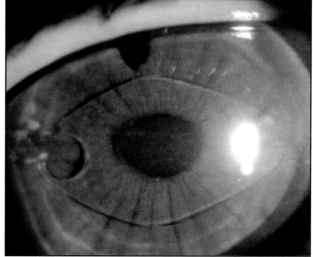

**Figure 9-26.** Severe exudative reaction 3 weeks after the operation, which is recovering under treatment. The 3-D picture shows that the crystalline lens is unaffected. If a severe reaction develops after posterior chamber phakic lens implant, the crystalline lens may be adversely affected.

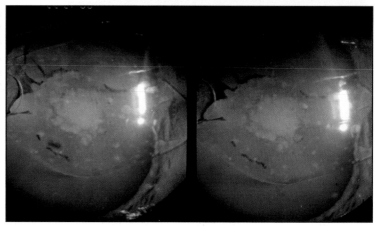

epithelium by perpetual rubbing by the phakic posterior chamber lens. A pigmentary glaucoma is a distinct possibility with this design years or decades later. If a patient develops diabetes mellitus, the pigment epithelium becomes even more liable to shedding

3. Cataract formation can result from friction/pressure between the crystalline lens and the implanted phakic posterior chamber lens. Adhesions can form between the artificial and the natural lens. The management lies in explantation and surgery for cataract on standard lines. Cataract formation, if it appears in presenile years, raises questions about the role of surgical trauma years or decades before, or the role of biophysical or biochemical changes due to the mere presence of the artificial lens (Figure 9-27)

4. Corneal decompensation can result from a natural fall in the endothelial cell density with time, to a critical level below 700 cells/mm². The decompensation can be hastened by a high cell loss at the time of surgery, or by an obvious acute or chronic inflammation, glaucoma or intermittent endothelial touch. Corneal decompensation is best avoided by a yearly recording of endothelial cell density. In the event of an abnormally high yearly loss of cells, even in the absence of any complication, it is best to explant, whatever the type of the lens

5. A posterior pigment epithelium sheet may grow along the pupillary margin and cover a variable area of the anterior surface of the iris. It does not seem to cause any problem. The start of any phakic lens complication shall be subtle, it may be perceived as irritation, pain redness and change of visual acuity. For every patient complaint, the eye shall have to be examined thoroughly to exclude its relationship to an implanted phakic IOL. Every instance of otherwise natural onset of cataract, glaucoma, uveitis, and a progressive endothelial disease shall be blamed squarely by the patient on the implanted phakic lens. The success of an alternative refractive technique—for example PRK to treat most refractive errors—may start a scramble toward lens explantation

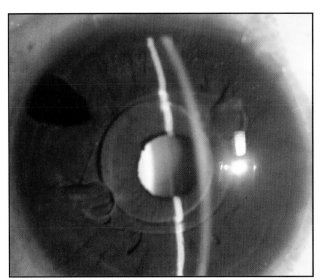

**Figure 9-27.** Age 35 years. Myopia lens of -20 D in both eyes 14 years postoperative. Cataract has developed in both eyes. A more severely affected eye is shown above. It is difficult to discount the effect of phakic lens implantation on the development.

## Rehabilitation

To overcome amblyopia patching of the better eye and pleoptic exercises for the amblyopic eye is started at the earliest opportunity. Active vision therapy[11] under expert care gives satisfying results.

## Outcomes

The refractive and visual results are excellent with most phakic lens implants. In experienced hands there is a high degree of safety with any type of IOL. It is only when a complication develops that a right or a wrong decision affects the future of the eye.

In our recent series of 54 phakic lens implants (Artisan-type) in hyperopes, the average age of the patients was 18 years. The average follow up was 12.5 months. Active vision therapy was given to amblyopic eyes. The average refractive error treated was +6.89 D with no surgical problems.

POSTOPERATIVE PROBLEMS

Severe early cell deposits or exudates: 3 cases. They all cleared with anti-inflammatory treatment. Endothelial cell loss at 6 months: average 3%. The study was done with Bioptics contact type specular endothelia microscope.

The visual results were as follows:

- Preoperative average BCVA: 20/120
- Postoperative average BCVA: 20/75
- 3 patients lost 1 line
- 25 patients had no gain or loss
- 8 patients gained 1 line
- 10 patients gained 2 lines
- 5 patients gained 3 lines
- 3 patients gained 4 lines

We gave up myopia phakic lens implant in favor of PRK in 1996. PRK with WASCA has been in use for myopia as well as hyperopia for over 1 year. The visual results in myopia have improved further. If hyperopia visual results, comparable to the present phakic lens implants are obtained, after a reasonable follow-up, an option shift in favor of laser refractive procedure might become inevitable.

# REFERENCES

1. Assetto V, Benedetti S, Pesando P. Collamer intraocular contact lens to correct high myopia. *J Cataract Refract Surg.* 1996; 22(5):551-6.

2. Baikoff G, Arne JL, Bokobza Y, Collin J. Angle-fixated anterior chamber phakic intraocular lens for myopia of -7 to -19 diopters. *J Refract Surg* 1998;14(3):282-93.

3. Fechner PU, Haigis W, Wichmann W. Posterior chamber myopia lenses in phakic eyes. *J Cataract Refract Surg.* 1996; 22(2):178-82.

4. Fechner PU, Singh D, Wulff K. Iris-claw lens in phakic eyes to correct hyperopia: preliminary study. *J Cataract Refract Surg.* 1998;24(1):48-56.

5. Menezo JL, Avino JA, Cisneros A, Rodrigues-Salvador V. Iris claw phakic intraocular lens for high myopia. *J Refract Surg.* 1997;13(6): 545-55.

6. Perez-Santonja JJ, Iradier MT, Benitez del Castillo JM, Serrano JM. Chronic subclinical inflammation in phakic eyes with intraocular lenses to correct myopia. *J Cataract Refract Surg.* 1996; 22(2):183-7.

7. Rosen E, Gore C. Staar Collamer posterior chamber phakic intraocular lens to correct myopia and hyperopia. *J Cataract Refract Surg.* 1998;24(5):596-606.

8. Sanders DR, Brown DC, Martin RG, Shepard J. Implantable contact lens for moderate to high myopia: phase 1 FDA clinical study with 6 month follow-up. *J Cataract Refract Surg.* 1998; 24(5):607-11.

9. Sanders DR, Martin RG, Brown DC, et al. Posterior chamber phakic intraocular lens for hyperopia. *J Refract Surg.* 1999; 15(3):309-15.

10. Trindade F, Pereira F, Cronemberger S. Ultrasound biomicroscopic imaging of posterior chamber phakic intraocular lens. *J Refract Surg.* 1998;14(5):497-503.

11. Verma A, Singh D. Active vision therapy for pseudophakic amblyopia. *J Cataract Refract Surg.* 1997; 23(7):1089-94.

12. Wiechens B, Winter M, Haigis W, Rochels R. Bilateral cataract after phakic posterior chamber top hat-style silicone intraocular lens. *J Refract Surg.* 1997;13(4):392-7.

13. Zaldivar R, Davidorf JM, Oscherow S, Ricur G, Piezzi V. Combined posterior chamber phakic intraocular lens and laser in situ keratomileusis: bioptics for extreme myopia. *J Refract Surg.* 1999; 15(3):299-308.

14. Zaldivar R, Davidorf JM, Oscherow S. Posterior chamber phakic intraocular lens for myopia of -8 to -19 diopters. *J Refract Surg.* 1998;14(3):294-305.

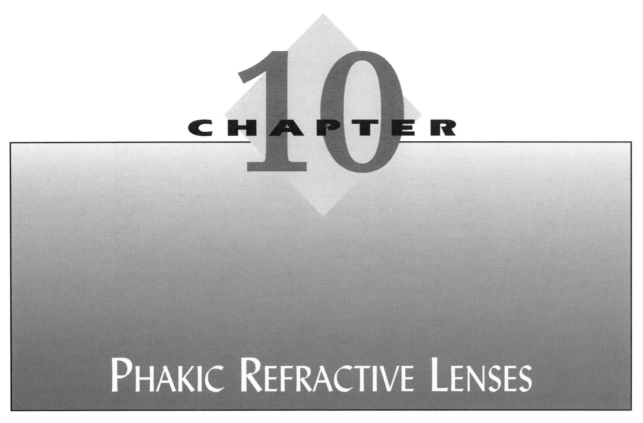

# Phakic Refractive Lenses

*Alexander Hatsis, MD, FACS and George Rozakis, MD, FACS*

## Introduction

Although the correction of ametropia dates back centuries, the modern era of refractive surgery began in the 1970s with the reintroduction of incisional keratotomy. For over 25 years, extensive numbers of radial and astigmatic keratotomies were successfully preformed. Although the overall outcome of these procedures resulted in good vision for most patients, there were limitations that inspired research into the development of alternative devices to reshape the cornea. One such device, the excimer laser spawned PRK, which was followed by LASIK and then LASEK. Over the last decade, we have continued to gain an appreciation for what excimer corneal refractive surgery does for vision—its benefits as well as its risks.

The understanding of the limitations of this procedure has led to the development of new devices for the intraocular correction of refractive errors. Among the benefits of intraocular vision correction is that the cornea and the ocular surface with its tear film, remain relatively undisturbed.

Various intraocular devices have evolved for correcting high myopia and hyperopia including the angle-fixated and iris-clip-supported anterior chamber phakic lenses as well as posterior chamber phakic implants. Refractive clear lens extraction with a mono- or multifocal IOL has also found a

niche as a refractive tool while new accommodating pseudophakic IOLs are currently being developed and studied. In this chapter we will be discussing the CIBA-Medennium (Irvine, Calif) posterior chamber *phakic refractive lens* called the PRL.

## History

The history of phakic refractive lenses dates back to Strampelli and Barraquer.[1] During the 1950s, they attempted the correction of ametropia using angle-supported anterior chamber implant lenses. Unfortunately, without today's understanding of endothelial physiology and the use of modern microsurgical techniques with viscoelastics, results were not encouraging. Research into phakic implants was abandoned until the 1980s when Fechner began applying the principals of the Worst pseudophakic iris-clip lens for the correction of high myopia.[2] Early results with this lens showed excellent long-term visual stability, however endothelial cell loss was still a concern. The Worst iris-clip lens has undergone several modifications including hyperopic and toric phakic implants and is currently being marketed as the Artisan lens (Ophtec BV, the Netherlands). US clinical studies are currently being conducted to determine the long-term safety and efficacy of the implant with its effect on the endothelium. Optically the results thus far have been excellent with high patient satisfaction.

Anterior chamber angle-fixed phakic implants were reintroduced in the early 1990s by Baikoff[3,4] and have since then undergone several modifications to reduce endothelial compromise and improve visual results.[5] The current ZS-AL-4 model (Morcher, Stuttgart, Germany) is a plano-concave PMMA angle-supported phakic implant 13.0 mm long. It differs from the previous models by incorporating a larger 5.5-mm optic with a transition zone and polished edges. These modifications have been developed to reduce light diffraction in an attempt to eliminate glare and improve night vision. Toric and foldable models are being developed and should be available in the near future. Visual results with this phakic implant are excellent and long-term endothelial studies are currently being conducted internationally to determine the long-term safety of the device.

Early work in the field of phakic posterior chamber implant lenses dates back to the 1980s when Fyodorov[6] began developing a foldable implant lens for the posterior chamber. He hypothesized that to prevent endothelial cell loss, as well as iris vascular compromise and ovalization of the pupil, the implant should be placed in the posterior chamber. Since then several implant design modifications have been made to prevent the 2 major concerns of placing a lens in close proximity to the anterior capsule and against the posterior iris surface (ie, is anterior subcapsular cataract and iris chaffing [with depigmentation and pigment glaucoma]).[7] Currently there are 2 phakic implants undergoing US clinical trials, the STAAR ICL (Monrovia, Calif) and the CIBA-Medennium PRL. In this chapter, we will be discussing the CIBA-Medennium PRL.

# PROPERTIES OF THE PRL

The CIBA-Medennium PRL has been designed as a posterior chamber lens for phakic intraocular implantation. Over the past decade it has evolved into a precise curvilinear plate haptic style lens that when implanted in the eye corrects either spherical myopia or hyperopia. It is produced from a proprietary highly polished vulcanized platinum based silicone having an index of refraction of 1.46. The central optic is situated on the anterior surface, the posterior surface is polished smooth, and the haptics are frosted to improve visualization during surgical implantation and to theoretically reduce glare.

## Hyperopic PRL

All hyperopic PRLs are 10.6 mm long by 6.0 mm wide. The optic maintains a constant 4.5-mm diameter throughout the full dioptric range from +3.00 to +15.00. Because the diameter of the optical button is constant the convexity and the radius of curvature determine the refractive power. The height of the hyperopic PRL optic and its center thickness are proportional to the dioptric power such that the optic height increases with the power. For example, the +4.00 D PRL has a center thickness of 200 μm while the + 10.00 D is 400 μm. The power range of the PRL extends from the lowest at +3.00, which corrects +3.00 D while the +15.00 PRL corrects +12.75 D of hyperopia.

## Myopic PRL

The myopic PRL is currently available in 2 lengths, 10.8 mm and 11.3 mm with a width of 6.0 mm. The haptics are frosted on the anterior surface while the posterior surface is smooth. The optic is on the anterior surface and its diameter varies from 4.5 mm to 5.5 mm according to the Dic power. For example, a -10.00 D PRL corrects -12.25 D of spherical myopia and has a 5.5-mm optic, a center thickness of only 50 μm and an optic ridge elevation of 600 μm. The -20.00 D PRL has a 4.5-mm diameter optic and corrects -24.50 D of myopia at the spectacle plane. The myopic PRL implant is available in powers from -3.00 to -20.00 correcting spherical myopia from -3.00 to -24.50 D. An extended PRL power range to -27.00 is currently being evaluated to correct spherical myopia to about -34.00 D.

## PRL Biomechanics

The unique features of the PRL are its biocompatibility and its ability to remain quietly centered in the posterior chamber away from the anterior lens capsule. We are concerned with 2 positions the PRL assumes in the eye, namely centration and anteriorization. Centration is the orientation of the optic relative to the pupil and anteriorization is the position the posterior surface of the PRL assumes relative to the anterior capsule of the natural lens of the eye. Some of the characteristics of the PRL that have been developed to maintain its position in the posterior chamber include its propriety surface finish, high index of refraction, specific gravity, light weight, strength, and hydrophobic nature. These entities unite to center the implant behind the pupil while maintaining a separation between the anterior capsule of the natural lens of the eye and the posterior surface of the PRL. It must be mentioned that as of this writing, statements regarding PRL centration and anteriorization are hypothetical and are currently being verified in clinical studies.

The PRL is not a vaulted implant and thus differs from other anterior and posterior chamber refractive devises. It does not rely on being a rigid structure fixed against any intraocular tissue such as the anterior chamber angle or the ciliary sulcus. Stable centration and anteriorization are accomplished without intraocular pressure points of any significance. Centration in the pupil appears to be accomplished by the length of the PRL relative to the internal diameter of the ciliary sulcus as well as the anterior flow of aqueous. Since the circumference of the eye is not a perfect

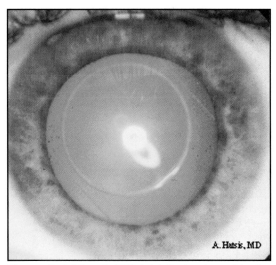

**Figure 10-1.** Myopic PRL initially implanted in the 180-degree axis has rotated to 120-degree axis.

sphere the internal diameter of the ciliary sulcus varies. We believe that once implanted the rectangular PRL, having little intraocular contact, will rotate to assume a position across the widest diameter of the sulcus. We frequently see a horizontally implanted PRL positioned diagonally or vertically on the first postoperative day, suggesting that the PRL has rotated to the widest point in the ciliary sulcus indicating very little intraocular contact (Figure 10-1). Once in place the implant appears to remain in position with no further rotation. For stability, at least 3 of the 4 implant corners are in gentle contact with the ciliary sulcus while the haptic edge remains at or is anterior to the zonules. The soft haptics, being about only 100 µm thin, are so flexible that if the PRL is slightly longer than the sulcus diameter they symmetrically plicate to accommodate the available space without exaggerated pressure on the sulcus tissue. The light weight of the PRL, as well as its hydrophobic nature, act together to distribute the flow of aqueous evenly across the smooth posterior haptic surface. It is believed that anteriorization is accomplished by the mechanism of aqueous flow coupled with its design. The PRL is pushed forward against the posterior iris surface as the haptics capture the current of aqueous moving away from the ciliary processes toward the anterior chamber. The constant flow of aqueous keeps the PRL positioned away from the anterior capsule while it nourishes the anterior cortex of the lens. This movement of aqueous across the posterior surface of the PRL and over the anterior capsule is what has been described as a ball bearing effect. As long as aqueous flow continues, it will pass between the anterior capsule and the PRL stabilizing the implant position away from the anterior capsule and nourishing the crystalline lens. Therefore centration and anteriorization can be maintained without excessive pressure of the PRL edge against intraocular tissue (ie, without vaulting).

# PATIENT SELECTION

Patient selection for a PRL is determined by the preference a surgeon has for each procedure as well as success with other treatment modalities. Concern with creating the post-LASIK oblate corneal surface is eliminated with intraocular refractive correction. Surgeons comfortable with corneal surgery for high refractive errors will continue with this approach while others may want to treat even low ametropia with an intraocular approach. There are patients who are clearly not candidates for corneal surgery due to either their degree of refractive error or the relationship between their refractive error and corneal thickness. For example, few refractive surgeons will consider LASIK to correct myopia greater than -12.00 D or hyperopia greater than +5.00 D. LASIK is also limited by corneal thickness and we would question the wisdom of correcting a -7.00 myope with a pachymetry of 490 µm. Additionally lower power patients with an irregular topography or an unusual posterior corneal curvature may be considered for PRL surgery with the goal of complete visual restoration without affecting the cornea. Extreme refractive errors can be corrected without changing the natural prolate corneal shape resulting in a better visual quality than that achieved with the laser. With the higher LASIK corrections the functional optical zone becomes limited reducing visual quality. Radial keratotomy taught us a lesson about the limits of a surgical procedure and not to push that limit. We should apply this knowledge to the excimer.

Candidates for PRL surgery should be limited to patients over 18 years of age with stable refractive errors for at least 1 year. The myopic PRL currently corrects from -3.00 to -24.50 spherical D. The hyperopic PRL corrects from +3.00 to + 12.50 spherical D. Although there is no upper age limit, our experience is with patients under 50 years old. We have thus far excluded older patients because of their natural tendency to develop cataract. This could compromise the validity of the ongoing PRL studies. Individuals who are not candidates for PRL include patients with large pupils, a shallow anterior chamber of <3.00 mm or an unusually narrow or excessively large limbus-to-limbus diameter. Correctopia, coloboma, or traumatized irregular pupils are excluded as well as patients with systemic autoimmune diseases, cataract, glaucoma, a history of any previous intraocular surgery or a history of uveitis. Patients with chronic blepharitis or rosacia must be completely treated prior to PRL surgery. The PRL does not currently correct astigmatic errors so astigmatic errors must be corrected with associated astigmatic keratotomy or the excimer laser.

Astigmatism of less than 2.00 D of cylinder can be corrected with astigmatic keratotomy at the time of PRL implantation. Any commonly used astigmatic nomogram that the surgeon is comfortable with can be used. If LASIK and PRL are planned as bioptics, then the flap should be created before the PRL surgery. Then 1 month later the LASIK astigmatic enhancement can be done. Currently, there have been no studies conducted to confirm the safety of creating a LASIK flap with a PRL in the eye. PRK on the other hand can follow the PRL once the <3.5 mm clear corneal surgical wound has stabilized. Internationally the PRL has been used to correct anisometropic amblyopia in children with early success. In a presentation in 1998, Dimitrii Dementev, MD, of Milan Italy, concluded that anisometropic amblyopic children had an overall improvement in their BCVA of the amblyopic eye after PRL implantation.[8] These children are being followed closely for long-term stability, complications and effectiveness including a reversal of the amblyopia. Additionally, the PRL has successfully corrected ametropia in stable keratoconus and stable form fruste corneal irregularities.[9]

## Preoperative Evaluation

Candidates for a PRL must have a complete ophthalmic exam including visual acuity, topography, anterior chamber depth and pupillometry. Because the PRL optic ranges from 4.5 mm to 5.5 mm, attention should be given to eliminate those patients with irregular or off-centered pupils or those patients with 6.5 mm or greater mesopic pupils. Glare and halo may reduce the effectiveness and success of the surgery and PRL implantation should be reconsidered. If the anterior chamber depth is under 3 mm, implantation of a PRL should also be reconsidered. After the current spectacle vision is taken, a manifest refraction is done to record the best spectacle corrected visual acuity. It is important to note that if the myopic refractive error is greater than -10.50 D a contact lens overrefraction must be done to reduce the vertex distance error for refractive precision. The selected PRL power is based on the refractive correction therefore precision is extremely important. As of this writing, the PRL power chosen to correct a given refractive error is being generated by the manufacturer Medennium, Inc. Kenneth Hoffer, MD, has been directly involved in determining the Dic power of the PRL and has created the principles of PRL implant power calculation.[10] After the manifest refraction a cycloplegic refraction should also be done with contact lens overrefraction, when the myopia is over -10.50 D to assure precision. A slit lamp exam with gonioscopy will rule out any anterior segment abnormality. Although there is no precise relationship between the corneal diameter (white to white) and the internal ciliary sulcus, this measurement is required to select either the 10.8 or 11.3 myopic PRL length and to exclude those hyperopic patients with small anterior segments of under 10.5 mm. Pachymetry is done as a general tool for checking corneal health and those candidates with axial measurements over 625 µm should have endothelial cell counts with morphology because this may imply poor

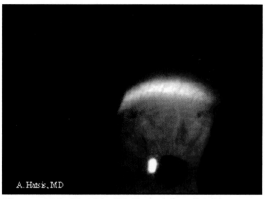

**Figure 10-2.** Double YAG peripheral iridectomy, note size and basal location.

endothelial function secondarily. An exam of the retina completes the required evaluation. It is beneficial to have an axial length recorded if a future lensectomy with IOL must be done. Interposing a PRL in the path of an ultrasound scan will distort the speed of the wave and alter the value.

# SURGERY

## Preparation of the PRL Patient

Bilateral PRL implantation has been accepted by some surgeons in the international community and is currently an option. In the United States, the standard of care permits intraocular PRL surgery 1 eye at a time separated by a minimum of 3 to 4 days.

The surgeon must decide if a double YAG iridotomy or an intraoperative surgical iridectomy is to be used (Figure 10-2). Generally, if the patient has a light iris the YAG should go smoothly but it requires an additional visit to the YAG laser suite. Dark-skinned patients with a deeply pigmented iris may be better candidates for an intraoperative iridectomy although the YAG laser iridotomy could be performed as well in just about all cases.

The advantage of the surgical iridectomy is that no YAG laser is needed, the patient has fewer visits to the clinic and only a single opening is needed. The disadvantages to the surgical iridectomy include intraoperative hemorrhage; the possible need to use a suture to close the paracentesis; the tendency to make the surgical PI larger than the double YAG causing glare and the additional patient time on the operating table. Advantages of the double YAG laser iridotomy are that both the size and position can be exactly adjusted preoperatively to be functional and less likely to cause glare. Furthermore, a cut-down type of corneal incision is needed to create the very peripheral iridectomy, which is more likely to leak. Surgery is less time consuming with no question as to the patency of the iridotomy. The disadvantages of the

YAG iridotomy are that it requires additional visits to the clinic, it may be difficult to create on the darkly pigmented iris and it leaves pigment in the trabecular meshwork.

## Peripheral Iridectomy

With the PRL situated in the posterior chamber, the pupil becomes occluded by the implant optic. Aqueous flow positions the PRL anterior and away from the lens capsule toward the posterior surface of the iris. This action results in pupil occlusion with pupillary block if an alternative pathway for the aqueous to pass into the anterior chamber is not available.[11] For this reason, a patent peripheral iridectomy is absolutely necessity to prevent a pupillary block.

## YAG Iridectomy

If the YAG laser technique is employed, a double PI should be done a minimum of 3 to 4 days before the PRL surgery. The 2 iridotomies should be made very basal (peripheral) on the iris under the upper lid to prevent glare Because most patients have been long-time contact lens wearers we frequently encounter limbal corneal neovascularization. We attempt to place the laser treatment between these peripheral vessels. An Abraham iridectomy contact lens facilitates the procedure by magnifying the iris crypts and stabilizing the globe. Prior to the YAG laser treatment, 1 or 2 drops of 1% pilocarpine drops can be given to put the iris on stretch. Each laser opening should be made at least 1.25 to 1.75 mm in diameter and placed in the supronasal and suprotemporal peripheral iris. Once the miotic wears off the diameter of the iridotomies decreases to about 1 mm and their position becomes even more peripheral. Two very peripheral YAG iridectomies are created because the nature of the PRL is to rotate into position after implantation. If the iridotomy communication is not peripheral enough, the haptic can rotate and block the opening. A high-frequency ultrasound image of the ciliary sulcus shows the relationship between the peripheral iris and the PRL. From this, we can see that if the iridectomy is peripheral enough the curved shape of the PRL will maintain its position away from the iris. With a properly placed peripheral opening, occlusion will be unlikely even after a rotation that directly places the implant under the opening. Bleeding that occurs from the YAG laser can be controlled either by applying direct pressure on the eye with the Abraham iridectomy contact lens during treatment or pressure patching after. The 2 patent iridotomies must be directly visualized by seeing the lens capsule through the openings before the patient is discharged. Visualizing a red reflex through the iris with retroillumination will not guarantee the openings are adequate. Upon discharge we recommend treatment with a topical antiglaucoma medication such as 1% iopodine or 0.5% timolol once to prevent a pressure spike and a topical anti-inflammatory drop QID for 3 days.

The single surgical iridectomy is usually performed through a vertical paracentesis incision after the viscoelastic has been removed and miosis induced by acetylcholine. Because the surgical iridectomy is more peripheral and usually much larger than the 1-mm YAG iridotomy, only one is needed. The surgeon must be careful not to disinsert the iris root when the iris tissue is withdrawn through the paracentesis with the forceps. The proper surgical maneuver would be to depress the limbus with the scissors toward the iris rather than to pull up on the iris tissue at its base of insertion. Bleeding from the iridectomy site can be controlled with tamponade pressure by over hydrating the anterior chamber with either BSS or viscoelastic. Once the bleeding stops the viscoelastic can be removed. It is obligatory that the surgeon directly visualize the patent iridectomy before patching the eye.

## Surgical Preparation

The eye is dilated with 1 drop of a sympathomemetic and 1 drop of a parasympatholytic (eg, 2.5% neosynephrine and 1% cyclopentolate). Additionally we recommend 3 applications of an NSAID such as 0.3% Flurbiprofen (Ocufen, Allergan Inc, Irvine, Calif) to maintain mydriasis during intraoperative manipulation of the PRL on the iris surface. Only a single preoperative application of each dilating drop is recommended because these young patients dilate easily and rapid reversal facilitates haptic capture after implant placement behind the iris. Although a preoperative antibiotic is suggested, it is not necessary and up to the surgeon's preference as are oral steroids such as dexamethasone 6 mg. If used, a fluroquinalone antibiotic has been shown to effectively reduce the flora of the ocular surface if given at least 90 min before surgery. A 5% Betadine (Seton Healthcare, Tex) surgical prep of the ocular surface, eyelid margins and lashes has also shown to significantly reduce the incidence of endophthalmitis after intraocular surgery.

During PRL implantation, the risk of anterior lens touch is considerable if the eye has any movement therefore topical anesthesia is contraindicated. Currently, we are recommending either retrobulbar or a deep peribulbar block to obtain complete akinesia and anesthesia. Once given, orbital pressure should be applied (eg, Honan Balloon device [Altomed, England]) for about 20 minutes to diffuse the anesthetic and deepen the anterior chamber by deturgessing the vitreous.

## Surgical Intervention

After an adequate 5% Betadine prep the lids and lashes are draped away as for intraocular surgery. If astigmatic incisions are to be used, they should be created at this time while the eye is firm. Following this a 2.8- to 3.5-mm temporal short tunnel CCI is made (Figure 10-3). A cohesive long-chain viscoelastic (Biolan [Allergan, Irvine, Calif], Univisc [CIBA Vision, Duluth, Ga], and Provisc [Alcon, Fort

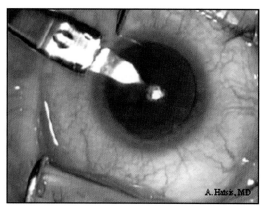

**Figure 10-3.** Forceps implantation of a myopic PRL using Hatsis horizontal opening technique and silicone-covered spatula.

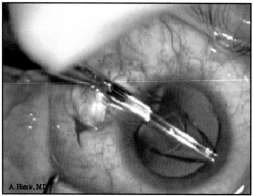

**Figure 10-5.** Forceps implantation of a myopic PRL using Hatsis horizontal opening technique and silicone-covered spatula.

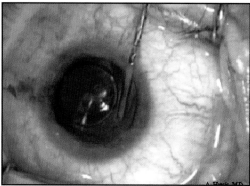

**Figure 10-7.** Tent and tack maneuver to position haptics under the iris.

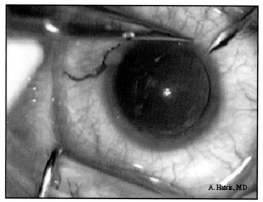

**Figure 10-4.** Forceps implantation of a myopic PRL using Hatsis horizontal opening technique and silicone-covered spatula.

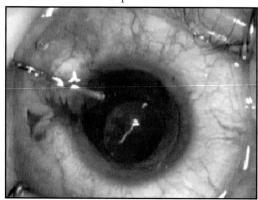

**Figure 10-6.** Tent and tack maneuver to position haptics under the iris.

Worth, Tex]) is injected toward the endothelium in the anterior chamber and allowed to float back onto the anterior capsule without over inflating. A 1.5-mm paracentesis is then made in either the supronasal or inferonasal limbus placing the paracentesis toward the nasal cornea on the limbus facilitates placement of the nasal haptic with the spatula (Figure 10-4). If a surgical iridectomy is to be done, then the paracentesis is always superior. Currently, the PRL is being

placed into the anterior chamber with a forceps although an injector system is currently available internationally. One feature of the PRL is that it is very soft, flexible, controllable, and does not roughly traumatize the intraocular structures (Figure 10-5). After placement into the viscoelastic filled anterior chamber, the PRL usually remains scrolled until it is slowly opened in a controlled fashion by injecting additional viscoelastic through the cannula. Once opened and flat on the iris surface a spatula is then employed to place the haptics under the iris by first plicating and then tucking them into position (Figures 10-6 and 10-7). Acetylcholine (Miochol, CIBA Vision, Duluth, Ga) is then used to induce miosis capturing the haptics behind the iris as the viscoelastic is completely removed (Figure 10-8). If a double YAG iridotomy was used, then centration of the PRL is verified as well as wound closure by hydrating the wounds (Figure 10-9) and the eye is patched with an antibiotic/steroid combination ointment. If an intraoperative iridectomy is to be performed, then the peripheral miotic iris is taken with a 0.12 forceps through the paracentesis wound and the limbus depressed to approach the captured iris. The peripheral iris is incised creating the iridectomy. Patency of the opening must be absolutely verified before patching the eye closed.

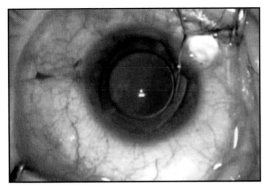

**Figure 10-8.** Miochol injected with 30G cannula while depressing the posterior wound lip to evacuate the viscoelastic.

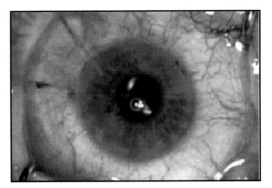

**Figure 10-9.** Miochol injected with 30G cannula while depressing the posterior wound lip to evacuate the viscoelastic.

Unless contraindicated the patient is given, either 250-mg tablet or a 500 mg-sequel acetazolamide (Diamox, Lederle, Inc., Pearl River, NY) and discharged to home until the next day.

## Postoperative Care of the PRL Patient

On day 1, the patch is removed and lids gently washed of the particulate matter that usually collects from the night before. Visual acuity is taken after the eye has a chance to adjust. We should expect the visual acuity to be in the 20/40 or better range at this exam for both the myopic and hyperopic PRL patients. The pupil may be somewhat dilated and slit lamp exam of the cornea may show a slight edema with a grade 1 cell and flare. There may be a dusting of pigment on the endothelium and the PRL with no iris transillumination while tonometry should be normal with both the paracentisis and primary wound closed. If the pupil is not too dilated, patency of the iridectomy should be verified. If the pupil is dilated, the PRL position should be documented to determine if a haptic has rotated into position under an iridectomy opening. If a surgical iridectomy was created, or the YAG iridectomy opening is peripheral and at least 1.0 mm, this rotation should not cause a problem. We begin treatment with a fluoroquinolone antibiotic, a 1% prednisilone acetate steroid and an ocular hypotensive such as Alphagan (Allergan, Irvine, Calif) which simultaneously maintains the intraocular pressure and reduces mesopic pupillary dilation. Oral 250 mg bid Diamox and 6 mg Decadron QID for 2 days has been recommended by some authors and is of course an option.

The next planned visit is at 1 week where the expected visual acuity is in the range of the preoperative best-corrected vision. The topical steroid is discontinued as well as the topical antibiotic. It would be rare to see a trace cell or flare of the anterior chamber at this visit; however, this is not impossible. If present the topical steroid should be switched to an NSAID to prevent an elevated IOP from prolonged steroid use. In this young ametropic population, this response seems to occur at a higher incidence than previously reported. It is the surgeons' preference to either discontinue the Alphagan or continue for its miotic effect on the pupil.

At 1 month, expect the patient to have an acuity equal to or better than their preoperative best corrected acuity. Many unilateral patients prefer the PRL vision to their fellow contact lens eye. An exam should reveal a quiet anterior chamber with a centered PRL and a normal IOP. The iridectomies should be patent and the round, regular, reactive pupil should be dilated to document any PRL rotation as well as to completely visualize the anterior lens cortex and peripheral retina. All medications should be terminated by this time.

# ASTIGMATISM

Since the PRL corrects the spherical component of the refractive error, coexisting astigmatism must be treated by either wound placement and size, intraoperative incisional keratotomy, or planned postoperative excimer laser treatment.

## Wound Placement

The PRL can be inserted into the eye through a clear corneal self-sealing 3-mm incision, which is astigmatically neutral in the hands of most surgeons. If the incision is enlarged to satisfy the coexisting cylinder and placed in the steep axis, the astigmatism will be reduced. For example, an incision sutured with 10-0 Vicryl will relax enough, once the sutures dissolve to reduce about 0.50 to 0.75 D of astigmatism.

## Astigmatic Keratotomy

Corneal and limbal incisional keratotomies have been shown to accurately correct up to 2.00 D of astigmatism with good stability. It is possible to correct the astigmatic refractive error by first performing the incisional keratotomy then proceeding to the PRL implantation. While most experienced refractive surgeons have developed their own refractive techniques various nomograms are available to indicate the length and position of the incisions. Treating coexisting astigmatism with incisional keratotomy at cataract surgery has thus far been the same as for PRL without modification.

## *Excimer Laser Correction of Astigmatism*

For cylinder greater than 2.50 D, the excimer laser can be used in association with the PRL to correct the high refractive error. The surgery should be planned in advance as either FLAP-PRL-LASIK or PRL-PRK. For either approach the excimer laser ablation should follow the PRL implantation. If LASIK is to be used, it is recommended that the flap be created prior to the PRL implantation without laser application (although LASIK has been performed after PRL these results have not been completely studied). After the PRL procedure has achieved refractive stability, then the flap can be lifted and the expected residual refractive error can be completely treated. To date, there are no clinical studies demonstrating the effect of a microkeratome pass over an implanted PRL.

# COMPLICATIONS[12]

## *Under- or Overcorrection*

As of this writing, our refractive results with the PRL have been precise. Most postoperative refractive errors have been limited to incorrect PRL power selection based on an inaccurate vertex distance adjustment. To select the proper PRL power for those patients over -10.50 D, the vertex distance error must be neutralized with a contact lens overrefraction. For significant under- or overcorrections, it is possible to exchange the PRL. The refractive result will be known by the 1 week visit and the initial incision can be used. Through a dilated pupil, the PRL can be prolapsed into the anterior chamber with a cohesive viscoelastic and then removed with the inserting forceps. For small errors, incisional refractive surgery or PRK should be done no sooner than 1 month.

## *Corneal Edema*

A low-grade corneal edema may be seen on the first postoperative day. This may be due to either endothelial touch from the instrument or aggressive viscoelastic washout. In-vitro studies performed at the Storm Eye Institute by Dr. David Apple's group have shown that static PRL contact with a viscoelastic-coated endothelium does not cause damage or loss of endothelial cells. It can also be a response to a transient overnight elevation of the intraocular pressure from retained viscoelastic, which has passed. This edema should resolve in a few days and no treatment is necessary.

## *Increased Intraocular Pressure*

One of the more common problems with PRL surgery is an increased IOP. These can be grouped into 3 categories:

first, occluded iridotomy with pupillary block; second, retained viscoelastic; and third, steroid response.

### PUPILLARY BLOCK

A reason for early postoperative eye pain would be an occluded iridotomy with pupillary block. The patient could develop eye pain from an increased IOP within 6 hours of surgery. The etiology of this is either the peripheral iridectomy wasn't patent to begin with or the PRL rotated into a position under a nonperipheral or incomplete iridotomy blocking it. Any postoperative pain should be examined immediately noting an exaggerated space between the PRL and the anterior capsule with shallowing of the anterior chamber and a high pressure. The pupil may or may not be responsive to light.

Treatment depends on reestablishing a communication between the anterior and the posterior chamber. The most definitive approach would be to immediately bring the patient back to the operating room and complete the iridectomy. Because there is a pressure gradient between the anterior and posterior chambers, tapping the anterior chamber to release aqueous would cause the chamber to shallow further allowing the PRL to advance forward with possible endothelial touch. A viscoelastic should be first placed into the anterior chamber by bluntly dissecting the viscocannula through the surgical wound. This prevents a shallowing of the anterior chamber as well as iris prolapse through the wound. A peripheral surgical iridectomy should then be performed. If an operating room is not immediately available, a YAG laser iridotomy could be attempted but if the iris is edematous it may not respond. Finally, a pupillary block can be temporized if the pupil is responsive to mydriasis. By dilating the pupil past the haptic edge, the pupillary block will be relieved. Dilating the pupil will reduce the IOP and allow time to subdue an inflamed eye until a definitive surgical treatment can be completed.

### RETAINED VISCOELASTIC

An elevated IOP no higher than the mid to upper 30s on the first postoperative day is most likely due to residual viscoelastic in the eye. This is more common with manual irrigation. There is usually a small amount of viscoelastic left between the PRL and anterior capsule and this can cause a temporary elevated IOP. Treatment is medical using oral Diamox (Wyeth, Madison, NJ) 500-mg sequel BID with the surgeons preferred topical glaucoma medications. The patient should be seen daily until the IOP has returned to normal.

### STEROID RESPONSE

The third commonly encountered reason for an elevated IOP is a response to prolonged use of steroids. This occurs no earlier than 1 week postoperative with an elevated pressure in the high 20s. It is for this reason that we routinely stop all steroid medications at 1 week and switch to NSAIDs if there is a low-grade prolonged iritis. Treatment consists of discontinuing all steroids, beginning an NSAID as well as a topical glaucoma medication of the surgeon's choice.

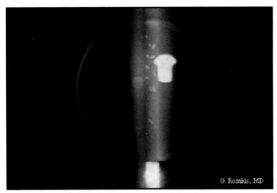

**Figure 10-10.** Rozakis fleck capsulotomy: visually insignificant focal anterior capsular opacifications seen post-myopic PRL implantation.

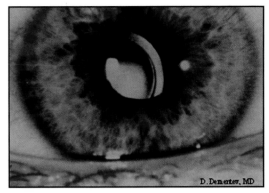

**Figure 10-11.** Decentered style II 10.8-mm myopic PRL treatment is exchanged with 11.3-mm style III.

## Cataract

There are a number of names given to an opacification of the natural lens of the eye. The most dense, which results in a loss of vision, is the anterior subcapsular cataract. This traumatic cataract results from instrument touch of the anterior capsule with disruption of the anterior cortical fibers at the time of implantation. With surgical experience, the incidence of traumatic anterior subcapsular cataract is eliminated. Chronic or long-term cataract are exceedingly rare with the PRL except in cases where overcorrected myopic patients were treated with prolonged miotics to reverse the induced hyperopia. It has been theorized that the exaggerated fixed miotic pupil caused either an intermittent touch of the PRL to the anterior capsule or a stagnation of the flow of aqueous across the anterior capsule with a lack of nutrition.

Localized small areas of "feathering" of the anterior cortex have been seen during the immediate postoperative period and were usually created by excessive intraocular manipulation by novice surgeons. These focal "feathered" areas have to date been nonprogressive and do not as a rule compromise vision. Nonprogressive spotted anterior capsular opacities have been rarely seen following PRL implantation and are thought to be due to retained viscoelastic between the implant and the lens capsule (Figure 10-10). They have been referred to as "fleck capsulopathy" by Dr. G. Rozakis. Any visually significant cataract will be noted within the first month of PRL implantation and should be treated by cataract extraction with implant using the pre-PRL biometry values. Long-term traumatic, cortical, nuclear, and posterior capsular cataract have not been reported as of the writing of this chapter.

## Decentered PRL

This is an uncommon finding since the introduction of the Style III PRL (Ciba-Medennium, Irvine, Calif). Previously the Style II myopic implant was a 10.8 mm long PRL that had a 15 % incidence of decentration (Figure 10-11). Since the introduction of the 11.3-mm PRL, the incidence of decentration is less than 1%. Although the PRL does not exert any significant internal pressure within the eye, it still needs at least 3 of its 4 corners in contact with the ciliary sulcus. If the PRL is too short for the eye, a decentration will be seen with complaints of poor vision, glare, and halo.

A more serious cause of PRL decentration is hypothesized to be zonular disruption from a traumatic insertion. The etiology of this is excessive pushing of the PRL under the iris into the ciliary sulcus with rupture of the zonules. If the decentration is small and not visually significant, then the patient can be observed for any further advancement of the decentration or phakodinesis. If the decentration appears to be progressive, then either the PRL should be rotated into a new position away from the disrupted zonules or completely removed.

## CONCLUSION

The overall value of an ideal surgical procedure is one that is minimally invasive, simplistic, functional, not distorting, and potentially reversible. We are aware of the benefits of the excimer laser in the lower myopes where the cornea is not disturbed significantly. However, there are still issues with creating the flap and permanently changing the ocular surface. The PRL seems to have solved the problems of correcting the high ametropias without altering the ocular surface. The soft, thin, flexible, and durable silicone makes it compatible with the internal structures of the eye. In Europe, there has been a 10-year follow-up while here in the USA there have been controlled studies for over 6 years. Controlled European studies have also included the PRL for correcting anisometropic amblyopia in children with satisfactory short-term results as well as treating accommodative esotropia in adults. We have become convinced that the PRL is currently an effective alternative to correcting moderate and high ametropia. Both the myopic and hyperopic PRLs have been approved in most countries internationally and is currently undergoing clinical trials in the United States.

# REFERENCES

1. Strampelli B. Supportalita di lenti acriliche in camera anteiore nella afachia e nai vizi di refrazione. *Ann Ottalmol Clin Oculista.* 1954;80:70-82.

2. Fechner PU. Intraocular lenses for the correction of myopia in phakic eyes: short-term success and long term caution. *Refract Corneal Surg.* 1990;6:242-44.

3. Baikoff G. Phakic anterior chamber intraocular lenses. *Int Ophthalmol Clin.* 1991;31:75-86.

4. Baikoff G, Joly P. Comparison of minus power anterior chamber intraocular lenses and myopic epikeratoplasty in phakic eyes. *Refract Corneal Surg.* 1990;6:252-60.

5. Baikoff G. Angle fixated anterior chamber lens for myopia of -7.0 to -19.0 diopters. *J Refract Surg.* 1998;14(30).

6. Fyodorov SN, Zuev VK, Aznabaev BM. Intraocular correction of high myopia with negative posterior chamber lens. *Ophthalmosurgery.* 1991;3:57-58.

7. Fyodorov SN, Zuyev VK, Tumanyan NR et al. Clinical and functional follow-up of minus IOL implantation in high myopia. *J Cataract Refract Surg.* 1993;19:352-55.

8. Tumanian E, Zuev VK, Koslova TV. Hydrodynamics before and after implantation of negative IOL in highly myopic phakic eye. *Ophthalmosurgery.* 1997;4:50-56.

9. Dementiev D. Silicone phakic posterior chamber intraocular lens (P-PCIOL) and the management of pediatric anisometropia. Presented at: ASCRS Annual Meeting; San Diego; 1998.

10. Avalos G. Silicone posterior chamber intraocular lens (P-PCIOL) in the management of LASIK complications. Presented at: ASCRS Annual Meeting; San Diego; 1998.

11. Hoffer KJ. Predicting silicone phakic posterior chamber IOL power in the management of high hyperopia. Presented at: ASCRS Annual Meeting; San Diego; 1998.

12. Rozakis G, Dementev D, Avalos G, et al. Complications of silicone phakic posterior chamber intraocular lens (P-PCIOL) for the correction of high ametropia. Presented at: ASCRS Annual Meeting; San Diego; 1998.

# CHAPTER 11

# INTACS: BREAKING THE PROLATE AND REFRACTIVE REVERSAL BARRIER

*JE "Jay" McDonald II, MD; Allyson Mertins, OD; and David Deitz, Research Assistant*

The introduction of *Intacs* in 1 fell swoop revolutionized the tool chest of the modern refractive surgeon. With the advent of this additive technology, we can now for the first time utilize a corneal refractive procedure that not only leaves the visual axis undisturbed, but also preserves its optically superior, naturally occurring prolate shape. Moreover, in sparing the removal of any tissue, we have ushered in a procedure that has proven titratable as well as reversible (Figure 11-1).

## ANATOMY

Two-thirds of the refractive the power of the eye resides in the cornea. The middle 90% of the cornea is composed mostly of nonliving collagen. Changing the corneal refractive power centers around altering the curve of the cornea by recontouring this relatively inert corneal lamellae. The Intacs neither subtracts or alters the condition or structure of the collagen. The inserted segments of PMMA while present behave in an inert manner. As long as the Intacs segments are positioned so as to leave adequate clearance above, corneal physiologic and neurologic activity continues to function within normal limits and remains stable. When removed, the cornea lamellae returns to its previous position, collapsing the tunnel occupied by the previously inserted Intacs. The corneal power returns to its original shape.[1]

## HISTORY

It seems only fitting that Gene Reynolds, OD, the inventor of the cornea scope (the forerunner of today's corneal mapping technology), was the same person who conceived of the idea of using concentric forces at measurable intervals from the anatomic center of the cornea to quantitatively modify the central corneal curvature. Reynolds' idea was to develop a procedure whereby the refractive surgeon would place a ring in the corneal stroma and by tightening and/or loosening it under real-time cornea keratoscope monitoring will steepen or flatten the central cornea, thus relieving any myopia or hyperopia (Figure 11-2).

After developing the ring and some preliminary tools for insertion and tightening, Dr. David Schanzlin, MD, became involved in this emerging technology and began to help evolve its potential through a series of investigations focused on biocompatibility and surgical technique refinements. Steepening of the cornea proved difficult to titrate and real time intrasurgical adjustment of a expanding contracting band proved impractical. What did emerge was the fact that the mere presence of the ring produced central flattening. Schanzlin discovered that varying the thickness of the ring without trying to expand or constrict it produced greater and lesser degrees of flattening that was much easier to consistently reproduce.

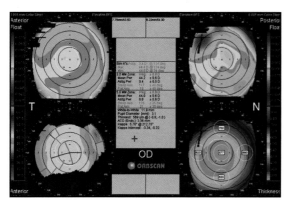

**Figure 11-1.** Intacs in an eye.

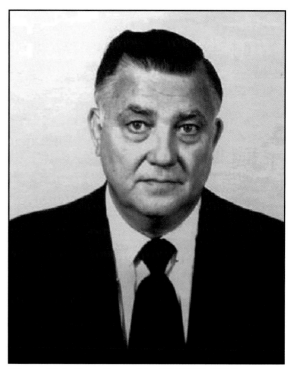

**Figure 11-2.** Gene Reynolds, OD (1921-1994).

In 1991, Professor Rubens Belfort Jr, in Sao Paulo, Brazil, placed the first corneal rings in blind eyes. His results were so encouraging that with in a few months he began placing them in sighted eyes with low myopia and achieved corresponding flattening as well as 20/30 visual acuities on day 1. In the same year, David Schanzlin, MD, began phase I corneal ring studies in blind eyes and found the same positive responses. Phase II studies began in 1993. During these trials, the technique of insertion with the 360 rings as well as some wound healing problems proved challenging, prompting Schanzlin's development of 2 segments each 150 degrees in length. Schanzlin's modification greatly simplified the surgical procedure and eliminated the wound healing issues caused by the continuous 360-degree band. Thus, the current iteration of 2-segment Intacs emerged as the platform of today's myopic Intacs surgery.

## MECHANISM OF ACTION

The symmetrical, circumferential Intacs segments inserted at the 7- to 8-mm OZ exerts its central flattening effect by elevating the overlying corneal tissue (Figure 11-3), thus lengthening the total distance the defined overlying corneal stromal fibers must traverse from limbus to limbus. The arc length shortens thus flattening the curve it subtends. This can be conceptualized as being analogous to pushing the sidewalls of a domed tent out from the inside of the tent. The curvature of the out side dome located above the circumferences one pushes out must flatten. In the cornea, the power of the cornea is decreased inducing a new more myopic state of the refractive eye. The chord length can be quantified by varying of the thickness of the Intacs thus giving a predictable reproducible effect. While present, the Intac acts a smaller diameter slightly elevated limbus, which induces corneal flattening all the while maintaining the natural prolate configuration (Figure 11-4).

## INDICATIONS FOR INTACS

KeraVision (Fremont, Calif) Intacs are intended for the reduction or elimination of mild myopia (-1.00- to -3.00-D spherical equivalent at the spectacle plane) in patients (-3.50 to -4.50 approval outside the United States):

✧ Who are 21 years of age or older
✧ With documented stability of refraction as demonstrated by a change of less than or equal to 0.50 D for at least 12 months prior to the preoperative examination
✧ Where the astigmatic component is +1.00 D or less

## CONTRAINDICATIONS FOR INTACS

KeraVision Intacs are contraindicated:

✧ In patients with collagen vascular, autoimmune or immunodeficiency diseases
✧ In pregnant or nursing women
✧ In the presence of ocular conditions, such as recurrent corneal erosion syndrome or corneal dystrophy, that may predispose the patient to future complications
✧ In patients who are taking one or more of the following medications: isotretinoin (Accutane, Roche, Nutley, NJ); amiodarone (Cordarone, Wyeth, Madison, NJ); Sumatriptan (Imitrex, GlaxoSmith-Kline, Research Triangle Park, NC)

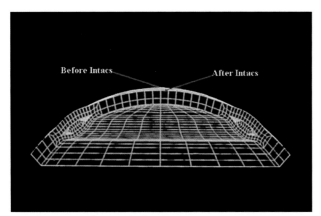

**Figure 11-3.** Before and after Intacs.

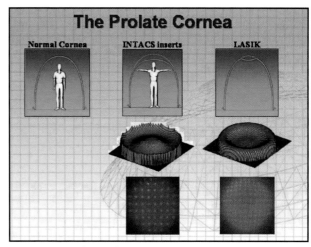

**Figure 11-4.** The prolate cornea.

# SURGICAL PROCEDURE

The Intacs surgical technique is as outlined in Figure 11-5.

## Preoperation

- ✧ 30 minutes before surgery
  - ✦ 10 mg of Valium (Roche, Nutley, NJ) orally
- ✧ In both eyes
  - ✦ Drop of proparacaine
  - ✦ Drop of alphagan
  - ✦ Drop of acular
  - ✦ Minutes before surgery
  - ✦ Drop of proparacaine
- ✧ 3 minutes before surgery
  - ✦ Drop of proparacaine
- ✧ 1 minute before surgery
  - ✦ Drop of proparacaine
  - ✦ Prep insert lid speculum
  - ✦ Drop of proparacaine

## Ambience

The surgery is performed in a clean minor surgical office room. The surgical team wears surgical scrubs, as well as masks and gloves. The patient dons a bonnet and lays on a small gurney with a special positioning pillow so as to position the iris plane parallel with the floor. A low power binocular microscope with moderate illumination is adequate.

Prior to the preparation, drape, and gloving, the eyelids are retracted with the index finger and thumb of the left hand and a central pachymetry reading is taken for both eyes. Ninety µm are subtracted from the central thickness reading. The resultant number will be used for the diamond knife setting for the singular incision. Alternatively, 68% of the pachymetry reading over the incision site can be used.

## Preparation

The patient is prepped by washing upper and lower lid and lashes with 5% povidone solution and then carefully blotting dry any residual moisture. The drying is extremely important as we use steri strips to isolate the lashes. Any moisture on the lid or lashes can prohibit the strips from sticking. Improper lash covering exposes the risk of the lashes coming into contact with an instrument or the Intacs themselves. Additionally, uncovered lashes can stroke across the wound and operative field and disseminate bacteria attached to the lashes or oily debris. Because we are inserting an inert object into a open channel in nonvascularized tissue, attention to a "no touch" technique is mandatory. Also, draping the lids in a manner as to isolate the lashes from the field is necessary.

The Intacs procedure has 6 primary steps: the marking of the geometric center, the incision, the creating of the pocket, the dissection of the channels, the insertion of the Intacs, and the closure of the wound.

## The Marking of the Geometric Center

The crossed hair marker is firmly placed centered over the anatomical limbus with the cross hairs lined with the 90- and 180-degree meridian (Figure 11-6). Taking care to line the horizontal wire intersecting the inner and outer canthus as well as squaring the vertical wire so that it appears to vertically bisect the upper and lower lid, prevents one from ending up with an incision that tilts nasally or temporally, or that rotates the incision nasally or temporally. Early on, I found the tendency to have my incisions more temporal than nasal. We now have a cross hair reference point for the incision marker, which is now applied having been coated with gentian violet. Keep in mind the orientation of the wire cross hair imprint on the cornea as you line up the "superior T" of the marking apparatus. It is relatively easy to get too much gentian violet on the marker and one can end up with

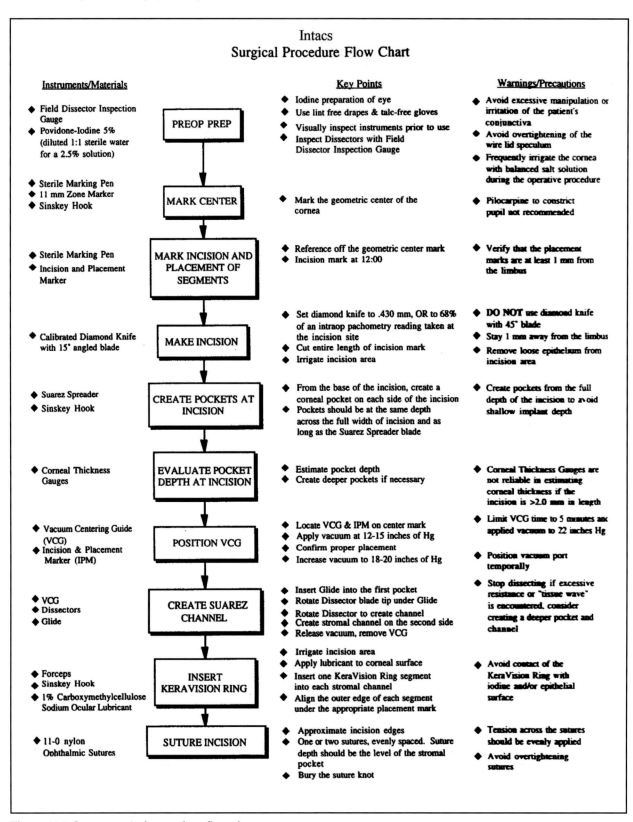

**Intacs**
**Surgical Procedure Flow Chart**

| Instruments/Materials | | Key Points | Warnings/Precautions |
|---|---|---|---|

**Instruments/Materials**

◆ Field Dissector Inspection Gauge
◆ Povidone-Iodine 5% (diluted 1:1 sterile water for a 2.5% solution)

◆ Sterile Marking Pen
◆ 11 mm Zone Marker
◆ Sinskey Hook

◆ Sterile Marking Pen
◆ Incision and Placement Marker

◆ Calibrated Diamond Knife with 15° angled blade

◆ Suarez Spreader
◆ Sinskey Hook

◆ Corneal Thickness Gauges

◆ Vacuum Centering Guide (VCG)
◆ Incision & Placement Marker (IPM)

◆ VCG
◆ Dissectors
◆ Glide

◆ Forceps
◆ Sinskey Hook
◆ 1% Carboxymethylcellulose Sodium Ocular Lubricant

◆ 11-0 nylon Ophthalmic Sutures

**Flow steps:**
PREOP PREP → MARK CENTER → MARK INCISION AND PLACEMENT OF SEGMENTS → MAKE INCISION → CREATE POCKETS AT INCISION → EVALUATE POCKET DEPTH AT INCISION → POSITION VCG → CREATE SUAREZ CHANNEL → INSERT KERAVISION RING → SUTURE INCISION

**Key Points**

◆ Iodine preparation of eye
◆ Use lint free drapes & talc-free gloves
◆ Visually inspect instruments prior to use
◆ Inspect Dissectors with Field Dissector Inspection Gauge

◆ Mark the geometric center of the cornea

◆ Reference off the geometric center mark
◆ Incision mark at 12:00

◆ Set diamond knife to .430 mm, OR to 68% of an intraop pachometry reading taken at the incision site
◆ Cut entire length of incision mark
◆ Irrigate incision area

◆ From the base of the incision, create a corneal pocket on each side of the incision
◆ Pockets should be at the same depth across the full width of incision and as long as the Suarez Spreader blade

◆ Estimate pocket depth
◆ Create deeper pockets if necessary

◆ Locate VCG & IPM on center mark
◆ Apply vacuum at 12-15 inches of Hg
◆ Confirm proper placement
◆ Increase vacuum to 18-20 inches of Hg

◆ Insert Glide into the first pocket
◆ Rotate Dissector blade tip under Glide
◆ Rotate Dissector to create channel
◆ Create stromal channel on the second side
◆ Release vacuum, remove VCG

◆ Irrigate incision area
◆ Apply lubricant to corneal surface
◆ Insert one KeraVision Ring segment into each stromal channel
◆ Align the outer edge of each segment under the appropriate placement mark

◆ Approximate incision edges
◆ One or two sutures, evenly spaced. Suture depth should be the level of the stromal pocket
◆ Bury the suture knot

**Warnings/Precautions**

◆ Avoid excessive manipulation or irritation of the patient's conjunctiva
◆ Avoid overtightening of the wire lid speculum
◆ Frequently irrigate the cornea with balanced salt solution during the operative procedure

◆ Pilocarpine to constrict pupil not recommended

◆ Verify that the placement marks are at least 1 mm from the limbus

◆ **DO NOT** use diamond knife with 45° blade
◆ Stay 1 mm away from the limbus
◆ Remove loose epithelium from incision area

◆ Create pockets from the full depth of the incision to avoid shallow implant depth

◆ Corneal Thickness Gauges are not reliable in estimating corneal thickness if the incision is >2.0 mm in length

◆ Limit VCG time to 5 minutes and applied vacuum to 22 inches Hg

◆ Position vacuum port temporally

◆ Stop dissecting if excessive resistance or "tissue wave" is encountered, consider creating a deeper pocket and channel

◆ Avoid contact of the KeraVision Ring with iodine and/or epithelial surface

◆ Tension across the sutures should be evenly applied
◆ Avoid overtightening sutures

**Figure 11-5.** Intacs surgical procedure flow-chart.

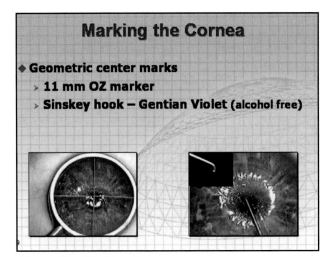

**Figure 11-6.** Marking the cornea.

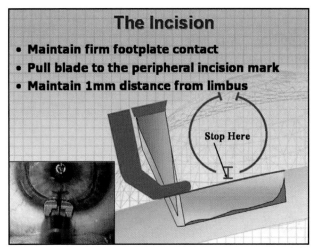

**Figure 11-7.** The incision.

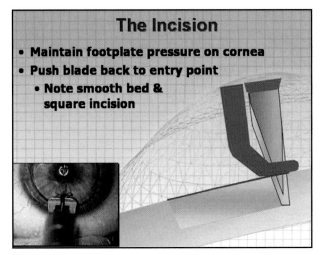

**Figure 11-8.** The incision (ctd.).

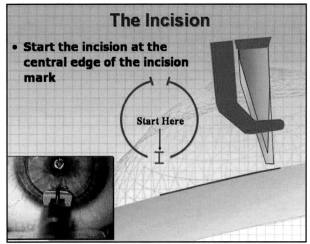

**Figure 11-9.** The incision (ctd.).

a wide smeared incision mark that is confusing when trying to decide on and make the incision.

## The Incision

The incision is made with a double-sided diamond corneal incisional blade.

I use a "dual track" knife to make the 1.8-mm radial incision. The same advantages gained by employing this knife in any corneal incision technique are appreciated. Namely, the ability to cut a square edged even depth incision while avoiding central encroachment (Figure 11-7) is expedited as shown in Figure 11-8. The making of the incision is one of the critical surgical steps that needs undivided attention to the following details (Figure 11-9).

The knife is held perpendicular and pressed firmly straight down until one sees and feels the foot plate indenting the cornea surface.

The knife is moved posteriorly 1.8 mm. Direct visualization of this end point is difficult if one keeps the knife perpendicular. For this reason, practice making this length of incision on some practicing media (a boiled egg works satisfactorily) and noting the relationship of the front of the diamond foot plates to an easily visualized landmark on the cornea marks. This way, you'll know that, for example, when the front edge of the footplate is halfway down the incision mark, one has made a 1.8-mm incision. When the front of the footplates reaches this mark, one had made a 1.8-mm length incision (Figure 11-9).

When the posterior destination with the diamond knife has been reached, the diamond is then pushed centroid until the dull part of the leading edges is stopped (Figure 11-10). One then knows that the endpoint of the incision traverse has been reached. This makes sure that one has a squared incision front and back and the incision is long enough to accept the glide guide as well as the glide dissectors.

The incision should never come closer than within 1 mm of the limbus.

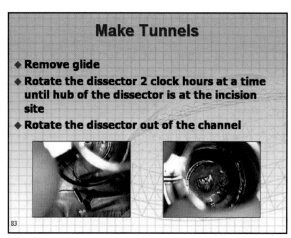

**Figure 11-10.** Making tunnels.

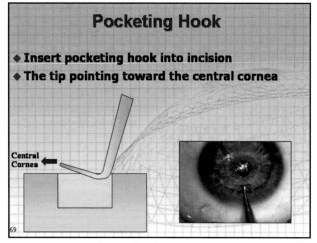

**Figure 11-12.** Pocketing hook.

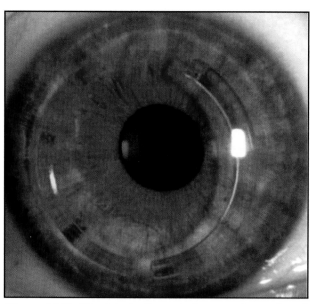

**Figure 11-11.** Rivulets in the anterior capsule produced during the capsulorrhexis in a patient with congenital aniridia.

## The Creation of the Pocket

Once an incision of proper depth and length is made, the creation of the pocket becomes the next focus. Most Intacs surgeons have moved to using the "prolate" system of intacs surgery. In doing so the awkward pocket dissector has been eliminated and we use the pocket hook (often referred to "a Sinskey on steroids") exclusively to create the pockets.

If the incision is of proper length, one should be able to place the pocket dissector directly into and to the base of the incision without using any torque or tilt. I slightly elevate the toe 10 degrees up so that I go directly down and can feel a real end point when the heal reaches the bottom of the incision. This confident end point reinforces the feeling that an adequate depth has been achieved. I now tilt the toe down from its elevated angle so that the pocket dissector is fully in contact with the bottom of the incision along its entire length (Figures 11-11 and 11-12).

One is now ready to create the semicircular "pocket" that will serve as the gateway for the channel dissectors to create the intac channel. I like to visualize the pocket and its subsequent right and left channels as the sleeve of a jacket or sport coat. If the entry way at the shoulder is adequate and easy access to the sleeve, finding the gateway with one's hand becomes easy, thus facilitating the sliding of one's arm down the sleeve with undue impediment. We have all experienced trying to put our arm in a coat whose sleeves are unduly awkward to get to or off-centered. The frustration of not being able to slide one's arm down the sleeve transforms the somewhat simple task of putting on a coat from a unconscious automatic task to a frustrating wrestling match often entailing stripping mechanical change and injury to the coat sleeve. This same aggravation can come to past in intacs sur-

### Incisional Issues

If the incision is too short, one will struggle with the proper depth and size of the pocket. One then gets tight strangulated guide passage with a subsequent torquing of the blades. This can be compounded by weak suction, and this can result in a decrease diameter of the optical zone. Also, one can get an elliptical appearing placement of the Intacs that will cause some undercorrection and/or induced astigmatism.

If the incision is too long, one can have induced astigmatism against the rule due to relaxation of the "annulus tension." Also, one can cut into the perilimbal blood vessels and end up with a pathway for vascular ingrowth.

If the incision is too shallow:

- *Mildly too shallow*—One can get under correction as the Intac does not support enough tissues at the periphery to get adequate peripheral lift and cord shortening to induce adequate flattening.

- *Significantly too shallow*—One gets photophobia, induced thinning over the segments and decreased effect. These Intacs need to be removed.

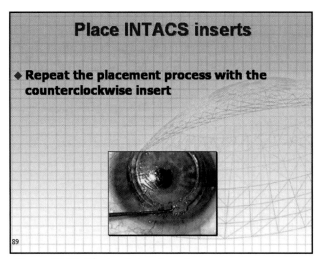

**Figure 11-13.** Placing Intacs inserts.

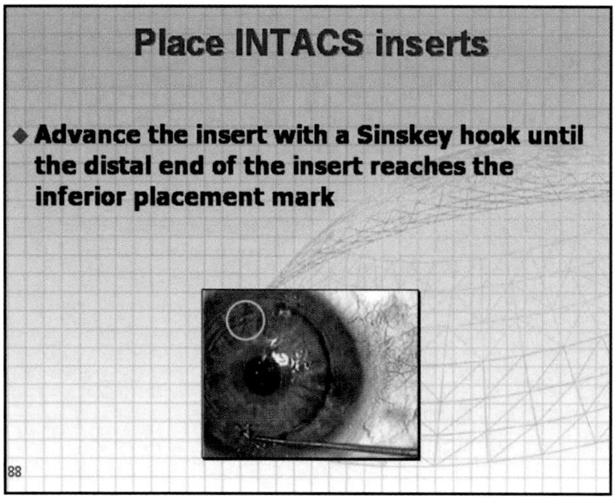

**Figure 11-14.** Placing Intacs inserts (ctd.).

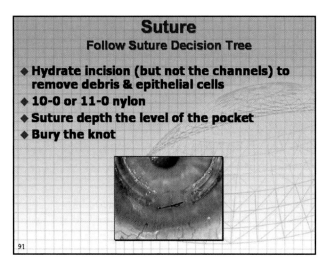

**Figure 11-15.** Suturing.

gery if one has an inadequate pocket down in which to slide the guide, dissector, and finally the intacs themselves.

Once the pocket dissector is parallel to the endothelium a twisting windshield wiper force is employed. This is effected by twirling the handle of the dissector between your fingers and your thumb. If some form of countertraction is not employed, the eye will simply move with you and your dissection will be inadequate.

Some surgeons use countertraction with a forceps to facilitate the dissection. However, I have found that having the patient look opposite of the direction in which I am attempting to make the dissection to be a most effective means establishing the necessary force. In addition, one does not stimulate a painful response from the patient that frequently occurs when one grasps the conjunctiva with toothed forceps for counter traction. I also come slightly posterior on each end of the arc so as to effect a pocket of 245 degrees.

## Intacs Insertion

The intacs are grasped with the special insertion forceps and slid into their respective channel. The final length is pushed away from the incision. It is critical that either segment end does not lie under the incision (Figures 11-13 and 11-14).

## Incision Closure

A single 10-0 nylon suture is placed to close the incision. The tightening knot should be buried. Avoid overtightening. The suture is removed from 1 to 4 weeks (Figure 11-15).

## Postoperative Care

Antibiotic steroid drops are used 4 times daily for 1 week. Additionally we use a non-steroidal anti-inflammatory drop 4 times daily for the first 72 hours. Oral analgesics are used the first evening of surgery as needed. Patients are encouraged to use light ice packs for 15 minutes out of each hour for the first 4 hours for additional discomfort.

## Outcomes

A comparison of the original FDA study group as well as over 900 eyes after approval is seen. Almost 80% of the patients achieved 20/25 or better visual acuity in both groups (Figure 11-16).

## Keratoconus and Ectasia

Joseph Colin, MD, reported success in using intacs to treat contact lens intolerant patients with keratoconus.

When the intac is inserted into the ectatic keratoconic cornea and a new limbus at the 8-mm corneal diameter is created. The arc length is shortened thus flattening the cornea as well as symmetrically uplifting the sagging corneal apex back toward its centroid position. When we next insert superiorly, the second intacs, the "fabric of the cornea" is "pulled" superiorly further rounding the cornea and moving the center of the apex of the cornea toward the optical axis. A new contour is induced, providing a more stable platform for contact lens fitting.

Intacs has also been used successfully to stabilize ectasia following LASIK and PRK.

## Intacs Removal

In the event the intacs must be removed, the patient is prepped and draped similar to the initial placement procedure, and inserts can be removed in just a few minutes. The corneal topography and refractive status returns to the original status stabilizing within 3 months.[2]

### THE INCISION

For inserts in place less than 6 months, re-open the original incision with a Sinskey hook by simple blunt dissection through the epithelial layer.

For inserts in place for longer than 6 months, or in individuals demonstrating aggressive incision healing, re-open the original incision to a depth of approximately 100 µm using a guarded diamond knife. A Sinskey hook can then be used to achieve blunt separation of the stromal layers to the full depth of the incision by gently stroking back and forth the full length of the incision until containing the original base.

### THE CHANNEL

Locate appropriate channel depth by gently depressing the floor of the incision with the Sinskey hook.

With the Sinskey hook at the incision floor, exert minimal pressure to one side of the incision by rotating the tip of the Sinskey hook to separate intrastromal layers previously delaminated. Perform this maneuver on both sides of the incision.

Bluntly separate the channel with the Sinskey hook while advancing along the channel toward the insert. (The Sinskey hook is the same position used to advance the inserts after initial placement.)

### LOCATING THE INTACS INSERTS

✧ "Clean" the presenting face of each insert to remove any re-apposed stromal tissue by carefully rotating the tip of the Sinskey hook 2 clock hours above and below each insert-positioning hole

✧ Engage the positioning hole with the tip of the Sinskey hook by placing the Sinskey hook underneath the insert and rotating the tip "up" into the positioning hold

✧ Gently begin to pull and rotate each insert out of its respective channel

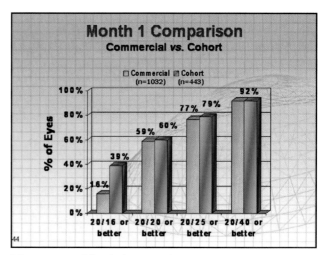

**Figure 11-16.** Month 1 comparison.

✧ If necessary, have patient move eye in opposite direction of intacs inserts rotation

✧ Repeat "cleaning" maneuver as necessary

### INCISION REPAIR

✧ Hydrate incision size and channel with BSS using an irrigating cannula

✧ Suture wound with single 10-0 nylon suture

✧ Remove suture after 2 weeks

This concept is under high power has the tectonic property of:

✧ Increase thickness generates increased corneal flattening

✧ Unique flattening as it shortens the corneal cord length and produce flattening across entire cornea

In contrast excimer causes preferential flattening in the center of the cornea. Intacs maintain the positive asphericity of the cornea. The central 3 to 4 mm of the cornea is still steeper than the midperipheral zone. Typically one sees a blue zone inside the edge of the segments with a zone that is slightly less blue just central to that.

## REFERENCES

1. Colin J, Cochener B, Savary G, et al. Intacs inserts for treating keratoconus. *Ophthalmology.* 2001;108:1049-14.

2. Clinch TE, Lemp MA, Foulks GN, Schanzlin DJ. Removal of intacs for myopia. *Ophthalmology.* 2002;109:1441-1446.

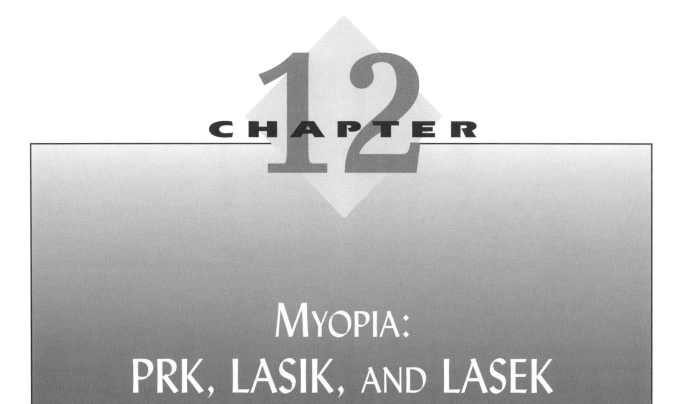

## MYOPIA: PRK, LASIK, AND LASEK

*Patricia Sierra Wilkinson, MD; David R. Hardten, MD;*
*Richard L. Lindstrom, MD; and Elizabeth A. Davis, MD*

## INTRODUCTION

The exiting field of refractive surgery has advanced geometrically over the past 25 years. This growth may be due to a combination of factors, while increased safety and precision are probably the most influential. Other contributing factors have increased consumer awareness; the increased number of refractive surgeons and laser centers, as well as the expanded approval of new technology and treatment modalities.

Because the surface of the cornea provides approximately two-thirds of the refractive power of the eye, changing its curvature provides the most common means of changing the eye's refractive error.

Refractive surgery for myopia can be divided into several categories. Incisional surgery includes those procedures that involve partial thickness incisions in the cornea such as RK and AK. Lamellar surgery involves removal of tissue parallel to the surface of the cornea to change its curvature. Intraocular surgery generally involves the introduction of a high refractive index lens into the anterior or posterior chamber with or without removal of the crystalline lens. This chapter will limit the discussion to lamellar surgery, namely LASIK, LASEK, and photorefractive keratectomy (PRK).

## ANATOMY

Myopia is a condition with an overall incidence of 25% in the general population.[1] In myopia, the parallel rays of light entering the eye are brought into focus at a location anterior to the retina. The total refractive power of the eye is greater than that required for emmetropia; this is due to either a steep cornea or a long eye. Correction of myopia with spectacles, contact lenses or refractive surgery allows the incoming rays to come into clear focus in the retina.

The normal cornea has a prolate shape (greater curvature centrally than peripherally) (Figure 12-1). Laser vision correction procedures reverse this natural prolate shape of the cornea and decrease the central corneal curvature (to create an oblate shape) (Figure 12-2).

## PATIENT SELECTION

Many patients arrive to the surgeon's office well informed about refractive surgery having read professional or lay literature. It is important for the surgeon to be able to provide the patient with current information for relevant procedures so that the appropriate procedure can be selected during the surgeon-patient interaction.

The first step in the evaluation should be to determine the goals that a patient has in seeking refractive surgery. Also

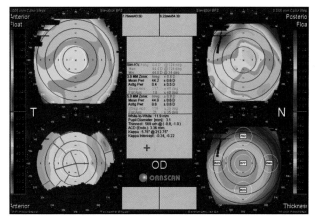

**Figure 12-1.** Normal corneal imaging with Orbscan (Bausch & Lomb, Rochester, NY). Note symmetry of the corneal anterior surface elevation, anterior surface curvature, posterior surface, and pachymetry.

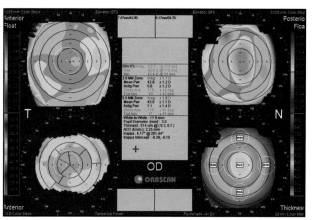

**Figure 12-2.** Post-LASIK corneal imaging with Orbscan. Note the symmetry of the flattening of the anterior curvature.

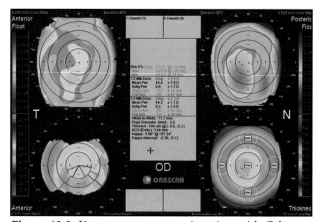

**Figure 12-3.** Keratoconus suspect imaging with Orbscan. Note the inferior steepening associated with inferior thinning and inferior elevation.

important is a review of ocular and systemic conditions. Visual acuity is measured using manifest and cycloplegic refraction. Pupil size, ocular dominance testing, and distance and near vision with and without correction should also be documented. Anterior and posterior segment examinations are performed to rule out other conditions that may adversely affect the surgical result. Glaucoma is more common among myopic patients than in the general population.[2] A careful assessment of the optic nerve and measurement of the intraocular pressure are also necessary.

Pachymetry measurements are performed to make sure that the cornea is of normal thickness. Computerized corneal topography is now used routinely in the assessment of preoperative and postoperative refractive surgery patients. This can help to screen for subclinical keratoconus or other corneal diseases (Figure 12-3). Extreme keratrometric values (flatter than 41.00 or steeper than 47.00) or abnormal corneal thickness should be identified. Rigid contact lens wearers should be out of their contact lenses for 3 to 4 weeks, and soft contact lens wearers need 2 weeks without lenses. Wavefront analysis is increasing in usage, as the ability to treat higher order aberrations improves.

The possibility of monovision should be discussed with patients near the presbyopic age. A discussion on glare and halos, the possibility of under and overcorrection, as well as any special considerations should take place with the patient. Appropriate reading materials are given to the patient for education.

This initial examination is a good occasion to counsel and assess the patient's goals to make certain they are realistic. Informed consent should include a discussion of the most frequent side effects and potential risks involved with the surgery.

# PRK

PRK was developed in the late 1980s as the first laser vision correction procedure. In October of 1995, PRK became the first FDA-approved laser treatment for the correction of myopia and eventually myopic astigmatism.

The excimer laser is used to reshape the surface of the cornea by removing anterior stromal tissue. The process by which the excimer laser removes corneal tissue is nonthermal ablative photodecomposition. Photons at extremely high energy are emitted towards the corneal tissue molecules and cause ejection of the fragments without thermal damage.[3]

Laser delivery patterns include broad beam, scanning slit, and flying spot. Broad beam lasers deliver a particular diameter beam of laser through a diaphragm that can expand or contract to modulate the beam size. Typically, the beam starts small and expands as the laser is delivered. The main advantage of broad beam lasers is a shortened operative time, which results in less time for stromal hydration to change throughout the procedure. The main disadvantage is that broad beam lasers resulted in central islands because the emitted laser plume masked the cornea from successive laser pulses. New laser software addresses this by applying more treatment to the central cornea. Scanning excimer lasers including scanning slit and flying spot provide a smoother ablation than the older broad beam lasers. Additionally, the profile can produce aspheric ablations and larger diameter ablations. Scanning lasers can achieve any ablation profile, which is an advantage for irregular or asymmetric corneas.[4] Some lasers such as the VISX (Santa Clara, Calif) system have a combination of mechanisms that allow for large and small treatment areas through a system termed *variable spot scanning*. This combines the advantage of a shorter treatment time by treating large areas all at once, as well as the flexibility of treating smaller areas asymmetrically when needed with a small diameter beam.

An important terminology in refractive surgery is the optical zone size and entrance pupil. The pupil that is seen when looking at an eye is termed the entrance pupil, which is approximately 0.5 mm anterior to and 14% larger than the real pupil.[5] It is a virtual image of the real pupil formed by the cornea. There is an ongoing debate within surgeons regarding the best point to use for centration during the refractive procedure. Some surgeons use the corneal intercept of the visual axis which is the point where the cornea meets the line joining the fixation point to the fovea while other use the entrance pupil or the corneal light reflex.[5]

Advancement in technology continues to improve refractive outcomes. Eye tracking devices rely on infrared lasers or cameras to follow small eye movements and move the laser ablation beam accordingly. Preliminary studies have shown better UCVA, BCVA, and centration with eye-tracking devices.[6,7] Corneal ablation patterns that may be different based on the specific optics of the eye in a manner more specific than sphere and cylinder are now becoming a reality.[8,9] Time will tell whether these formats will provide better visual results.

The best results with the lowest incidence of complications occur in the lower ranges of myopia and astigmatism.[10] In Phase III trials for PRK with the Summit ExciMed UV200LA laser (Summit Technology, Waltham, Mass), approximately two-thirds of the patients had 20/20 or better uncorrected acuity, >90% were 20/40 or better uncorrected, and 77.8% had postoperative refractions within 1.00 D of the target outcome.[11]

The higher the refractive error, the greater the chance of regression and corneal haze.[12] The depth of the ablation that is required to achieve a given refraction result for myopia is defined by the Munnerlyn equation:[13]

- Equation 1: depth (mm) = [diameter (mm)] 2 x 1/3 power (D)

Smaller OZs are associated with greater degrees of regression, as well as haze.[14] The optical zone size and depth must be optimized to avoid excessive wound healing that occurs in deep ablations and the excessive haloes, edge glare, and irregular astigmatism found with small optical zones.[15]

PRK has been supplanted by LASIK as the predominant refractive procedure. However, there are situations where PRK may be preferred to LASIK. These situations include patients with anterior basement membrane dystrophy (ABMD), corneal thinning, small and deep-set orbits, superficial corneal scars, very steep or flat keratometry values, anterior scleral buckles, glaucoma patients after trabeculectomy, optic nerve disease, risky occupation or activity, and corneal ectasia.

## Indications

The principles applicable to patient selection for excimer laser PRK are no different than those for any other refractive procedure. Two fundamental criteria are:

- Realistic expectations, motivation, and awareness of potential complications and side effects
- Stability of preoperative refractive error

Excimer laser photorefractive keratectomy results appear to be more reproducible for patients who have lower amounts of myopia.[16,17]

## Contraindications

Laser vision correction has a higher risk in patients with collagen vascular, autoimmune, or immunodeficiency diseases; women who are pregnant or nursing; patients with signs of keratoconus and patients taking isotretinoin (Accutane, Roche, Nutley, NJ) or amiodarone (Cordarone, Wyeth, Madison, NJ).

Other conditions with potential adverse outcome include: ophthalmic *herpes simplex* or *herpes zoster*, or other systemic diseases likely to affect healing such as diabetes and atopic disease.[18] In patients with progressive myopia or astigmatism, the results will not be stable.

## Surgical Treatment

PRK is performed under topical anesthesia with the patient under the microscope. The patient should be relaxed but not oversedated. Communicating to the patient what will occur during the procedure will alleviate much of the patient's anxiety. Preoperatively, the patient may receive antibiotic, corticosteroid, nonsteroidal, and anesthetic drops. The contralateral eye is taped shut so that the patient does not crossfixate. A speculum is used to keep the eyelids open.

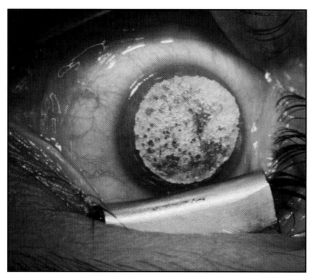

**Figure 12-4.** Cellulose sponge disc with alcohol is placed over the cornea for 20 to 60 seconds to loosen the epithelium before removal for PRK or LASEK.

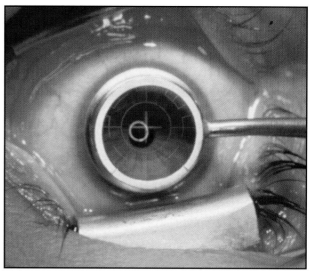

**Figure 12-5.** Optical zone marker can also be used to hold alcohol before epithelial removal with PRK or LASEK.

### EPITHELIAL REMOVAL TECHNIQUE

Quick and precise epithelial removal is critical for a good PRK result. The central corneal epithelium can be removed by a variety of available techniques, including manual scraping, mechanical rotating brushes, laser ablation combined with manual scraping (laser-scrape), or laser ablation alone (transepithelial approach). Debridement should take as little time as possible to avoid corneal hydration changes that may affect the outcome.

1. *Alcohol removal* is our current preferred technique. Absolute alcohol is mixed with balanced saline solution to dilute to 20% and is applied to the corneal epithelium on a 7 to 10 mm cellulose sponge disc for 20 to 120 seconds (Figure 12-4). The epithelium can then be removed without resistance. A metal 7 to 10 mm optical zone marker can alternatively be used to hold the alcohol within the marker followed by irrigation to help lift the epithelium (Figure 12-5).

2. *Mechanical debridement* consists of removing the epithelium bluntly with a blade, or disposable excimer spatula (Figure 12-6). A relatively blunt instrument helps prevent cutting Bowman's membrane.

3. *Laser-scrape technique* uses the laser to remove 40 mm of the epithelium followed by the use of a blade or excimer spatula to remove the remaining debris.

4. *Transepithelial laser removal* uses the excimer laser set to a depth of approximately 50 mm (200 pulses) with the beam set to its widest aperture. There is evidence that the incidence of haze is less with this method.[6] Many lasers do not allow this option for large treatment diameters.

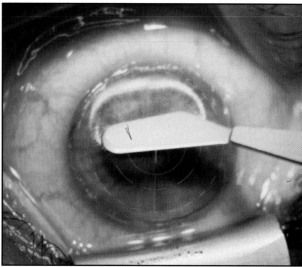

**Figure 12-6.** Mechanical debridement of corneal epithelium using PRK spatula.

5. Rotary brushes are 6.5 and 9 mm in diameter and are used to remove epithelium.

The surgeon should always verify the entered computer data before starting the ablation (Figure 12-7). For PRK, the spectacle correction is adjusted to the corneal plane to take into account the vertex distance. The microscope should be focused on the corneal surface. The patient should be instructed to fixate on the target light and adequate centration over the pupil should be maintained at all times. This centration is essential in order to achieve the expected visual results (Figure 12-8). Tracking systems are now incorporated in most excimer lasers, which aid in the maintenance of centration.

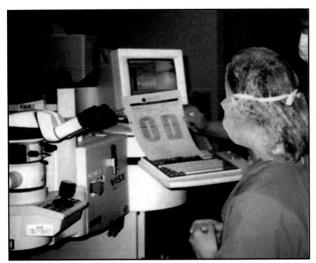

**Figure 12-7.** Surgeon verifies the computer data before the ablation. (Courtesy of Benjamin F. Boyd, MD, FACS.)

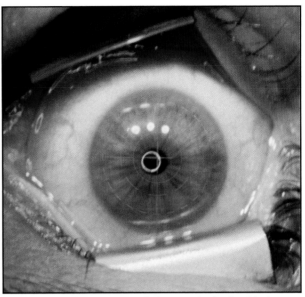

**Figure 12-8.** Centration with laser reticule. In this image, note that the reticule is not perfectly centered on the pupil, but the reticule makes it easy to verify proper adjustments needed to be well centered.

If excess fluid is detected during the ablation, the procedure is halted temporarily and the excess fluid removed by using a cellulose sponge to dry the cornea, taking care to ensure even hydration.

After laser ablation, chilled balanced salt solution may be applied to the cornea, followed by a drop of a nonsteroidal agent, an antibiotic, and a steroid. A disposable bandage contact lens is then placed over the cornea and the speculum is removed.

## Postoperative Management

PRK can cause significant discomfort to the patient despite the placement of the bandage contact lens so adequate pain control should be provided to all patients. It is important to monitor the extent of the epithelial defect. The contact lens should be left in place for at least 4 days or until re-epithelialization is complete. Discomfort and pain can be reduced with the use of an NSAID. Systemic analgesics can be used if necessary.

Antibiotic and corticosteroid medications are administered 4 times a day. The antibiotics can be discontinued once the epithelium is healed. Typically, mild corticosteroid drops are used 4 times per day for the first month, followed by a slow taper to 3 times a day for 1 month, twice a day for 1 month, and once a day for the last month.

## Complications of PRK

Photorefractive keratectomy is a complex surgical procedure that achieves high quality results. Attention to detail, an appropriate relationship between physician and patient (with careful patient counseling), and meticulous postoperative care are essential in order to obtain the desired results. Unfortunately, no surgical technique can be entirely without complications.

In higher levels of correction, haze or regression may reduce patient satisfaction. Helmy et al demonstrated a better accuracy of refractive results as well as a decreased incidence of complications in patients who underwent LASIK for myopia between -6.00 D and -10.00 D, as compared to surface PRK.[12]

*Delayed epithelial healing.* Typically the epithelial surface is intact after 4 days. Aggressive lubrication should be emphasized to minimize this complication. If there is a long delay in healing, corneal scarring may be more common. The doctor should ensure that the patient is not self-medicating with anesthetic drops if there is no response to aggressive lubrication. Control of other ocular surface problems such as blepharitis will also improve epithelial healing. Rarely, a tarsorrhaphy may be required.

*Loss of BCVA.* Visual acuity should start to improve after re-epithelialization has occurred. After this initial period, causes of loss of BCVA usually include epithelial irregularity, central islands, corneal haze, or a decentered ablation.

*Central islands* are small central elevations in the corneal topography, which may occur for a variety of reasons.[19,20] Beam profile abnormalities, increased hydration of the central corneal stroma, or particulate material falling onto the cornea may block subsequent laser pulses. A flat ablation beam may direct stromal fluid into the central area of ablation, and the hydrated tissue is ablated at a slower rate. This is more common with broad-beam lasers.[21] Laser software can add extra pulses in the central cornea to compensate for this. Typically, these central islands resolve with time as epithelial remodeling fills in the surrounding area.

*Decentration* can result from poor fixation and alignment, eye movement during the laser procedure, or asymmetric hydration of the cornea (Figure 12-9). The higher the myopic correction, the greater the risk of decentration.[12] It may result in visual aberrations, glare, halos, irregular astigmatism, and decrease in BCVA.[5,22] Low-contrast visual acuity is a more sensitive measurement of visual function after PRK than high-contrast Snellen acuity and can be used to assess these patients more accurately.[23] Decentration may be decreased with the use of current lasers with incorporated eye tracking systems, yet careful attention must still be paid to patient fixation.[24]

Corneal haze is greater in patients treated for more than 6.0 D of myopia as compared with patients with low to moderate myopia.[16,25,26] Low levels of haze are clinically insignificant, representing the normal healing response following treatment. Severe haze interfering with refraction is frequently associated with myopic regression, loss of BCVA, and a greater tendency to present in the other eye if treated.[16]

*Under- and overcorrection* may result from errors of refraction, improper surgical ablation, malfunctioning of the excimer laser, abnormal corneal hydration status, or an excessive or inadequate wound healing response. It is crucial to maintain consistent hydration of the cornea because excessive fluid on the cornea results in an undercorrection. If desiccation of the corneal stroma is present, then overcorrection and haze may occur. An enhanced wound healing response can cause regression that results in undercorrection and possibly scarring. Often the regression can be asymmetric, leading to an appearance not unlike a decentration. No or minimal tissue healing may sometimes lead to overcorrection.[3]

*Sterile corneal infiltrates* have been reported to have an incidence of approximately 0.4%.[27] Usually they present within the first 2 days following laser therapy and can be related to recruitment of leukocytes, presenting as an immune ring or stromal melting. These are typically subepithelial, multiple, and negative for organisms on cultures and Gram stain.

*Infectious keratitis* after PRK has been reported to occur in 0.1% to 0.2% of cases.[28] Virtually all cases have been associated with the use of soft therapeutic contact lenses. It usually presents as a single white infiltrate with associated pain and photophobia. Corneal cultures should be performed as soon as possible. The contact lens should also be removed and sent for cultures and drug sensitivities. Corneal infections should be treated aggressively with frequent fortified antibiotics.

*Steroid-related ocular hypertension* is most likely to occur if potent steroids such as prednisolone acetate 0.25% or dexamethasone 0.1% are used. If a significant IOP increase is detected after surgery, cessation or at least reduction of the

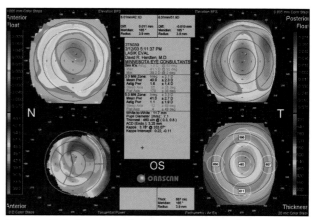

**Figure 12-9.** Decentered ablation on corneal topography. Note the asymmetry of the elevation and the curvature. The top image is the corneal curvature, and the bottom image shows the corneal elevation.

topical steroid should be made, supplemented with the concurrent use of a topical beta-blocker.

### Results

Previous studies have demonstrated better results in those patients undergoing PRK with less than -6.00 D of myopia.[11,12,16,17,25,26,28,29] A high percentage (93%) of these eyes achieve corrections within 1.00 D of emmetropia.[17] Gartry et al reported correction within 1.00 D of attempted correction in 95% of eyes within -2.00 D of myopia undergoing PRK.[30]

Other reports showed that in patients with moderate myopia, approximately 74% obtained correction within 1.00 D of attempted correction at 6 months.[31,32]

Of patients enrolled in the Summit (Waltham, Mass) and VISX (Santa Clara, Calif) Phase III studies, 78% to 79% respectively, were within 1.00 D of emmetropia at 1 year.[33] The refractive outcome appeared to stabilize by the sixth month after surgery for most patients except those with higher myopia. Results do not appear to be as reproducible with higher levels of myopia, and with correction of -6.00 to -7.00 D, only 20% of eyes were corrected within 1.00 D of attempted at the 1-year follow-up.[25,34-36]

# LASIK

LASIK combines lamellar corneal surgery with the accuracy of the excimer laser. LASIK was first reported by Pallikaris et al in 1990.[37] It is an increasingly popular technique for correcting refractive errors. It involves the excimer laser ablation of the corneal stroma beneath a hinged corneal flap that is created with a microkeratome.

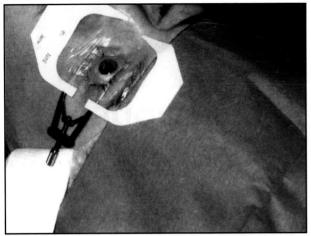

**Figure 12-10.** Adequate exposure is necessary with all of the refractive procedures. (Courtesy of Benjamin F. Boyd, MD, FACS.)

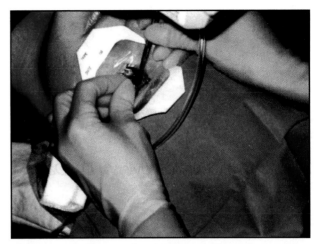

**Figure 12-11.** Bimanual technique used to place suction ring. Adequate exposure facilitates this process. (Courtesy of Benjamin F. Boyd, MD, FACS.)

## Patient Selection

As mentioned earlier, refractive surgery patients should have realistic expectations of the outcome of the surgery. Patients should understand the risks, benefits, and alternatives of the LASIK procedure. A stable refraction is important, and most surgeons now limit the upper range of correction to -12.00 D of treatment, even though the lasers are capable of treating higher corrections.

It is thought that leaving at least 250 µm of residual stroma untouched posteriorly may reduce the incidence of corneal ectasia.

According to the Munnerlyn formula mentioned above, each SE diopter of myopic correction performed at 6-mm OZ, will ablate 12 µm of tissue.[15] However, each excimer laser ablates a different amount of stromal tissue per diopter of refractive correction. This is due to the differences in the ablation zone diameters and ablation characteristics.

The average central cornea thickness is approximately 550 µm. Because the flap thickness is generally between 160 to 180 µm, the average corneal will have 370 to 390 µm of posterior stromal bed left after the flap creation. The maximal correction that may be performed on a patient depends on the degree of correction, the ablation zone diameter, the corneal thickness, and the ablation characteristics of the laser used.

As with PRK, patients with abnormal corneal topographies or with ocular abnormalities as well as systemic conditions that are likely to affect wound healing should be approached with caution.

## Microkeratomes

Several different microkeratomes are available for use in LASIK. The main differences among these microkeratomes are the method of assembly, the location of the corneal flap's hinge, and automated or manual translation across the cornea during the procedure.

Alternatives to blade containing microkeratomes, include the use of high-speed water jet and laser technology.[38,39]

## Operative Technique

The surgeon should help the patient understand the LASIK procedure before the surgery. Approximately 5 to 10 minutes before the procedure, 5 mg of diazepam are given to the patient to alleviate the anxiety of undergoing the procedure and to help them sleep postoperatively.

The patient is then positioned under the microscope, with the head carefully aligned to make sure the iris is perpendicular to the laser beam. Careful centration with the eye aligned in the $x$, $y$, and $z$ planes is crucial.

Topical anesthesia is then applied to the eye. The eyelids are prepared with dilute povidone-iodine solution and a lid speculum is inserted to open the eyelids. Eyelashes should be kept away from the surgical field by the use of adhesive drapes or a closed bladed lid speculum (Figure 12-10). The contralateral eye is taped shut to prevent cross-fixation and drying.

The microkeratome should be inspected for any defects in the blade or function of the moving parts. It is also vital to confirm that the excimer laser will be able to deliver treatment after the corneal flap is reflected.

The cornea can be marked with ink before creating the corneal flap with the microkeratome to more easily realign the corneal flap in the event that a free flap is created.

The suction ring is placed using a bimanual technique where the shaft of the suction ring is held in the fingers of one hand and a finger from the other hand provides additional support on the ring itself (Figure 12-11). Once adequate placement has been achieved the suction is engaged by foot control (usually done by the technician). Adequate IOP

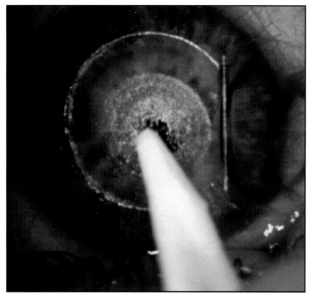

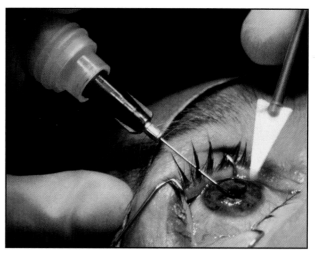

**Figure 12-13.** Irrigation under the flap can remove debris from the interface. Care must be taken not to over irrigate as this can increase the risk of flap striae from over hydration. (Courtesy of Hardten DR. *Operative Techniques in Cataract and Refractive Surgery.* 1998;1[1]:32-39. Reproduced with permission of WB Saunders Company.)

**Figure 12-12.** Excess moisture should be removed with a cellulose sponge. Note that the central portion of this cornea has a sheen that reveals excess moisture centrally. Close visual monitoring with the ring light of the laser remaining on can facilitate the identification of areas of relative excess or under hydration. (Courtesy of Hardten DR. *Operative Techniques in Cataract and Refractive Surgery.* 1998;1[1]:32-39. Reproduced with permission of WB Saunders Company.)

(above 65 mm Hg) is then verified, with one useful method being an applanation lens (Barraquer tonometer). When adequate suction is achieved, the patient will confirm the temporary loss of visualization of the fixation light.

Before the pass of the microkeratome, several drops of artificial tears are placed on the cornea. This lubrication reduces the likelihood of a corneal epithelial defect occurring during the microkeratome pass. If using a 2-piece microkeratome, the head is slid onto the post of the suction ring and advanced until the gear on the microkeratome head engages the track. It is important to again verify that the suction ring is still firmly attached to the globe at this point by gently lifting the suction ring upward, making sure that the suction is not lost. The surgeon then activates the microkeratome using forward and reverse foot controls, the suction is turned off after the microkeratome pass and the suction ring can then be carefully removed. Prompt attention at this point is extremely important in the case that a free cap or buttonhole has been created. In cases where the stromal bed is too small or irregular for a good result, the laser ablation should not be performed, and the flap is placed carefully back into position.

Before lifting the flap, a wet cellulose sponge is used to remove any cells, debris, or excess fluid from getting onto the stromal bed. Using a flat cannula, iris sweep or a smooth forceps, the flap can be lifted and directed toward the hinge.

A dry cellulose sponge is then used to carefully remove any excess fluid from the stromal surface. Hydration of the stromal bed needs to be adjusted evenly and consistently in all cases (Figure 12-12). It is important at this point to minimize the procedure time in order to prevent stromal dehydration and subsequent overcorrection. Uneven hydration can lead to central islands and/or irregular astigmatism. Excess pooling of fluid can often be found near the hinge after folding back the flap and should be wicked away.

The patient is then asked to fixate on the alignment target. The laser and eye tracker are activated. The surgeon should maintain his dominant hand over the laser joystick and maintain adequate centration. If fluid starts accumulating over the stromal surface, the laser ablation can be halted and the fluid should be removed with a cellulose sponge. The hinge should be protected if within the ablation zone.

After the ablation, the flap is the repositioned onto the bed using an irrigation cannula or an iris sweep. Saline solution is used to remove debris from the interface (Figure 12-13). A wet cellulose sponge is then used to realign the flap. Sweeping movements should be performed from the hinge toward the periphery of the flap (Figure 12-14).

Good adhesion of the flap is verified by stretching the flap towards the gutter. If good adhesion is present, there is minimal space in the gutter, and no movement of the flap occurs when stroking the flap with a dry sponge. When the flap is felt to be securely in position, a drop of an antibiotic, a steroid, and a lubricating agent may be applied to the cornea before removing the speculum. If bilateral LASIK will be performed, the operated eye is covered and the procedure

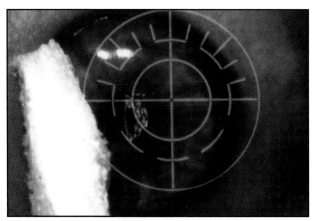

**Figure 12-14.** Aligning the flap is a critical step in the LASIK procedure. The gutter should be symmetric and as tight as possible at the completion of the procedure. (Courtesy of Hardten DR. *Operative Techniques in Cataract and Refractive Surgery.* 1998;1[1]:32-39. Reproduced with permission of WB Saunders Company.)

repeated in the contralateral eye. Both eyes are then protected with transparent plastic shields until the following day.

## Postoperative Care

The patient is placed on topical prophylactic antibiotics and topical steroids 4 times per day for the first week. Preservative-free, lubricating drops are helpful in most patients for the first several weeks after surgery and frequent use should be encouraged.

The patient may resume most activities if the postoperative examination is normal. Instructions not to rub the eyes or swim underwater should be reinforced in order to prevent flap displacement or infectious keratitis.

## Intraoperative Complications

*Incomplete flap* is created due to premature termination of the microkeratome advancement. If resistance is met during the forward passage of the keratome or the keratome comes to a stop, the surgeon should stop and examine the field for any obstruction. Usually lids and lashes, drapes, or the speculum can cause interference with the keratome pass. If this is not successful in allowing the microkeratome to pass forward, then the microkeratome should be reversed and removed from the eye. One should never reverse the microkeratome and then go forward. This can result in the blade penetrating to a deeper level than the initial pass. In case of an incomplete pass, if there is not enough room beneath the flap to perform the ablation, then the surgeon should reposition the flap and conclude the surgery. Typically a new flap can be created 6 to 12 months after the original procedure.

*Thin flaps* are usually due to poor suction. An extremely thin flap is more difficult to reposition and more likely to wrinkle. If the flap is complete enough to cover the ablated

area without a buttonhole, then the ablation portion of the case can proceed.

Should a *buttonholed flap* occur, ablation should not be performed through the remaining epithelium. The flap should be repositioned and smoothed in to place. Treatment of the second eye is not advisable at the same setting, as the same complication is likely to happen in the presence of a steep cornea or poor suction. Epithelial ingrowth or haze may occur in the area of the buttonhole, and may require further intervention. A waiting period of over 6 months should ensue prior to attempting to create a new flap to reduce the occurrence of a connection between the first and subsequent flaps.

*Full-thickness resection* can occur with entry into the anterior chamber during the creation of the flap. This can occur if the plate is not properly positioned during the assembly process or if it is not tightened into place. Newer microkeratomes, which use a fixed plate should reduce or eliminate the possibility of entry into the anterior chamber.

A *free cap* can occasionally occur and the surgeon should be prepared to deal with this problem. In these situations, the cap is typically placed on the conjunctiva with the epithelial side down during the photablation. Care must be taken to reposition the cap into the same orientation after the ablation. Adequate drying time should be allowed for the cap to adhere without sutures. The most frequent cause of a free cap is a flat or small cornea in which there is less tissue to be brought forward into the microkeratome. Poor suction can also cause small free flaps.

*Epithelial defects* can be prevented with adequate lubrication of the cornea before the microkeratome pass. Also, toxic anesthetics should be kept to a minimum before the procedure. If an epithelial defect occurs, typically the course is minimally changed from normal. A contact lens can be placed over the cornea if the defect is likely to cause significant discomfort to the patient. An epithelial defect may lead to greater cap edema with poorer adherence in the area of the defect, increasing the risk of epithelial ingrowth and diffuse lamellar keratitis.

## Ablation Complications

*Central islands* typically resolve more slowly after LASIK than after PRK. If resolution has not occurred by 3 months, the flap can be lifted, and the island can be retreated to reduce irregular astigmatism.

*Decentration* (see Figure 12-9) of the refractive excimer laser ablation can result in glare, irregular astigmatism, and a decrease in BCVA.[40] Typically if the ablation is more than 1 mm decentered, the irregular astigmatism that occurs is symptomatic. Current lasers utilize active eye tracking, which should decrease the rate and severity of decentration. Management of decentration by treatment based on wavefront or topographic information may decrease symptoms in patients with an unsatisfactory outcome with the first procedure.[41]

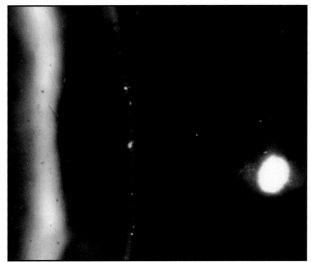

**Figure 12-15.** Interface debris can occur in LASIK, and is usually not visually significant. (Courtesy of Hardten DR. *Operative Techniques in Cataract and Refractive Surgery.* 1998; 1[1]:32-39. Reproduced with permission of WB Saunders Company.)

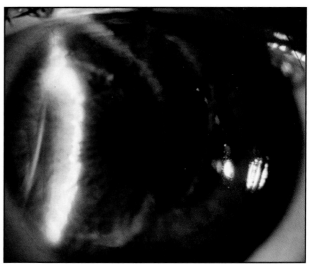

**Figure 12-16.** Displaced flap can occur, and requires repositioning to reduce the striae and decreased vision that results. (Courtesy of Hardten DR. *Operative Techniques in Cataract and Refractive Surgery.* 1998;1[1]:32-39. Reproduced with permission of WB Saunders Company.)

## Postoperative Complications

*Interface debris* is common even with aggressive interface irrigation (Figure 12-15). Most frequently, it is meibomian gland material that comes from the lids and is trapped in the interface. Careful cleaning of the interface with BSS before and after the flap is floated into position can help to reduce the incidence of this problem.[42] Preoperative treatment of blepharitis with lid hygiene, antibiotic ointments, and oral tetracyclines may reduce the occurrence of this complication.

*Flap displacement* usually occurs in the first 24 hours postoperatively (Figure 12-16). When a flap displacement occurs, it should be lifted and repositioned.[43] The epithelium at the flap edge grows remarkably fast to cover the stromal bed. Care must be taken to clean the bed and back of the flap of debris and epithelial cells. Stroking the cap slightly with a moist cellulose sponge can minimize persistent folds in the flap and properly line up the cap with the bed.

*Punctate epithelial keratopathy* can be seen after LASIK. It is more common in patients with preexisting dry eye or blepharitis. The corneal nerves are severed during LASIK and this may increase the susceptibility to keratopathy.[44,45] Treatment involves frequent lubrication of the ocular surfaced with artificial tears. Management of any eyelid disorder may also be of benefit. Punctal plugs may also be employed to assist in the management of this common problem.

*Diffuse lamellar keratitis* (DLK), also known as Sands of Sahara, is an interface inflammatory process that occurs in the early postoperative period after LASIK (Figure 12-17).[42] Patients are usually asymptomatic and often have no visual impairment. A fine granular appearing infiltrate that looks like dust or sand typically presents initially in the interface periphery. The inflammation, if left untreated, can progressively worsen and may lead to corneal scarring with resultant irregular astigmatism. In the typical cases, on the second postoperative day, the cells can progress to cover the pupil. On the third day, they may begin to clump and, with the release of inflammatory mediators, can result in a stromal melt by day 4 or 5. The cause of DLK is likely multifactorial. Bacterial toxins or antigens, debris on the instruments, eyelid secretions, or other factors may play a role.[46-49] Treatment involves frequent topical steroids. In cases in which inflammation progresses to where the cells clump centrally on day 3 or 4, the flap must be lifted to irrigate the interface.[50,51]

*Over- and undercorrections.* As with PRK, under and overcorrection can occur with LASIK. The etiology and management are similar.

*Flap striae and microstriae* are a common complication after LASIK. Most striae are asymptomatic and can be visualized if the flap is carefully examined with retroillumination (Figure 12-18).[42] When microstriae occur over the pupil or when macrostriae exist, irregular astigmatism with visual aberrations and monocular diplopia may result. In such cases, the flap should be relifted, hydrated, and stretched back into position.

*Epithelial ingrowth* into the interface between the cap and the stromal bed occurs in 2% to 3% of myopic LASIK sur-

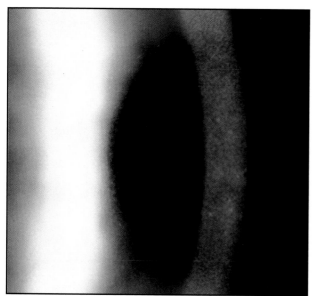

**Figure 12-17.** Diffuse lamellar keratitis (DLK). This is Stage II DLK, and identification of this should be followed by increased topical steroid administration, and close follow-up. If the cells begin to clump centrally with Stage III DLK, then interface irrigation is appropriate. (Courtesy Hardten DR. *Operative Techniques in Cataract and Refractive Surgery*, 1998; 1[1]:32-39. Reproduced with permission of WB Saunders Company.)

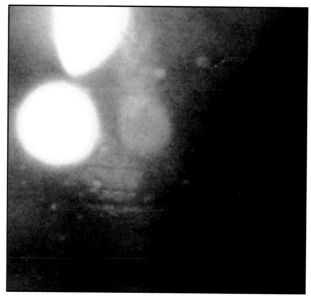

**Figure 12-18.** Flap striae can be fairly subtle, and may not be visually significant as in this eye. (Courtesy of Hardten DR. *Operative Techniques in Cataract and Refractive Surgery*. 1998; 1[1]:32-39. Reproduced with permission of WB Saunders Company.)

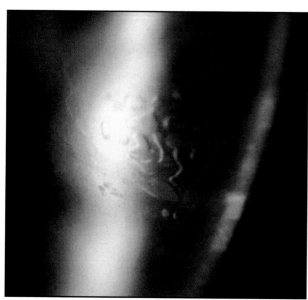

**Figure 12-19.** Epithelial ingrowth under the flap. Progression towards the center with visual significance is an indication for removal of the epithelium. (Courtesy of Hardten DR. *Operative Techniques in Cataract and Refractive Surgery*. 1998;1[1]:32-39. Reproduced with permission of WB Saunders Company.)

geries, and is more common when an epithelial defect has occurred or after enhancements (Figure 12-19).[52] Rarely, the epithelial growth progresses into the central visual axis causing irregular astigmatism and loss of BCVA. In some cases, the epithelial cells will block nutritional support for the overlying stroma and lead to flap melt.[42] If this is the case, the flap should be lifted and careful scraping of the epithelium should be performed at the stromal bed as well as under the flap.

*Results*

Many surgeons find that adjusting the amount of treatment using a nomogram based on their actual surgical results improves their refractive outcomes.

Accuracy appears to be greater for lower degrees of myopia. In one study of 130 eyes with an average preoperative spherical equivalent of -3.61 D followed for 12 months after LASIK, 98% obtained a correction within ±1 D from target and 93% obtaining 20/40 or better UCVA.[53]

Another study showed that in low myopia (-0.75 D to -6.00 D of myopia and 0 to 0.75 D of preoperative astigmatism) 50% were 20/25 or better and 90% were 20/40 or better at 1 month postoperatively and the SE was between ±1.00 D of emmetropia in 89% of the patients. In high myopia (-6.00 to -20.00 D of myopia and 0 to 4.5 D of preoperative astigmatism) at 1 month, 35% were 20/25 or better and 71% were 20/40 or better and the mean SE was within ±1.00 D of emmetropia in 63%.[54] Results if this and other studies suggest more predictable results in low myopia without astigmatism than in high myopia correction or in eyes requiring astigmatic correction.[51,52,55,56]

Preliminary data obtained from multicenter trial results on wavefront guided LASIK ablations are very promising. Ninety-eight percent of eyes achieved 20/20 UCVA and 71% were at 20/16 or better uncorrected. What is even more impressive is the fact that postoperative UCVA was better than the preoperative best corrected results in 47% of patients.[57]

# LASEK

With the increasing popularity of refractive surgery over the past 2 decades, surgeons have continued their search for improved procedures in order to provide better and more consistent results, rapid recovery and safer profiles.

As mentioned previously, PRK and LASIK are currently the most popular procedures in refractive surgery. PRK is a relatively safe procedure and its major limitations are postoperative pain, subepithelial haze and prolonged visual rehabilitation. On the other hand, LASIK offers a rapid recovery but a potential for flap related complications.

LASEK is considered a blend of PRK and LASIK that provides relatively quick visual recovery while potentially reducing some of the complications inherent to both procedures. In one study, late-onset corneal haze was not found as a problem, even in the higher refractive errors, which is an extremely promising aspect of LASEK.[58]

## *Indications*

LASEK appears to be a good alternative for patients with thin corneas and large corrections; small palpebral fissures or deep-set eyes; and in those whose job or recreational activities increase their risk of corneal trauma. In patients who experience recurrent corneal erosions and are therefore poor LASIK candidates, LASEK may also reduce the incidence of recurrent erosions.[56]

The same preoperative assessment as mentioned for PRK and LASIK should be performed for patients undergoing LASEK. Patient should have a clear understanding of the risks, benefits, and alternatives of undergoing LASEK versus LASIK or PRK.

Patients with systemic contraindications for LASIK or PRK may also have a higher complication rate with LASEK.[59]

## *Surgical Technique*

The cornea is anesthetized with a topical anesthetic and the same initial preparation for lids and lashes as described earlier should be performed. A lid speculum is placed to separate the eyelids. The cornea may be marked to help realign the epithelial flap after the ablation. Using a 9-mm OZ

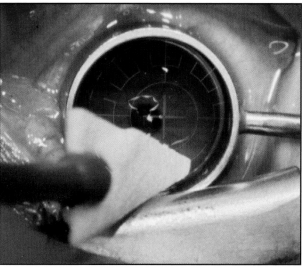

**Figure 12-20.** Alcohol is absorbed from the well with a cellulose sponge to avoid getting alcohol on the remaining epithelium or conjunctiva.

marker centered over the pupil, the epithelium is delineated and pressure is applied on the cornea while the barrel of the optical zone marker is filled with 2 drops of 20% ethanol (see Figure 12-5). After 20 to 60 seconds, the ethanol is absorbed with the use of a dry cellulose sponge (Figure 12-20). The viability of the epithelium following alcohol exposure is under investigation and other materials are being tried to find a balance between loss of viability versus ease of removal of the epithelium.[60,61]

The arm of a jeweler's forceps is then inserted under the epithelium and traced around the delineated margin of the epithelium, leaving 2 to 3 clock hours of intact margin for a hinge. Using a microhoe or a dry cellulose sponge, the loosened epithelium is then peeled as a single sheet leaving the hinge still attached (Figure 12-21).

The stromal bed is then carefully inspected for residual areas of moisture or epithelium and wiped with a dry cellulose sponge to achieve even hydration.

The laser ablation should proceed in the same manner as described for the LASIK procedure. The epithelial flap should then be hydrated using BSS and replaced on the stroma (Figure 12-22). Care should be taken to align the epithelium flap using the previous marks and to avoid epithelial defects. The flap is the allowed to dry for 1 to 5 minutes. This is followed by a drop of a nonsteroidal agent, an antibiotic, and a steroid. A disposable bandage contact lens is then placed over the cornea and the speculum and drapes are removed.

Immediate postoperative management includes topical nonsteroidal, an antibiotic and a steroid 4 times a day. The contact lens is left over the eye until the epithelium is completely healed, which is usually within 1 to 3 days. The steroid should be continued for 3 to 4 months.

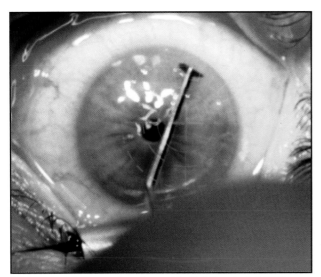

**Figure 12-21.** Retracting the epithelial flap in LASEK.

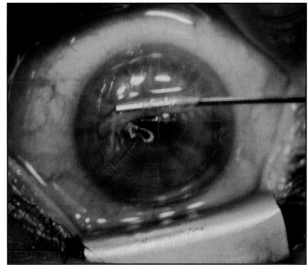

**Figure 12-22.** Lifting the epithelial flap during LASEK.

## Complications

LASEK was developed as a blend of the positive aspects of PRK and LASIK. It eliminates the microkeratome and flap related complications and in some situations, provides a faster recovery as compared to PRK.[59]

The most frequent complications of LASEK are probably related to difficulties during the epithelial flap creation and lifting. Claringbold reported the need for additional exposure to ethyl alcohol solution in 16% of his cases to facilitated lifting of the epithelial flap and recommended additional alcohol exposure in the second eye in these patients.[58]

Difficulties creating the flap can result in extension of the incision at the site of the epithelial hinge with subsequent *dislocation of the flap* or a free epithelial flap. *Buttonholes of the flap* can be created in areas of increased epithelial attachment. Care must be taken to scrape and remove these epithelial islands before the laser ablation.

*Delayed epithelial healing* should be managed with aggressive lubrication as described for PRK.

*Ablation complications* can also occur and adequate centration should always be carefully assessed during the excimer laser ablation.

Subepithelial or late-onset *corneal haze* may be less frequent with LASEK than with PRK. In his series, Claringbold reported that none of his 84 patients demonstrated appreciable haze at 12 months. However, more long-term data is necessary to confirm his series.

*Steroid induced ocular hypertension* can be a potential complication due to the prolonged use of steroids and intraocular pressure should always be monitored.

## Results

In 1996, Azar reported the first series of LASEK procedures in the United States, obtaining UCVAs of 20/40 or better in all eyes after 1 week. His postoperative data demonstrated epithelial defects in 63% of the eyes on day 1 and 9% of the eyes on day 3. UCVAs of 20/25 or better was achieved in 64% of eyes at 1 week and 92% at 1 month. Postoperative spherical equivalent of ±0.50 D was attained by 58% of the eyes at 1 month and 100% at 12 months. There were no reports of recurrent epithelial defects.[57]

In the series by Lee et al, who compared LASEK performed in 1 eye and PRK in the other, subjective pain scores were significantly decreased in eyes that underwent LASEK. At 1 week, UCVA was 20/25 or better in 37% of PRK treated eyes as compared to 59% of those who underwent LASEK.[62] After treating 249 patients, Camellin reported 80% of preoperative BCVA achieved in 90% of patients 10 days postoperatively.[63]

Results at this point, while extremely encouraging, represent early experience with the LASEK procedure. Further prospective investigations are needed to support these studies.

## SUMMARY

Over the last 10 years, excimer laser lamellar refractive surgery techniques (PRK, LASIK, or LASEK) have emerged as the procedures of choice for correcting the majority of myopic refractive errors. A comprehensive and solid knowledge of these procedures enables the surgeon to offer a variety of options based their patient's individual needs.

As the techniques continue to improve and advances such as wavefront-guided technology become widely introduced, refractive surgery will continue to evolve and will continue to change the way we assess our refractive expectations and outcomes.

# REFERENCES

1. Sperduto RD, Seigel D, Roberts J, et al. Prevalence of myopia in the United States. *Arch Ophthalmol.* 1983;101(3):405-7.

2. Landers J, Goldberg I, Graham SL. Analysis of risk factors that may be associated with progression from ocular hypertension to primary open angle glaucoma. *Clin Experiment Ophthalmol.* 2002;30(4):242-7.

3. Hardten DR. Excimer laser photorefractive keratectomy. In: Yanoff M, Duker JS, eds. *Ophthalmology.* London; Mosby International; 1999.

4. Fiore T, Carones F, Brancato R. Broad beam vs. flying spot excimer laser: refractive and videokeratographic outcomes of two different ablation profiles after photorefractive keratectomy. *J Refract Surg.* 2001;17(5):534-41.

5. Uozato H, Guyton DL. Centering corneal surgical procedures. *Am J Ophthalmol.* 1987;15(103 [3 Pt 1]):264-275.

6. Tsai YY, Lin JM. Ablation centration after active eye-tracker-assisted photorefractive keratectomy and laser in situ keratomileusis. *J Cataract Refract Surg.* 2000;26(1):28-34.

7. Mrochen M, Eldine MS, Kaemmerer M, et al. Improvement in photorefractive corneal laser surgery results using an active eye-tracking system. *J Cataract Refract Surg.* 2001;27(7):1000-6.

8. Wu HK. Astigmatism and LASIK. *Curr Opin Ophthalmol.* 2002;13(4):250-5.

9. Manns F, Ho A, Parel JM, et al. Ablation profiles for wavefront-guided correction of myopia and primary spherical aberration. *J Cataract Refract Surg.* 2002;28(5):766-74.

10. Stein R. Photorefractive keratectomy. *Int Ophthalmol Clin.* 2000;40(3):35-56.

11. Hersh PS, Stulting RD, Steinert RF, et al. Results of phase III excimer laser photorefractive keratectomy for myopia. The Summit PRK Study Group. *Ophthalmology.* 1997; 104(10):1535-53.

12. Helmy SA, Salah A, Badawy TT, Sidky AN. Photorefractive keratectomy and laser in situ keratomileusis for myopia between 6.00 and 10.00 diopters. *J Refract Surg.* 1996;12(3):417-21.

13. Munneryn CR, Koons SJ, Marshall J. Photorefractive keratectomy: a technique for laser refractive surgery. *J Cataract Refract Surg.* 1988;14(1):46-52.

14. Morris AT, Ring CP, Hadden OB. Comparison of photorefractive keratectomy for myopia using 5 mm and 6 mm diameter ablation zones. *Refractive Corneal Surg.* 1996;12:S275-7.

15. Barraquer JI. Keratomileusis. *Int Surg.* 1967;48:103-17.

16. Sher NA, Hardten DR, Fundingsland B, et al. 193-nm excimer photorefractive keratectomy in high myopia. *Ophthalmology.* 1994;101(9):1575-82.

17. Talley AR, Hardten DR, Sher NA, et al. Results one year after using the 193-nm excimer laser for photorefractive keratectomy in mild to moderate myopia. *Am J Ophthalmology.* 1994;118(3):304-11.

18. Rapuano CJ. Excimer laser phototherapeutic keratectomy. *Int Ophthalmol Clin.* 1996;36(4):127-36.

19. Gris O, Guell JL, Muller A. Keratomileusis update. *J Cataract Refract Surg.* 1996;22(5):620-3.

20. Gomes M. Laser in situ keratomileusis for myopia using manual dissection. *J Refract Surg.* 1995;11(3 Suppl):S239-43.

21. Kremer FB, Dufek M. Excimer laser in situ keratomileusis. *J Refract Surg.* 1995;11(3 Suppl):S244-7.

22. Amano S, Tanaka S, Shimizu K. Topographical evaluation of centration of excimer laser myopic photorefractive keratectomy. *J Cataract Refract Surg.* 1994;20(6):616-9.

23. Verdon W, Bullimore M, Maloney RK. Visual performance after photorefractive keratectomy. A prospective study. *Arch Ophthalmol.* 1996;114(12):1465-72.

24. Pineros OE. Tracker-assisted versus manual ablation zone centration in laser in situ keratomileusis for myopia and astigmatism. *J Refract Surg.* 2002;18(1): 37-42.

25. McCarty CA, Aldred GF, Taylor HR, and the Melbourne Excimer Laser Study Group. Comparison of results of excimer laser correction on all degrees of myopia at 12 months postoperatively. *Am J Ophthalmol.* 1996;121(4):372-83.

26. Rogers CM, Lawless MA, Cohen PR. Photorefractive keratectomy for myopia of more than -10 diopters. *J Refract Corneal Surg.* 1994;10(2 Suppl):S171-3.

27. Sher NA, Kruegger RR, Teal P, et al. The role of topical steroidal and nonsteroidal anti-inflammatory drugs in the etiology of stromal infiltrates after excimer photorefractive keratectomy. *J Refract Corneal Surg.* 1994;10:587-588.

28. Maguen E, Machatt JJ. Complications of photorefractive keratectomy, primarily with the VISX Excimer Laser. In: Salz JJ, ed. *Corneal Laser Surgery.* St Louis: Mosby; 1995.

29. Stark WJ, Chamon W, Kamp N, Enger CL, et al. Clinical follow up of 193-nm ArF excimer laser photokeratectomy. *Ophthalmology.* 1992;99:805-812.

30. Gartry DS, Kerr Muir MG, Marshall J. Excimer laser photorefractive keratectomy. 18-month follow-up. *Ophthalmology.* 1992;99(8):1209-19.

31. Dougherty PJ , Lindstrom RL, Hardten DR. Effect of refractive surgery experience on outcomes after photorefractive keratectomy. *J Refract Surg.* 1997;13(1):33-9.

32. Sher NA, Chen V, Bowers RA, et al. The use of the 193-nm excimer laser for myopic photorefractive keratectomy in sighted eyes: a multicenter study. *Arch Ophthalmol.* 1991;109(11): 1525-30.

33. Thompson KP, Steinert RF, Stulting RD. Photorefractive keratectomy with the Summit excimer laser: the phase III U.S. results. In: Salz JJ, ed. *Corneal Laser Surgery.* St Louis, Mosby-Yearbook; 1995; 57-63.

34. Seiler T, McDonnell PJ. Excimer laser photorefractive keratectomy. *Surv Ophthalmol.* 1995;40(2):89-118.

35. Snibson GR, Carson CA, Aldred GF, et al. One-year evaluation of excimer laser photorefractive keratectomy for myopia and myopic astigmatism. Melbourne Excimer Laser Group. *Arch Ophthalmol.* 1995;113(8):994-1000.

36. Kaskaloglu M. Results of photorefractive keratectomy for myopia with the Technolas Keracor 116 excimer laser. *J Refract Surg.* 1996;12(2):S255-7.

37. Pallikaris IG, Papatzanaki ME, Stathi EZ, et al. Laser in situ keratomileusis. *Lasers Surg Med.* 1990;10(5):463-8.

38. Krueger RR, Parolini B, Gordon EI, et al. Nonmechanical microkeratomes using laser and waterjet technology. In: Pallikaris IR, Siganos DS, eds. *LASIK.* Thorofare, NJ: SLACK Incorporated; 1998:81-105.

39. Ratkay-Traub I, Juhasz T, Horvath C, et al. Ultra-short pulse (femtosecond) laser surgery. Initial use in LASIK flap creation. *Ophthalmol Clin North Am.* 2001;14(2):347-55.

40. Moreno-Barriuso E, Lloves JM, Marcos S, et al. Ocular aberrations before and after myopic corneal refractive surgery: LASIK-induced changes measured with laser ray tracing. *Invest Ophthalmol Vis Sci.* 2001;42(6):1396-403.

41. Mrochen M, Krueger RR, Bueeler M, et al. Aberration-sensing and wavefront-guided laser in situ keratomileusis: management of decentered ablation. *J Refract Surg.* 2002;18(4):418-29.

42. Davis EA, Hardten DR, Lindstrom RL. LASIK complications. *Int Ophthalmol Clin.* 2000;40(3):67-75.

43. Lin RT, Maloney RK. Flap complications associated with lamellar refractive surgery. *Am J Ophthalmol.* 1999;127(2):129-36.

44. Wilson SE, Ambrosio R. Laser in situ keratomileusis-induced neurotrophic epitheliopathy. *Am J Ophthalmol.* 2001;132(3):405-6.

45. Nng RT, Dartt DA, Tsubota K. Dry eye after refractive surgery. *Curr Opin Ophthalmol.* 2001;12(4):318-22.

46. Kaufman SC. Post-LASIK interface keratitis, Sands of the Sahara syndrome, and microkeratome blades. *J Cataract Refract Surg.* 1999;25:603-4.

47. Kaufman SC, Maitchouk DY, Chiou AG, Beuerman RW. Interface inflammation after laser in situ keratomileusis. Sands of the Sahara syndrome. *J Cataract Refract Surg.* 1998;24:1589-93.

48. Chao CW, Azar DT. Lamellar keratitis following laser-assisted in situ keratomileusis. *Ophthalmol Clin North Am.* 2002;15(1):35-40.

49. Shah MN, Misra M, Wihelmus KR, Koch DD. Diffuse lamellar keratitis associated with epithelial defects after laser in situ keratomileusis. *J Cataract Refract Surg.* 2000;26(9):1312-8.

50. Linebarger EJ, Hardten DR, Lindstrom RL. Diffuse lamellar keratitis: diagnosis and management. *J Cataract Refract Surg.* 2000;26:1072-7.

51. Linebarger EJ, Hardten DR, Lindstrom RL. Diffuse lamellar keratitis: identification and management. *Int Ophthalmol Clin.* 2000;40:77-86.

52. Wang MY, Maloney RK. Epithelial ingrowth after laser in situ keratomileusis. *Am J Ophthalmol.* 2000;129(6):746-51.

53. Ruiz LA, Slade SG, Updegraff SA, Doane JF, Moreno ML, Murcia A. A single center study to evaluate the efficacy, safety and stability of laser in situ keratomileusis for low, moderate, and high myopia with and without astigmatism. In: Yanoff M, Duker JS. *Ophthalmology.* 1st ed. London: Mosby International; 1999.

54. Lindstrom RL, Hardten DR, Chu YR. Laser in situ keratomileusis (LASIK) for the treatment of low, moderated and high myopia. *Trans Am Ophthalmol Soc.* 1997;95:285-96; discussion 296-306.

55. Perez-Santonja JJ, Bellot J, Claramonte P, et al. Laser in situ keratomileusis to correct high myopia. *J Cataract Refract Surg.* 1997;23(3):372-85.

56. Lyle WA, Jin GJ. Laser in situ keratomileusis with the VISX Star laser for myopia over -10.0 diopters. *J Cataract Refract Surg.* 2001;27(11):1812-22.

57. Koch D. Six-month results of the multi-center wavefront LASIK trial. Paper presented at: American Society of Cataract and Refractive Surgery Annual Symposium and Congress; June 1-5, 2002; Philadelphia, PA.

58. Claringbold II TV. Laser-assisted subepithelial keratectomy for the correction of myopia. *J Cataract Refract Surg.* 2002; 28(1):18-22.

59. Azar DT, Ang RT, Lee JB, et al. Laser subepithelial keratomileusis: electron microscopy and visual outcomes of flap photorefractive keratectomy. *Curr Opin Ophthalmol.* 2001;12(4):323-8.

60. Chen CC, Chang JH, Lee JB, et al. Human corneal epithelial cell viability and morphology after dilute alcohol exposure. *Invest Ophthalmol Vis Sci.* 2002;43(8):2593-602.

61. Dreiss AK, Winkler Von Mohrenfels C, Gabler B, et al. Laser epithelial keratomileusis (LASEK): histological investigation for vitality of corneal epithelial cells after alcohol exposure. *Klin Monatsbl Augenheilkd.* [Abstract]. 2002;219(5):365-9.

62. Lee JB, Seong GJ, Lee JH, et al. Comparison of laser epithelial keratomileusis and photorefractive keratectomy for low to moderate myopia. *J Cataract Refract Surg.* 2001;27(4):565-70.

63. Camellin M, Cimberle M. LASEK technique promising after 1 year of experience. *Ocular Surgery News.* 2000;18(1)14-17.

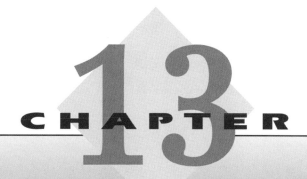

*Michael Küchle, MD; Nguyen X. Nguyen, MD;*
*Achim Langenbucher, PhD; and Berthold Seitz, MD*

## INTRODUCTION

Presbyopia remains one of the great unsolved challenges in ophthalmology. Ever since von Helmholtz, much research has been conducted concerning mechanisms of accommodation, presbyopia, and potential solutions.

Despite excellent restoration of visual acuity and good biocompatibility of presently used posterior chamber intraocular lenses (PCIOL), there is no accommodation in pseudophakic eyes so that patients usually remain presbyopic after cataract surgery. This problem has only partly been solved by the introduction of diffractive and bifocal PCIOL. Thus, efforts are being undertaken to develop PCIOL that restore accommodation. A new accommodative PCIOL (1 CU, HumanOptics, Erlangen, Germany) has been designed after principles elaborated by Hanna. As of October 2002, this PCIOL has been implanted in over 100 human eyes in our department.

## DEFINITIONS

In the literature, various terms such as accommodation, pseudoaccommodation and apparent accommodation are being used interchangeably with regard to pseudophakic eyes. We define *pseudophakic accommodation* as dynamic change of the refractive state of the pseudophakic eye caused by interactions between the contracting ciliary muscle and the zonules—capsular bag—IOL, resulting in change of refraction at near fixation. Furthermore, we define *pseudophakic pseudoaccommodation* (apparent accommodation) as static optical properties of the pseudophakic eye independent of the ciliary muscle, resulting in improved uncorrected near vision.

## ANATOMY AND DESCRIPTION OF THE 1 CU ACCOMMODATIVE INTRAOCULAR LENS

Several studies using impedance cyclography, ultrasound biomicroscopy, and magnetic resonance imaging have shown that the ciliary body retains much of its contractility in older patients. Furthermore, modern technology allows refined finite element computer methods to simulate the changes of the ciliary body-zonular lens apparatus during accommodation. Based on concepts by Hanna and on finite element computer simulation models, a new acrylic hydrophilic foldable single-piece PCIOL has been designed and manufactured (1 CU) (Figure 13-1). The 1 CU PCIOL is designed to allow transmission of the contracting forces of the ciliary body into anterior movement of the lens optic to achieve pseudophakic accommodation. This optic shift principle

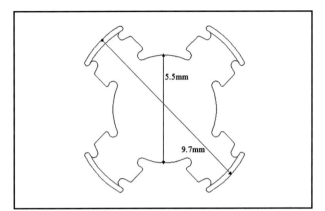

**Figure 13-1.** Schematic drawing of the 1 CU accommodative IOL.

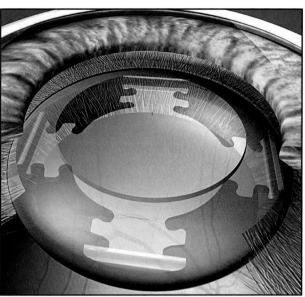

**Figure 13-2.** Localization of the 1 CU accommodative IOL in the capsular bag.

should allow a defined amount of accommodation, theoretically 1.6 D to 1.9 D per 1 mm anterior movement of the PCIOL optic (Figures 13-2 and 13-3). The spherical optic has a diameter of 5.5 mm, with total diameter of the PCIOL of 9.7 mm. The lens haptics are modified with transmission elements at their fusion with the lens optic. In earlier laboratory studies in porcine eyes and human donor eyes not suitable for corneal transplantation, we have refined methods for intraocular implantation of this PCIOL. The 1 CU PCIOL is CE-approved.

# INDICATIONS AND CONTRAINDICATIONS

At present, only patients with cataract (ie, clinically manifest and visually disturbing lens opacities) are candidates for lens exchange with implantation of the 1 CU accommodative IOL. Up to now, only patients older than 30 years have undergone this surgical option. In our opinion, there is no upper age limit.

Up to now and until there is more experience with 1 CU PCIOL and longer follow-up, we carefully observe exclusion criteria including manifest diabetic retinopathy, previous intraocular surgery, previous severe ocular trauma involving the lens, the zonules or the ciliary body, visible zonulolysis, phacodonesis, pseudoexfoliation syndrome, glaucoma, uveitis, high myopia, and high hypermetropia.

Furthermore, this kind of surgery will not result in satisfying clinical results in patients with severe ARMD or marked glaucomatous optic atrophy.

In case of problems during cataract surgery such as radial tears of the capsulorrhexis, diameter of capsulorrhexis >5.5 mm, zonulolysis, rupture of the posterior capsule, or vitreous loss, the 1 CU accommodative IOL should not be implanted and surgery should be converted to implantation of a conventional PCIOL.

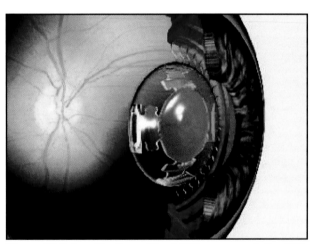

**Figure 13-3.** Localization of the 1 CU accommodative IOL in the capsular bag.

# SURGICAL TECHNIQUES

Generally, any of the modern small-incision phacoemulsification techniques may be used to remove the lens nucleus and lens cortex before the 1 CU accommodative intraocular lens is to be implanted.

## Anesthesia

Surgery may be safely performed under local or topical anesthesia. The surgeon may choose the methods that he is most comfortable with for cataract surgery. No specific modifications of anesthesia are necessary for implantation of the 1 CU accommodative IOL.

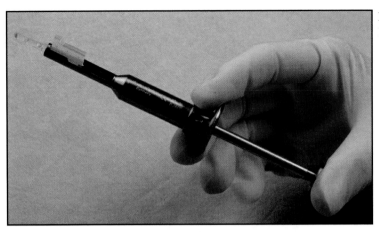

**Figure 13-4.** Injector used for implantation of the 1 CU accommodative IOL.

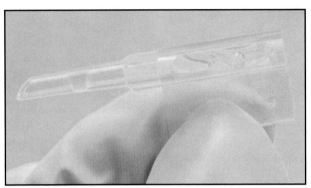

**Figure 13-5.** Cartridge used for implantation of the 1 CU accommodative IOL.

## Procedure (General)

Phacoemulsification of the lens nucleus and cortical cleaning is not much different from routine cataract surgery. The surgeon may choose the incision and phacoemulsification technique that he routinely uses for cataract surgery. Either a clear cornea or a sclerocorneal incision may be used. If possible, the incision should be placed in the steepest corneal meridian to reduce any preexisting corneal astigmatism. The capsulorrhexis is of great importance; it should be small enough (maximum 5.0 mm) to safely and circularly cover the peripheral optic of the IOL (diameter 5.5 mm). In addition, the capsulorrhexis should be round and well centered to allow for the elastic forces of the zonules and lens capsule to be equally distributed. Meticulous removal of all lens cortex and polishing of the posterior lens capsule is important to reduce the risk of capsular fibrosis and posterior capsular opacification. Any of the commercially available viscoelastic agents may be used.

## Procedure (Specifics)

Implantation and placement of the 1 CU accommodative IOL is the main step of the surgical procedure. It differs in

some aspects from implantation of standard IOLs but is relatively easily accomplished. IOL implantation is best performed with a cartridge and an injector (Figures 13-4 and 13-5). Folding and implantation with a forceps is also possible but may be associated with an increased risk of damaging the thin and delicate lens haptics. An incision width of 3.2 mm is usually sufficient. The 1 CU accommodative IOL is placed into the cartridge with the edges of the haptics pointing upward/anterior. When folding the lens inside the cartridge, care should be taken to avoid damage to the haptics. After completely filling the anterior chamber and the capsular bag with a viscoelastic agent, the lens is then implanted into the anterior chamber or directly into the capsular bag. In case the lens optic is placed in front of the capsular bag, it may be easily pressed down into the capsular bag with a cannula or a spatula. Then the 4 lens haptics are unfolded inside the capsular bag with a push-pull hook or an iris spatula. The viscoelastic agent should be completely removed also from behind the lens to prevent development of capsular block or capsular distension syndrome that might theoretically develop otherwise because of the relatively small size of the capsulorrhexis. The lens haptics should be placed at the 12-, 3, 6-, or 9-o'clock positions.

## Postoperative

Postoperative care and medications are similar to that of routine cataract surgery. Postoperative medication usually includes topical antibiotics, topical corticosteroids, and topical short-acting mydriatics such as tropicamide.

Our current postoperative regime includes combined antibiotic and corticosteroid eye drops (dexamethasone sodium phosphate 0.03% and gentamicin sulfate 0.3%) twice daily and tropicamide 0.5% twice daily. After 5 days, the combined antibiotic/steroidal eye drops are discontinued and changed to prednisolone acetate 1% eye drops 5 times a day for 4 weeks. The tropicamide eye drops are also discontinued after 4 weeks. No atropine is used.

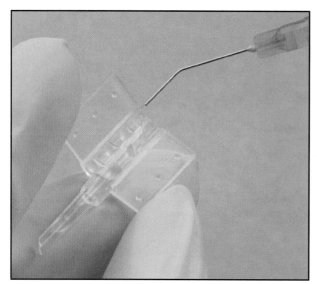

**Figure 13-6.** Cartridge and injector used for implantation of the 1 CU accommodative IOL.

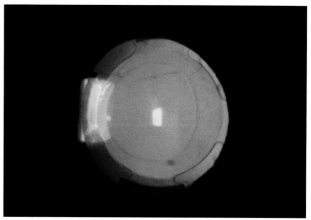

**Figure 13-7.** Transillumination photograph of 1 CU localized in the capsular bag 1 year after implantation.

## Outcomes

### Safety

Pilot studies have shown that the 1 CU PCIOL is safe for at least up to 2 years. We observed very little postoperative breakdown of the blood-aqueous barrier. No lens-specific complications were seen. No signs of decentration or dislocation were detected (Figure 13-6). The rate of posterior capsular opacification appears to be low (ie, not higher than in other types of PCIOL made of hydrophilic acrylate).

### Stability

Prospective studies that followed patients with the 1 CU PCIOL showed that refraction, anterior chamber depth, and accommodative range all remained stable without signs indicating a systemic trend toward myopia, hypermetropia, PCIOL dislocation, or regression of accommodative properties. Thus, the 1 CU accommodative PCIOL provides stable refraction, accommodation, and PCIOL position also for longer time periods for at least up to 1 year (Figure 13-7).

### Accommodation

We used several objective and subjective methods to measure pseudophakic accommodation after implantation of the 1 CU PCIOL.

1. Measurement of movement of the 1 CU lens optic with the IOL Master (Zeiss, Germany) after stimulation or relaxation of the ciliary muscle with eye drops. After pilocarine eye drops, a mean anterior movement of the lens optic of 0.63 ±0.16 mm in contrast to 0.15 ±0.05 mm in conventional control PCIOL was measured. Following relaxation of the ciliary muscle with cyclopentolate eye drops, a mean posterior movement of the 1 CU optic of 0.42 ±0.18 mm was determined versus 0.11 ±0.06 mm in control PCIOL. These findings indicate the proof of concept of the optic shift principle of this accommodative PCIOL.

2. Determination of accommodative range. We used several methods to measure pseudophakic accommodation. These methods included near point determination with an accommodometer (a), defocusing with minus lenses (b), and retinoscopy during near and distance fixation (c). Six-month results with the 1 CU PCIOL showed mean accommodative ranges of 1.83 D (a), 1.85 D (b), and 0.98 D (c). In comparison with a control group with conventional PCIOL, accommodative range was significantly greater in the 1 CU group, the difference being 0.67 D (a), 1.21 D (b), and 0.81 D (c).

3. Near visual acuity. Uncorrected or distance-corrected near visual acuity alone as the main outcome measure is problematic. Near visual acuity is severely influenced by a large number of factors. Determination of near visual acuity is troubled by inadequate bedside screening charts such as the Rosenbaum chart and the availability of several versions of inaccurate near reading charts. On most of these near reading charts, the optotypes are not scaled properly to the Snellen system, resulting in overestimation of near visual acuity by the Jaeger system. We use for standardized testing Birkhäuser reading charts in 35 cm and best distance correction. With this method, median near visual acuity with the 1 CU PCIOL was 0.4 versus 0.2 in control PCIOL.

## Future Research

After very encouraging results of pilot studies, presently a prospective multicentric randomized masked study is being conducted comparing accommodative and near vision results of the 1 CU PCIOL with those of a control PCIOL (Rayner RaySoft, East Sussex, United Kingdom).

Future research should be directed to further improving the optical and accommodative results of this new generation of accommodative PCIOL.

# BIBLIOGRAPHY

Bacskulin A, Gast R, Bergmann U, Guthoff R. Ultraschall-biomikroskopische Darstellung der akkommodativen Konfigurationsänderungen des presbyopen Ziliarkörpers. *Ophthalmologe.* 1996;93:199-203.

Glasser A, Kaufman PL. The mechanism of accommodation in primates. *Ophthalmology.* 1999;106:863-72.

Horton JC, Jones MR. Warning on inaccurate Rosenbaum charts for testing near vision. *Surv Ophthalmol.* 1997;42:169-74.

Kommerell G. Strichskiaskopie: Optische Prinzipien und praktische Empfehlungen. *Klin Monatsbl Augenheilkd.* 1993;203:10-8.

Küchle M, Gusek GC, Langenbucher A, Seitz B. First and preliminary results of a new posterior chamber intraocular lens. *Online J Ophth.* Available at http://www.onjoph.com/deutsch/artikel/pciol.html. Retrieved November 12, 2003.

Küchle M, Gusek-Schneider GC, Langenbucher A, Seitz B, Hanna KD. Erste Ergebnisse der Implantation einer neuen, potenziell akkommodierbaren Hinterkammerlinse—eine prospektive Sicherheitsstudie. *Klin Monatsbl Augenheilkd.* 2001;218:603-8.

Küchle M, Nguyen XN, Langenbucher A, Gusek-Schneider GC, Seitz B, Hanna KD. Implantation of a new accommodative posterior chamber intraocular lens. *J Refract Surg.* 2002;18:208-16.

Küchle M, Nguyen NX, Langenbucher A, Gusek-Schneider GC, Seitz B. Erste Sechs-Monats-Ergebnisse der Implantation einer neuen akkommodativen Hinterkammerlinse (1 CU). *Spektrum Augenheikd.* 2001:15:260-6.

Küchle M, Nguyen NX, Langenbucher A, Gusek-Schneider GC, Huber S, Seitz B. Stabilität von Refraktion und Akkommodation während eines Jahres nach Implantation der akkommodativen Hinterkammerlinse 1 CU. *Ophthalmologe.* 2002;99(Suppl 1):S 184.

Langenbucher A, Huber S, Nguyen XN, et al. Measurement of accommodation after implantation of a new accommodative posterior chamber intraocular lens (1CU). *J Cataract Refract Surg.* 2002.

Ludwig K, Wegscheider E, Hoops JP, Kampik A. In vivo imaging of the human zonular apparatus with high-resolution ultrasound. *Graefe's Arch Clin Exp Ophthalmol.* 1999;237:361-371.

Nguyen NX, Langenbucher A, Seitz B, Küchle M. Short-term blood-aqueous barrier breakdown after implantation of the 1 CU accommodative intraocular posterior chamber intraocular lens. *J Cataract Refract Surg.* 2002;28:1189-94.

Rohen J. Akkommodationsapparat. In: Velhagen K, ed. *Der Augenarzt.* Bd 1. Leipzig: Thieme, 1969:51-69.

Strenk SA, Semmlow JL, Strenk LM, Munoz P, Gronlund-Jacob J, DeMarco JK. Age-related changes in human ciliary muscle and lens: a magnetic resonance imaging study. *Invest Ophthalmol Vis Sci.* 1999;40:1162-1169.

Swegmark G. Studies with impedance cyclography on human ocular accommodation at different ages. *Acta Ophthalmol.* 1969; 47:1186-206.

von Helmholtz H. Über die Akkommodation des Auges. *Graefe's Arch Klin Exp Ophthalmol.* 1855;1:1-74.

Weale R. Presbyopia toward the end of the 20th century. *Surv Ophthalmol.* 1989; 34:16-30.

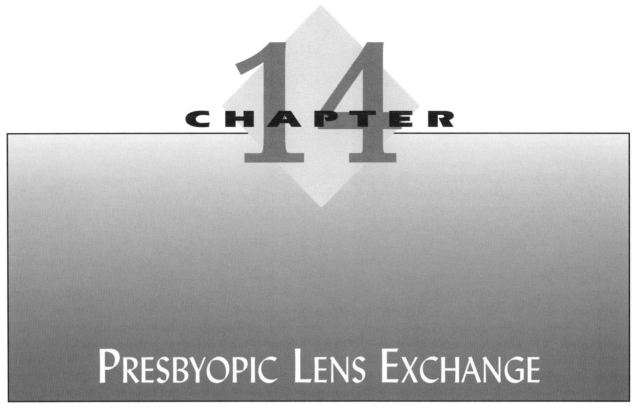

# CHAPTER 14

# PRESBYOPIC LENS EXCHANGE

*Kevin L. Waltz, OD, MD and R. Bruce Wallace III, MD, FACS*

## INTRODUCTION AND BACKGROUND

Modern cataract surgery has become a refractive procedure. Our patients expect the removal of the cataract and insertion of the lens without complications as a matter of course. They have recently come to expect a very specific refractive outcome—they want to be independent of their glasses. They must now be counseled that their expectations are probably unreasonable and may not be obtainable. The patient may be willing to live with reading glasses after their cataract surgery, but the surgeon who routinely leaves the patient with significant refractive error for distance vision will see a steady decrease in surgical volume.

Laser vision correction surgery is faced with unhappy patients who have distance vision of 20/20 or better without correction after their refractive surgery.[1] Sometimes these patients have uncorrected or iatrogenic higher order aberrations. However, these patients were commonly low myopes and have developed symptomatic presbyopia because of surgical correction of their myopia. We all tell these patients they will need reading glasses after their corrective surgery. Some of the patients are still surprised and very upset by their loss of near vision in exchange for their distance vision.

The modern ophthalmic surgeon tries to handle these challenging situations in various ways. Monovision is the most common method of maintaining near acuity. Monovision essentially under-treats 1 eye to minimize the negative effects of a successful treatment of both eyes for distance vision. Monovision works well in most patients who try it. But a significant percentage of patients who try monovision will not accept it and will need surgery to reverse the monovision. Another aspect of monovision that is frequently overlooked is the need to have the distance eye perfect. Because only 1 eye is focused for distance, the patient is very unforgiving of any blur. The patient can effectively optimize the near eye by moving a near object farther or closer to improve its focus. This increases the enhancement rate for the distance eye while decreasing it for the near eye. Surgical monovision has also been implicated in the possible permanent reduction of stereoscopic vision.

Another option is pseudoaccommodative IOLs. A pseudoaccommodative IOL corrects the distance vision in the usual manner as a monofocal IOL. It also has some mechanisms to allow for additional focal points in the near range. These mechanisms include a multifocal IOL optical design such as the Array Multifocal IOL (Advanced Medical Optics, Santa Ana, Calif) or a mechanical anterior-posterior translation of the lens such as the Crystalens (Eyeonics, Aliso Viejo, Calif). Since the mid to late 1990s, most markets in the world have had at least 1 lens option to simulate accommodation while correcting distance refractive error. The

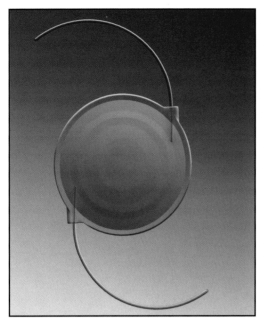

**Figure 14-1.** Array Silicone MIOL.

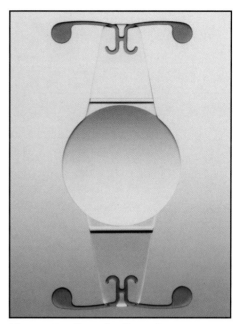

**Figure 14-2.** Eyeonics Crystalens.

Array Multifocal IOL (Figure 14-1) was approved by the FDA in the fall of 1997 for use in cataract patients over the age of 60. It subsequently received the CE mark from the European Union for the indication of correcting presbyopia in November 2001. There are other pseudoaccommodative IOLs pursuing approval for cataract indications in the US and Europe, including the Eyeonics CrystaLens (Figure 14-2), and the Alcon multifocal lens, the MA60D3 (Fort Worth, Tex). There are other pseudoaccommodative IOLs pursuing approval in the European Union, including the Human Optics 1CU Lens (Erlangen, Germany).

A safe, effective, and predictable treatment for presbyopia is the current "Holy Grail" of cataract and refractive surgery. All of the current options, including monovision and pseudoaccommodative IOLs, have significant risks and compromises that the surgeon and the patient need to understand to be successful.[2-6] Monovision with laser vision correction can be used to give many patients good distance and near vision. However, lens surgery is not reversible. The advantage of lens surgery is that it can correct almost any lower amount of order aberrations[7-9] and some of the higher order aberrations in 1 procedure. By removing the lens, you remove the higher order aberrations of the natural lens and replace them with the higher order aberrations of a manufactured lens. With lens surgery, you may also be preventing the development of cataracts and their associated morbidity later in life.

PRELEX stands for *PRE*sbyopic *Lens EX*change.[2] It is the surgical removal of the natural lens, replacing it with an artificial lens that has a pseudoaccommodative mechanism such as a multifocal optic and/or an anterior posterior translation of the optic to simulate the natural process of accommoda-

tion. In our view, PRELEX is a procedure that is independent of the presence or absence of a cataract. PRELEX is a procedure to treat presbyopia whether that presbyopia is surgically induced by the cataract surgeon or naturally occurring by the passage of time. While the PRELEX procedure has been performed with several different types of IOLs, our personal experience is mostly limited to the use of the Array Multifocal IOL. Therefore, unless otherwise indicated the remainder of this discussion will be devoted to PRELEX with a multifocal IOL.

## PATIENT SELECTION

PRELEX patients want to be less dependent on glasses after their surgery. They understand they will still need to wear glasses for some things, perhaps for most of their daily chores, but these patients want us to make every effort to decrease their dependence on their glasses or contacts. This means that the typical PRELEX patient is from 40 to 80 years old. Few patients younger that 40 would need or consider lenticular surgery and few patients older than 80 feel the need to be less dependent on their glasses. The typical age for a refractive PRELEX patient who is having the surgery for mostly refractive surgery reasons is about 53 years old. The typical age for a cataract PRELEX patient who is having the surgery primarily to correct cataracts is 62 years old (unpublished data).

When discussing treatment options with potential PRELEX patients, we emphasize several points. The surgery is irreversible. While the IOL can be exchanged, the natural lens cannot be replaced. The patient has the risk of a poten-

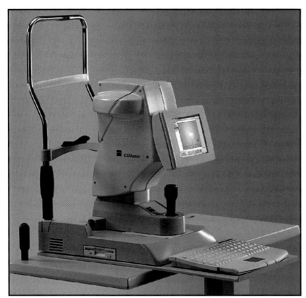

**Figure 14-3.** Zeiss-Humphrey IOL Master (Dublin, Calif).

tially devastating intraocular infection. Patients with eyes longer than 24 mm probably have an increased risk of retinal detachment. The patient will see halos after the surgery. The perception of the halos will decrease with time, but the halos will never go away. The patient will require some time to adapt to the new visual system. Most patients will experience most of this adaptation in the first 3 months but it can take more or less time depending on the individual patient.[2,3]

Patients who are hyperopic are usually better candidates for PRELEX than patients who are myopic or emmetropic. The concept of refractive lensectomy for hyperopia has been with us for some time.[7-10] Hyperopic patients usually have axial lengths less than 24 mm. Eyes with axial lengths less than 24 mm are not associated with an increased risk of retinal detachment associated with intraocular surgery.[11] Hyperopic patients frequently see halos preoperatively, so they are less bothered by the halos postoperatively. Hyperopic patients tend to have limitations of their visual systems that are similar to distance dominant multifocal optics systems; they have more challenges with their near vision than their distance vision.[3]

Most surgeons and optometrists think there are many more myopes in the world than there are hyperopes. PRELEX works best in hyperopes. Therefore, many ophthalmic surgeons think there is not much of a market for PRELEX for hyperopic presbyopes. Contrary to many surgeons' perceptions, there are many more hyperopic patients than myopic patients. Approximately 50% of the adult population of developed countries is hyperopic, 20% is emmetropic, and 30% is myopic.[11,12] While the typical 50-year-old myope is bothered by the need for glasses, he can still function at near without them. The typical 50-year-old hyperopic patient is very bothered by the need to wear glass-

es and cannot function without them for any visual task and his visual problems are progressively growing worse with every passing year. The typical presbyopic hyperope consistently meets our primary criteria for PRELEX. They desperately want to be less dependent on their glasses.

## PREOPERATIVE TESTING FOR PRELEX

The critical preoperative tests for PRELEX are those used to determine the correct IOL power. If the correct IOL power is achieved on the first attempt, the remainder of the process is much easier for the surgeon and the patient. Classic preoperative biometry includes tests for axial length and corneal curvature. They account for the majority of the preoperative variability. The most accurate determination of axial lengths is done by immersion A-scan biometry or optical coherence biometry (Figure 14-3). Routine applanation biometry is not consistently accurate enough to achieve the refractive results sought by the surgeon and the patient. The surgeon can use either manual keratometry or corneal topography to determine the corneal curvature. However, corneal topography is usually required to obtain the best results with astigmatic surgery at the time of lenticular surgery.[13,14]

There are other preoperative measurements that can be helpful in determining the best IOL power. For axial lengths less than 22 mm, predicting the size of the anterior chamber relative to the total eye length becomes more important. The depth of the anterior chamber relative to the total length of the eye predicts the effective lens position or the actual position of the lens relative to the overall length of the eye. The effective lens position assumed by many IOL calculation formulas tends to become less and less accurate in eyes less than 22 mm in length.

If you use an IOL formula that does not calculate the effective lens position accurately, the formula can be a source error. The Holladay II formula is one of the formulas that accurately accounts for the effective lens position. Unfortunately, the Holladay I formula, which comes installed on the IOL Master (Zeiss-Humphrey, Dublin, Calif), does not. This problem is most commonly seen with shorter eyes that have relatively normal anterior chamber depths. In these cases, you will get a hyperopic surprise if you do not take into account the depth of the anterior chamber. The magnitude of the error can be as much as several diopters in eyes with a very short axial length or very deep anterior chamber.

## PREOPERATIVE COUNSELING

Preoperative counseling is the key to a successful outcome with PRELEX. While it is mandatory to have a safe, uneventful procedure that securely places the IOL in an intact capsule, the patient must understand what will happen postoperatively before they can decide to have the surgery. The patient must not only be motivated to improve their visual system with PRELEX, they must be prepared to deal with the expected and unexpected challenges that can be created by the procedure.[15-17]

It is important to be realistic with the patient about potential visual outcomes after PRELEX. Assuming the refractive target has been achieved with the surgery, the patient can expect to have excellent unaided distance vision during the day. PRELEX patients frequently report that their unaided distance vision during daylight hours is the best it has been during their entire life.

Distance vision at night is usually less satisfying than the distance vision during the day. When the pupil dilates at night, it creates a significant increase in unwanted visual sensations in all human optical systems. These unwanted visual sensations can be manifest as increased starbursts, halos, and/or glare. Most PRELEX patients will experience an increase in these sensations after their surgery. They need to be made aware of this issue preoperatively and allowed to weigh this against the anticipated benefits of the surgery.[15-17]

Near vision after PRELEX is usually best in dimmer illumination. Bright lights usually make it more difficult to see at near, but not always. There are 2 optimal pupil sizes for near vision with the Array Multifocal IOL—1.9 mm and 3.4 mm. It is important to understand the smaller pupil size depends on the pinhole effect and the larger pupil size depends on the Array optical system for their effect on near vision.

When the pupil is 1.9 mm in diameter, the patient benefits from the pinhole effect. There is a minimum amount of diffraction-related vision loss. The central distance dominant zone of the Array IOL is 2.1 mm in diameter. As the pupil size becomes smaller than 2.1 mm, the human optical system becomes diffraction limited. Diffraction progressively limits the acuity of the eye as the pupil becomes smaller than 2 mm. When the pupil is this size or slightly larger, it effectively excludes any effect of the Array near zone. These patients tend to read best in brighter light that constricts their pupils.

The optical add of the Array IOL is best at a pupil size of 3.4 mm. At this pupil size, the relative light distribution of the Array favors the near vision. Almost 50% of the light is devoted to the near focal point. These patients tend to perform near visual tasks best in dimmer light. However, if they have larger pupils naturally they may choose to increase the light intensity when they read to constrict their pupils closer to the 3.4 mm optimum for the Array optics.

Some PRELEX surgeons prefer to routinely dilate the pupils of older patients at the time of surgery. This practice can create challenges for the patient and the surgeon. The quickest, most reliable way to increase a patient's higher order aberrations is to increase their pupillary diameter. This is also true when implanting the Array IOL. If a patient has very small pupils, less than 2.0 mm in the undilated state, it may be better to implant the Array without dilating the pupil. After the procedure evaluate the patient's distance and near vision. Most likely the patient will have excellent near vision from the pinhole effect and will not need further intervention. When leaving a patient with small pupils, it is helpful to also leave them slightly myopic, approximately -0.50 D.

The normal physiological responses of potential PRELEX patient can predict who will be the best candidates for the procedure. Let's examine 2 potential patients who are losing their accommodation. One is hyperopic and one is myopic. Their reaction to PRELEX can be predicted based on this information. Let's assume the hyperopic patient is wearing +2.00 D spheres in his glasses and the myopic patient is wearing -2.00 D spheres in her glasses.

Every hyperopic patient's visual system is stressed by the need to constant need to accommodate. The hyperopic patient must use his accommodation to see objects clearly at distance and even more for objects at near. Glasses probably correct the manifest hyperopia, but not the latent hyperopia. The patient's total hyperopic correction, the manifest plus the latent hyperopia, is probably closer to +3.00 D.

The patient allows the actual accommodative effort to lag behind the accommodative demand to decrease the stress on the visual system. This creates a constant blur for the hyperope that becomes progressively worse with the greater accommodative demand of near objects. It is exacerbated even further by the onset of cataracts. Glasses also create base-out prism. Base-out prism makes it more difficult for a patient to converge their eyes, thereby further stressing the hyperopic visual system.

The hyperopic patient benefits the most from PRELEX. The patient no longer needs to overcome the base-out prism in their glasses (try this in a trial frame for personal experience). Shortly after surgery, distance vision is good with the Array but near vision is more challenging to learn.

Unlike the hyperope, the myopic patient likes to over-accommodate at distance. Refractionists call this "eating the minus." The patient with -2.00 D in her glasses probably has only -1.50 D of myopia. The myopic patient tends to not overaccommodate at near. The myope tends to very nearly match the accommodative demand of near vision with the effort, giving the typical myopic patient excellent corrected and uncorrected near vision. The myope also has base-in prism in his glasses. The base-in prism assists the myope in their convergence effort, thereby decreasing the stress on the myopic visual system.

Therefore, the myope benefits the least from PRELEX. The distance vision is similar preoperatively and postoperatively. However, the near vision is often not as good postoperatively for the myope as it was preoperatively with the natural lens. Most patients notice the loss. The patient also loses the base-in prism of glasses and must exert more effort in convergence. The typical unwanted visual sensation for the

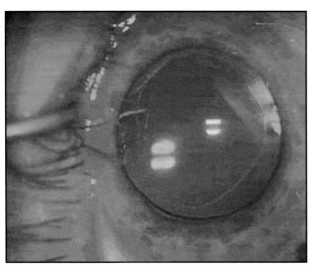

**Figure 14-4.** Alcon diffractive MIOL (Fort Worth, Tex).

myope is starbursts. When they see halos they are more symptomatic than hyperopes because they are not used to seeing halos in everyday life.

# THE PRELEX PROCEDURE

The PRELEX procedure is lenticular surgery. With PRELEX cases done for refractive reasons, the surgery is similar to the removal of a very soft cataract. PRELEX is unforgiving surgery. It should only be attempted by very experienced lenticular surgeons. For this reason, we anticipate the reader will already be an expert at lenticular surgery and we will concentrate on particular points of the procedure that may be different from routine lenticular surgery. The primary difference between a PRELEX procedure and a routine lenticular surgery is an intense effort to correct the preexisting corneal astigmatism. For optimal vision, the PRELEX patient needs to have less than 0.75 D of astigmatism after the procedure.

We generally prefer to correct the patient's preexisting astigmatism with CRIs at the time of the surgery.[18] CRIs are predictable, safe, and effective up to about 2.00 D. With astigmatism greater than 2.00 D, the CRIs become less predictable, but are still safe and effective. The surgeon may consider staging the PRELEX procedure with laser vision correction to treat astigmatism greater than 2.00 D. The reader is referred to the references for details on performing CRIs or laser vision correction (LVC) to treat astigmatism.

LVC to treat astigmatism can be performed before or after the lenticular portion of the procedure. It is also possible to stage the creation of a flap prior to the lenticular procedure, lift the flap after the procedure, and apply any required laser treatment at that time. If you are planning to treat the astigmatism with laser vision correction prior to the procedure, it is very helpful to have pre-LVC topography and

post-LVC topography. You can then adjust the corneal curvature measurements for the Array IOL calculation. The adjustment is technique dependent so it needs to be customized like an A-constant for an IOL. The change in corneal curvature from the pre to the post-LVC topography should be multiplied by 0.72 to correct for the new corneal curvature. For example, if you have decreased the corneal curvature with LVC by 2.00 D, you would multiply 2.00 x 0.72 to arrive at 1.44 D. You would then add 1.44 D to the originally calculated IOL power to arrive at the new IOL power.

We prefer to use sterile sponges soaked in a cocktail of anesthetic, antibiotic, and dilating drops preoperatively. We find that using sterile sponges soaked in our preoperative drops minimizes the deleterious effects of the preservatives on the corneal surface and keeps the patient more comfortable during and after the surgery. The sponge technique also dilates the eyes better than the drops. Sometimes the pupil will be dilated asymmetrically toward the prior position of the sponge in the inferior cul-de-sac. We find this a minimal annoyance.

The surgeon will want to minimize the impact of the surgery on the endothelium. There are many available viscoelastics to keep protect the cornea form the minimal ultrasound energy used during a typical PRELEX procedure. A capsulorrhexis slightly smaller than the lens optic is created centered on the apex of the cornea (Figure 14-4). We believe the anterior capsular opening should be between 5.5 mm and 4.5 mm. By covering the optic edge with the capsule, you will enhance the predictability of the refractive outcome and discourage posterior capsule opacification.

Maintaining a centered multifocal IOL is critical to the success of the PRELEX procedure. It is necessary to meticulously clean the posterior capsule, but not the anterior capsule. Once the capsular bag has been adequately cleaned and inflated with viscoelastic, the IOL is implanted. After IOL implantation, the viscoelastic is removed. After the viscoelastic is removed, the IOL is rotated in the capsular bag 2 full rotations. This rotation helps the surgeon clean the fornices of the capsular bag of residual viscoelastic. It also helps identify any lenticular remnant in the capsular bag.

Some PRELEX surgeons have reported occasional late decentration of the Array IOL. We believe this is related to retained viscoelastic within the capsular bag. If the viscoelastic is not completely removed, it prevents equal circumferential adhesion of the capsule and allows late dislocation of the IOL as the capsule contracts. Surgeons who have added 2 full rotations of the IOL after in-the-bag implantation have virtually eliminated late IOL dislocations.

PRELEX patients are very sensitive to the Maddox rod effect of a wrinkled posterior capsule. It is helpful to rotate the lens haptics into a position to create a vertical fold in the posterior capsule. The vertical fold serves several purposes. The Maddox rod effect of a vertical capsular fold is horizontal. We have found that a horizontal Maddox rod effect is less symptomatic than a vertical Maddox rod and much less symptomatic than an oblique Maddox rod effect. It confirms that both haptics are in the bag and the bag is intact. It also confirms the haptics are in the best position to allow the optic to stay centered in case there is a slight nasal decentration of the capsule. A 0.50-mm nasal decentration of the capsular bag is a relatively common late finding.

# REFERENCES

1. Holladay JT, Dudeja DR, Chang J. Functional vision and corneal changes after laser in situ keratomileusis determined by contrast sensitivity, glare testing, and corneal topography. *J Cataract Refract Surg.* 1999;25:663-69.

2. Fine IH, Hoffman RS, Packer M. Clear-lens extraction with multifocal lens implantation. *Internat Ophthalmol Clin.* 2001; 41:113-121.

3. Waltz KL, Wallace RB. PRELEX: surgery to implant multifocal intraocular lenses. *Ophthalmic Practice.* 2001;19(8):343-346.

4. Dick HB, Krummenauer F, Schwenn O, et al. Objective and subjective evaluation of photic phenomena after monofocal and multifocal intraocular lens implantation. *Ophthalmology.* 1999;106:1878-1886.

5. Pieh S, Weghaupt H, Skorpik C. Contrast sensitivity and glare disability with diffractive and refractive multifocal intraocular lenses. *J Cataract Refract Surg.* 1998;24:659-662.

6. Haring G, Gronemeyer A, Hedderich J, de Decker W. Stereoacuity and anisekonia after unilateral and bilateral implantation of the Array refractive multifocal intraocular lens. *J Cataract Refract Surg.* 1999;25:1151-56.

7. Siganos DS, Pallikaris IG. Clear lensectomy and intraocular lens implantation for hyperopia from +7 to +14 diopters. *J Refract Surg.* 1998;14:105-113.

8. Kolahdouz-Isfahani AH, Rostamiam K, Wallace D, Salz JJ. Clear lens extraction with intraocular lens implantation for hyperopia. *J Refract Surg.* 1999;15:316-323.

9. Fink AM, Gore C, Rosen ES. Refractive lensectomy for hyperopia. *Ophthalmol.* 2000;107:1540-1548.

10. Osher RH. Controversies in cataract surgery. *Audiovis J Cat Implant Surg.* 1989;5:3.

11. Verzella F. Refractive surgery of the lens in high myopes. *Refract Corneal Surg.* 1990;6:273-275.

12. Katz J, Tielsch JM, Sommer A. Prevalence and risk factors for refractive errors in an adult inner city population. *Invest Ophthalmol Vis Sci.* 1997;38:334-340.

13. Sorsby A, Leary GA, Richards MJ. Correlation ametropia and component ametropia. *Vision Res.* 1962;2:309-318.

14. Zaldivar R, Shultz MC, Davidorf JM, Holladay JT. Intraocular lens power calculations in patients with extreme myopia. *J Cataract Refract Surg.* 2000;26;668-74.

15. Holladay JT. How to prevent refractive surprise. *Review of Ophthalmology.* 1999 April;97-101.

16. Featherstone KA, Bloomfield JR, Lang AJ, et al. Driving simulation study: bilateral array multifocal versus bilateral AMO monofocal intraocular lenses. *J Cataract Refract Surg.* 1999; 25:1254-1262.

17. Steinert RF, Aker BL, Trentacost DJ, et al. A prospective study of the AMO Array zonal-progressive multifocal silicone intraocular lens and a monofocal intraocular lens. *Ophthalmology.* 1999;106:1243-1255.

18. Gills JP, Gayton JL. Reducing pre-existing astigmatism. In: Gills JP, Fenzl R, Martin RG, eds. *Cataract Surgery: The State of the Art.* Thorofare, NJ: SLACK Incorporated. 1998:53-66.

# BIBLIOGRAPHY

Dick HB, Gross S, Tehrani M, Eisenmann D, Pfeiffer N. Refractive lens exchange with an array multifocal intraocular lens. *J Refract Surg.* 2002;18(5):509-518.

Steiner RF, Post CT, Brint SF, et al. A progressive, randomized, double-masked comparison of a zonal-progressive multifocal intraocular lens and a monofocal intraocular lens. *Ophthalmology.* 1992;99:853-861.

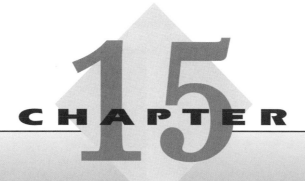

# CHAPTER 15

# SURGICAL REVERSAL OF PRESBYOPIA

*Gene W. Zdenek, MD*

## INTRODUCTION

Perhaps the most exciting development in this field of ophthalmology is understanding the pathophysiology of presbyopia. Dr. Ronald Schachar's theory refuting Hermann von Helmholtz's theory of accommodation has created the most enthusiastic discussion thus far.

### Anatomy

Leaving this battle to the theorists, simply put, the human lens grows continuously at the rate of 20 μm a year (Figure 15-1).

This growth has little impact on lens accommodation until the person reaches the approximate age of 40. At this time the space between the lens equator and the ciliary muscle has decreased sufficiently to begin lessening the zonular pull effect that results in accommodation.

The unpleasant aging process called presbyopia presents itself when the lens growth crowds the ciliary space. The treatment of presbyopia is to expand the ciliary space by scleral expansion.

As clinicians understanding Schachar's new theory, we can now approach the treatment of presbyopia. Inconsistencies in the Helmholtz theory have prevented the proper clinical approach to the treatment of presbyopia (Figure 15-2).

To further validate Schachar's theory, 3 completely different surgical techniques are being investigated by 3 independent groups of clinicians. All of the procedures rely on the expansion of the sclera, which increases the space between the ciliary muscle and the lens equator in order to restore accommodation. With the confidence that the scleral expansion theory is correct, clinicians are working toward perfecting a surgical approach to the restoration of accommodation.

Dr. Spencer Thornton has headed the radial sclerotomy approach for accommodative restoration (ACS—anterior ciliary sclerotomy). Thornton led a multicenter study to investigate the effect of scleral expansion on accommodation (Figure 15-3).

Dr. Hideharu Fukasaku has performed most of the work. Results from the first 2 years of the study demonstrated that scleral expansion could improve the lost accommodation that occurs in presbyopia. Due to a decreased effect after 6 months, Fukasaku placed silicone implants within the sclerotomies and sutured them in place to prevent regression. James Hayes, MD, has tried placing titanium "T" implants in the incisions, in order to minimize scaring with the resulting decrease in effect (Figure 15-4).

The second procedure under investigation involves use of an erbium laser to form radial sclerotomies in the same manner as ACS. Ronald A. Schachar, MD, PhD, originally developed the ACS approach.

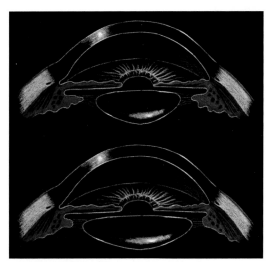

Figure 15-1. Lens growth over 60 years.

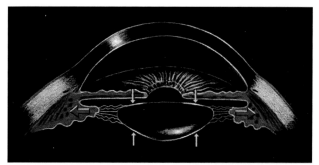

**Figure 15-2.** Schachar's theory. Peripheral flattening and central steepening of the lens during accommodation.

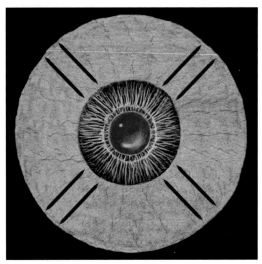

Figure 15-3. Anterior ciliary sclerotomy.

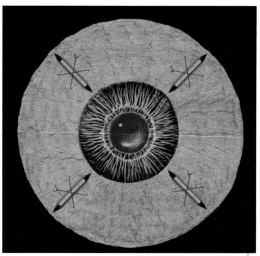

**Figure 15-4.** Anterior ciliary sclerotomy with sutured silicone implants.

The third procedure, currently in FDA trials, by Refocus Group, Inc. called the scleral spacing procedure (SSP) for the surgical reversal of presbyopia (SRP) (Figure 15-5).

In this procedure, 4 small, arched PMMA implants are tunneled through the sclera overlying the ciliary body (Figure 15-6).

## Evaluation (Preoperative)

The ideal candidate is between 40 to 70 years of age with minimal distance refractive error. If patients are in need of refractive surgery, it is recommended that they have their distance vision corrected first followed by scleral spacing procedure (SSP) approximately 4 to 6 months later. Generally it is preferable to performed LASIK before the SSP. A proper add should be determined for near vision. The proper add is to a larger extent determined by the persons age. Age 40 to 45 generally requires a +1.00. Age 50 to 55 generally requires a +2.00 and age 60 to 65 generally requires a +2.50 to +3.00.

In the preoperative evaluation of the patient include the following:

1. Distance visual acuity with correction in place
2. Visual acuity at 40 cm, 30 cm, and 20 cm
3. Visual acuity starting at 70 cm and bringing the eye chart closer until the smallest line read starts to blur (this test gives you the diopters of accommodation that the patient has—the formula to measure this is 1/distance in centimeters times 100 (ie, if the patient is able to read the line clearly up to 50 cm, the formula applied would be 1/50 x 100 = 2.00 D of accommodation)
4. Axial length measurement and corneal topography

Step 3 listed above is also important in the postoperative evaluation to measure the amount of accommodation gained. When repeating this step postoperatively, it is important that the patient use the same line he was able to see preoperatively (even if it was only 20/200). Have the eye chart brought in toward the patient as before to find the gain in accommodation. To illustrate (continuing from the example in step 3): if the patient is able to clearly see the same line on the eye chart when brought up as close as 20 cm, this would

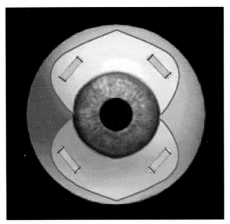

**Figure 15-5.** Four implants in place.

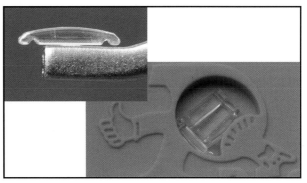

**Figure 15-6.** SSP implants in package and close-up on channel forcep.

result in 5.00 D of accommodation. These measurements are obviously more subjective than objective. There are a number of new techniques being developed to better objectively access accommodation.

The results in step 4 should not be affected as a result of the surgery. Corneal topography may show induced astigmatism immediately postoperatively. In all cases, this astigmatism disappears within 3 months. At this writing, SSP with scleral expansion band (SEB) implants have completed FDA Phase I Trials. Included in the trial data were the corneal topography and axial length readings. Upon the acceptance of SSP, these tests will not be necessary. Recently, CIBA Vision/Novartis (Duluth, Ga) developed a method in conjunction with ultrasound to more accurately predict the ideal implant placement for each individual patient. This will provide anatomical verification for the proper implant location. Previously, the implant location was one of the variables in the procedure, and its location is important because the implants render the maximum effect if they are placed within 200 μm posterior to the lens equator of the individual patient. Before this measurement system, the surgical placement of the implants have relied on the surgical limbus as a reference point. Two major placement obstacles accompanied this approach. First, the surgical limbus is not clearly defined, making its reference inconsistent from surgeon to surgeon. Second, the lens equator varies from patient to patient. The following is an illustory explanation of this method. This method provides a mechanism for marking the lens equator on the sclera surface at the time of surgery. The advantage and accuracy of this method is that the optical axis rather than the surgical limbus is the reference point. It is surgically evident that the optical axis is many times more accurate and precise that the surgical limbus. Ultrasound plays an integral role in this method. Axial length, lens thickness, anterior chamber depth, and corneal thickness are relied upon to determine the location of the lens equator relative to the sclera surface within the surgical field.

# INDICATIONS AND CONTRAINDICATIONS

Patients who are more than +1.00 hyperopic may not attain enough accommodation to satisfy their near vision needs. Depending on the expectations of your patient, this may or may not be satisfactory. Since the procedure is performed with the intention of giving as much accommodation as is physiologically possible, the variability lies within the patient's own anatomy as well as surgeon skill.

SSP may be considered an optional, cosmetic procedure with the same inherent issues. Therefore, it may not be for everyone. Patients need to be aware of the need to exercise and work at strengthening the muscle for several months after the procedure to gain optimum effects. The SSP patient's eyes will be quite red for a few weeks following the surgery. Postoperative expectations given prior to the procedure are extremely important.

When taking the patient's history, the physician should note the following contraindications:

- Insulin-dependent diabetes mellitus
- Severe hypertension
- Blood dyscrasias
- Chronic or recurrent uveitis, iritis, scleritis, *herpes simplex*
- Previous eye surgery (including cataract, corneal transplant, glaucoma filtering surgeries, retinal detachment repair)
- Patients on Heparin (Alcon, Fort Worth, Tex) or Coumadin (DuPont, Wilmington, Del)
- Sjörgren's Syndrome
- Chronic systemic disease (ie, subacute lupus erythematosus, Crohn's disease, collagen vascular disease, rheumatoid arthritis)

# SURGICAL TECHNIQUES

## Anesthesia

This procedure may safely be performed under local and topical anesthesia. The addition of light sedatives is beneficial to the comfort and well being of the patient. If the surgeon feels more secure with the assistance of an anesthetist, he should remember the benefits of minimal sedation so as to incorporate the patient's assistance by looking in various directions during the case. This will allow exposure of the quadrant of the eye being operated on. The only anesthesia that I now use in all my cases is 4% Xylocaine (AstraZeneca, Waltham, Mass) placed on a pledget and applied to each quadrant prior to performing surgery on that quadrant. Alphagan eye drops administered 15 to 30 minutes prior to beginning the procedure helps decrease operative bleeding. Light sedation may be achieved in a couple of different ways. Lorazipam 1 to 2 mg or diazepam 10 to 20 mg may be given PO about an hour before the procedure is started.

Letting the patient know in advance what he or she can expect are during the surgical procedure (and why they are not being put to sleep) will greatly enhance their ability to cooperate. General anesthesia and its inherent risks are not indicated because of the effectiveness of topical anesthesia. In addition, local injectable anesthesia should be avoided due to conjunctival swelling and reactive hyperemia. I have tried many different topical/local anesthesia techniques and found the aforementioned the most successful.

## Procedure (General)

After the instillation of 0.5% proparacaine, the patient should have his or her eyes marked with a skin scribe or marking pen at the 12-o'clock position. It is documented that up to 10 to 15 degrees of torsion or eye movement can occur when the patient is in a supine position as compared to the upright position. If this mark is not placed accurately, the implants may be off by as much as 20 degrees. This inaccuracy in positioning may be sufficient to compromise the anterior circulation of the eye. Anterior segment ischemia is a complication that could arise if implant placement is not accurate.

## Procedure (Specifics)

There are 8 basic steps to the surgical reversal of presbyopia procedure.

1. Oblique quadrant or axis marking
2. Opening the conjunctiva
3. Hemostasis
4. Scleral marking
5. Sclerotomy
6. Belt loop formation

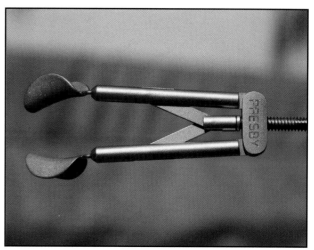

**Figure 15-7.** Eyelid speculum.

7. Implant insertion
8. Conjunctival closure

Each of these steps with appropriate clinical pearls will be discussed in detail. With the recent addition of the optional PresVIEW Drive (CIBA Vision, Duluth, Ga), steps number 3 to 6 are streamlined. The PresVIEW Drive will be discussed in detail later in the text.

After appropriate positioning of the patient in the supine position, the operative site is prepped and draped in the usual sterile fashion. Although the trend seems to be a bilateral procedure, there are occasions where a single eye may be operated on. If doing a bilateral case, I usually operate on the dominant eye first. If there is a reason not to progress on to the second eye, the dominant eye should attain better results.

The eyelid speculum (Presby PY ES 5 [Refocus Group Inc, Dallas, Tex]) is used to open the eye for maximum exposure (Figure 15-7).

## Axis Marking

With the proparacaine on board, the axis or quadrant marker (Presby PY AM 3) is inked and used to mark the 45-degree meridians (Figure 15-8).

The handle of the marker should be placed at the 12-o'clock position, thus assuring that the marks are delivered accurately at the oblique meridians. The marks will not necessarily be made directly onto the limbus. Most likely they will be about 2 mm posterior. Their purpose is to delineate the axis for the placement of the belt loop, not the limbus location (Figure 15-9).

You may need to re-ink any of the marks that you feel may fade by the time you are ready to use them.

Also remember that you are going to be creating a flap in the conjunctiva and you want your marks to be visible. This may necessitate remarking closer to the limbus. What you should see after appropriate marking is 12 separate spots in groups of 3. They are centered on the 45-degree meridians

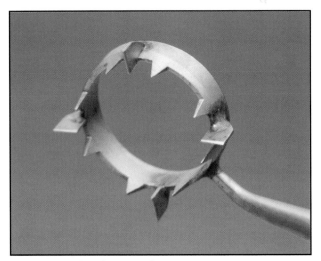

**Figure 15-8.** Quadrant marker.

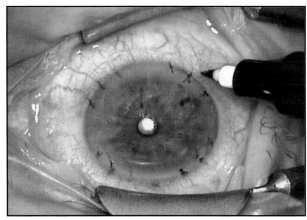

**Figure 15-9.** Quadrant marks and remarking.

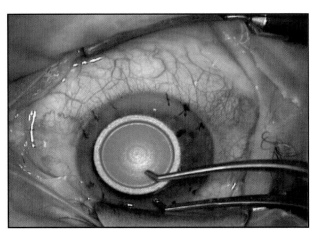

**Figure 15-10.** Corneal shield in place.

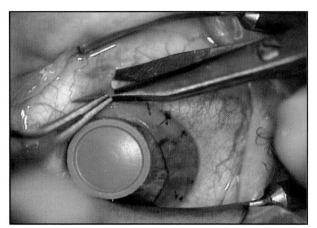

**Figure 15-11.** Conjunctival dissection.

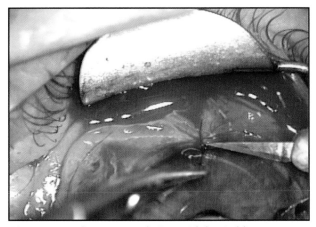

**Figure 15-12.** Suture completion with buried knot.

that will be marked. Straddling those will be 2 marks that are 4 mm apart (the length of the belt loop).

A corneal shield is then placed on the cornea with viscoelastic or viscous artificial tear (Figure 15-10).

This shield is placed after the quadrant marks have been made to insure stable ink markings, which could be interfered with by the viscous fluid.

## Opening the Conjunctiva

When using the PresVIEW Drive unit, the method of exposure is to make a 360-degree peritomy with relaxing incisions at the 3- and 9-o'clock positions.

The technique used in the manual approach incorporates a T-shaped conjunctival incision for exposing enough sclera for a pair of implants. This conjunctival approach involves a 5 clock hour limbal peritomy with a conjunctival relaxation incision at the 6- and 12-o'clock positions extending approximately 4.0 to 6.0 mm posteriorly and perpendicular to the limbus (Figure 15-11).

For closure, single sutures are used at the limbus, making sure to include a little of underlying sclera and bury the knot beneath the conjunctiva (Figure 15-12).

I recommend performing surgery on the inferior quadrants first for the following reasons. The time to perform the surgery will be longer than the anesthetic's (Xylocaine)

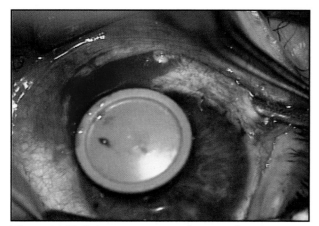

**Figure 15-13.** Strip cautery over sclerotomy location.

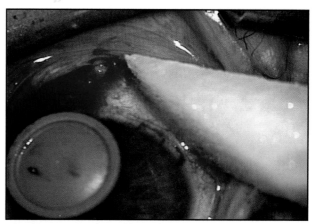

**Figure 15-14.** Applying 4% Xylocaine with pledget on sclera.

effect. After the topical anesthetic wears off, in many patients there is a reactive hyperemia and/or a postanesthesia hyperesthesia. These conditions make further anesthesia more difficult to attain. While anesthetizing the superior quadrants, the anesthetic pools in the lower quadrants. By the time the surgeon approaches the lower quadrants, they have already gone through the cycle of anesthesia, as mentioned above. When deciding between the 2 inferior quadrants, choose the quadrant with the least amount of bleeding to operate on first. By the time you approach the second quadrant, natural hemostasis should have occurred. The conjunctival approach involves a 5 clock hour limbal peritomy with a conjunctival relaxation incision at the 6-o'clock position extending approximately 4.0 to 6.0 mm posteriorly, perpendicular to the limbus.

## Hemostasis

I do not cauterize in preparation of these incisions, because this will shrink the conjunctiva and make reapproximation less accurate leading to poorer coverage. I make the 6-o'clock relaxing conjunctival incision first so as to not lose track of the exact 6- or 12-o'clock position. The conjunctiva peritomy should be extended approximately 1.0 mm farther than the last quadrant marker.

The conjunctiva is then grasped at the corner of the peritomy and the relaxing incision lifted and folded back posteriorly. Tenon's is then visualized and dissected posteriorly with Castroviejo scissors.

Since the implants are placed 3.5 mm posterior to the limbus and are 1.5 mm wide, one should plan on resecting Tenon's approximately 5.0 to 6.0 mm. I do not perform any cautery at this time. I then proceed to the adjacent quadrant, again lifting the conjunctiva and folding it backward and resecting Tenon's posteriorly. Whichever quadrant is bleeding the least will be the quadrant where I will begin. That will allow me to deliver a minimal amount of cautery. The quadrant with more bleeding will have time to stop without the use of cauterization. Bipolar pencil-style cautery is used

very sparingly only to enhance visualization, but not to totally blanch the sclera. One must remember that the sclera anterior to the implant is the area that is important for scleral expansion. Avoid cautery in this part of the quadrant. When using the automated technique with the PresVIEW Drive, cautery should not be necessary (Figure 15-13).

The only cauterization that I routinely use is what I refer to as strip cautery, and this is only in the area in which the sclerotomy is to be placed.

One can be slightly more liberal when cauterizing posterior to where the implant is going—in the region 5.0 to 6.0 mm posterior to the limbus. Depending on the patient's comfort level, after tucking back the conjunctiva, I once again place the 4% Xylocaine pledget underneath the conjunctiva on top of the sclera to enhance anesthesia in this area (Figure 15-14).

## Scleral Marking (Manual Method)

After proper exposure, the next step is marking for the sclerotomies. The 4-pronged marker (Presby PY SM 6) is used to place marks on the sclera in preparation for the next step of the procedure. This marker has been nicknamed "La Mesa" or table top, because of its appearance. One pair of prongs is pointed. This pair is 4 mm apart (the width of the belt loop) and are to be placed on the limbus (Figure 15-15).

The points assist with fixation during the marking process. The other 2 prongs are 1.5 mm wide, which is the width of the belt loop. The distance between the pointed and wide prongs is 3.5 mm, which is the distance between the limbus and the anterior portion of the belt loop. Violet dye is put on the tips of the 2 wide prongs so as to facilitate visualization of the exact area for the sclerotomy (Figure 15-16).

The technique that I like best in marking is as follows. The pointed pair of prongs are placed on the limbus in alignment with the quadrant marks placed at the beginning of the case. The conjunctiva is pushed back with a cellulose spear to absorb moisture and gain exposure. The 2 wide prongs are then placed on the limbus. One should place the 4-pronged

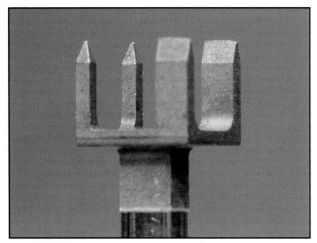

**Figure 15-15.** Four-prong scleral marker.

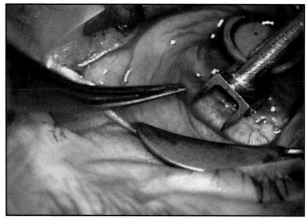

**Figure 15-16.** Four-prong scleral marker in position.

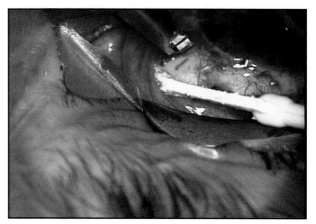

**Figure 15-18.** Scleral reference mark for location of the sclerotomy.

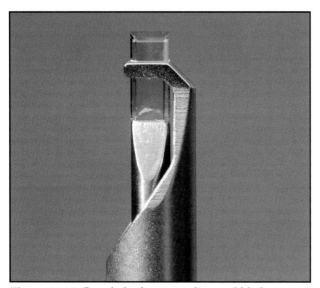

**Figure 15-17.** Guarded sclerotomy diamond blade.

marker on the limbus with the posterior legs of the 4-pronged marker tilted up so as not to touch the conjunctiva or the sclera. Once the limbal placement is satisfactory and good fixation established, one can then rock this 4-pronged marker posteriorly.

At the same time remove any conjunctiva that may be underneath the marker, rotating it until the prongs meet the sclera. The accurate placement of these marks may be confirmed using the scleral belt loop marker (Presby PY BL 3.5-4). This is a double-ended marker with 1 end measuring 4 mm and the other 3.5 mm.

I have found this technique serves to not only fixate the eye during marking, but enhances the control and accuracy of the marks. Globe rotation is prevented, because there are 2 prongs fixating 4.0 mm apart at the limbus. The marks that are on the sclera can be seen in the photograph and dia-

gram precisely representing the placement of the sclerotomy, which is the next surgical step.

## Sclerotomy (Manual Method)

The incisional diamond blade (Presby PY P 15)—guarded blade sclerotomy knife—is then used to make 2 sclerotomies. The guard allows the sclerotomy to be no more than 300 µm deep (Figure 15-17).

The lamella diamond blade (Presby PY P 9) is 1.5 mm wide, which is the exact width of the belt loop. It is of the utmost importance that the 2 sclerotomies be placed in the exact location of the markings. They will be parallel to each other—slightly off perpendicular to the limbus. Once the sclerotomies are made, the surgeon is now ready to create the belt loop using the lamella diamond blade (Figure 15-18).

## Belt Loop Formation (Manual Method)

I have frequently asked new surgeons which step of SSP they feel would be the most difficult. Nearly all of them have felt that making the belt loop would be the most challeng-

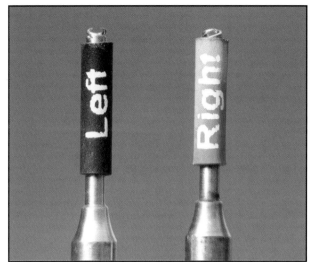

**Figure 15-19.** Left and right rotating scleral twist pick fixators.

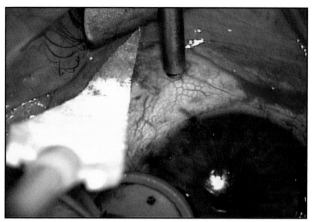

**Figure 15-20.** Twist pick placement in reference to belt loop exit.

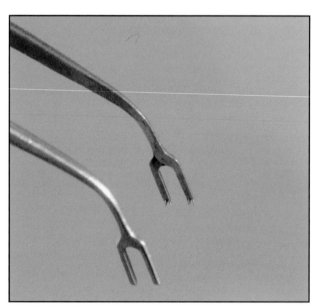

**Figure 15-21.** 0.12 dual fixation forcep.

ing. However, upon completion of their first case, most agree that implant insertion is potentially the most difficult. For this reason, anxiety should not exist related to the creation of the belt loop. Even though belt loop formation is relatively easy, depth and alignment are responsible for the most common errors in technique.

One of the biggest challenges of this procedure is fixation of the globe. Counterpressure is necessary when forming the belt loop and more counterpressure is needed during SEB insertion. I use 3 different fixating devices and will describe each briefly.

The most popular device is the scleral fixator (Presby PY SF2R or 2L) which I refer to as the twist pick (Figures 15-19 and 15-20).

The drawback in using the twist pick is that ocular rotation may occur. However, the advantage is that the pick can be placed just distal to the exit site. With depression, the sclerotomy created earlier will be forced open allowing visibility of the exit for the diamond blade. Following the current discussion on fixation, more details will be given regarding belt loop formation.

A second alternative fixation device is Arrowsmith 0.12 dual fixation forceps by Katena (Denville, NJ). The 2 pair of teeth are separated by 3.0 mm, which allows for easy passage of the 1.5-mm wide lamella diamond blade to pass between these 0.12 forceps and for the implants to be positioned (Figure 15-21).

Countertraction is an obvious necessity during belt loop formation and implant insertion. With the 2 fixating points being 3.0 mm apart, there is a decrease in ocular rotation that can occur with the countertraction. A disadvantage to using the dual fixation forceps is that sometimes, due to the force of countertraction when inserting the implant, this device will not be strong enough to fixate the sclera.

The placement of the fixation device is very important. One should place the fixation device approximately 1.0 to 2.0 mm away from the exit sclerotomy, but centered in line with it. This location makes countertraction more efficient. Additionally this position accompanied by pressure creating scleral indentation can facilitate the exit of the lamella blade or the exit of the SEB implant. The exit of the belt loop will become fishmouth in shape when this indentation is properly performed.

Prior to fixation, one should assess which would be the entrance and the exit portion of the sclerotomy. This determination should be made based on the surgeon's manual dexterity and the exposure of the surgical field.

These 2 issues are factors when deciding which sclerotomy will be used as the entrance for the belt loop formation and implant insertion. Once this has been decided it should be established as a reference during this surgical procedure.

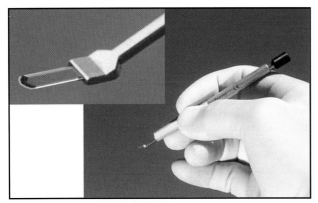

**Figure 15-22.** Lamella diamond blade.

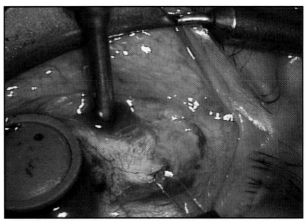

**Figure 15-23.** Lamella diamond blade beginning the belt loop formation.

There are 2 approaches when starting the belt loop with the lamella diamond blade. One approach appears to be intuitively correct, but I believe it results in too shallow of a belt loop. It may, however, be a good beginner's approach. This technique involves placing the lamella blade on the sclera, depressing, and beginning the belt loop by applying a straightforward pressure of the blade through the sclera. This intuitively appears correct, because one is taking advantage of the 300-μm depth of the sclerotomy. When depressing the sclera with the lamella blade flat against the sclera and going straight across, the depth should theoretically be at 300 μm (Figure 15-22).

However, I find the best technique to use to attain an accurate 300+ μm depth is to begin with the blade at about a 30-degree angle with some scleral depression. As soon as the blade has entered the sclera, level out and head toward the exit sclerotomy (Figure 15-23).

In both of these approaches the first assistant has a very important role to clear the small amount of blood that pools near the belt loop area and exit site. This allows visibility permitting greater accuracy and precision when creating the belt loop.

One of the most important steps in this procedure is assuring the depth of the belt loop. In this region the scleral thickness is 530 μm plus or minus 140 μm. Many clinicians believe that there is a marked variance in the thickness of the sclera and also believe that the depth of the implant may be proportional to the resultant accommodation. That is, we have seen that with more superficial implants (ie, thinner belt loops, there tends to be less effect in reference to the amplitude of accommodation gained postoperatively). I have found that the best way to monitor the depth of the belt loop is as follows. As one is passing the lamella blade through the sclera it is best to reflect on our previous cataract techniques. In the 1980s and early 1990s, we were forming scleral pockets in preparation for cataract surgery. It was then taught that as one makes the scleral pocket, the blade should barely be visualized through the sclera and this would assure that we are at approximately one-third the depth of the scle-

ra, this being approximately 200 μm. Although this was fine for the scleral pocket of cataract surgery, it is too superficial for scleral expansion. It seems reasonable that, if there is a thin belt loop when the implant pulls up on the sclera, the sclera will have a greater tendency to stretch rather than exert a pulling force. When there is a deeper (thicker) belt loop, the implants seem to be more stable and may even yield a larger gain in their amplitude in accommodation. Consequently, when passing the lamella diamond blade from the entrance sclerotomy to the exit sclerotomy, the blade should not be visualized. However, if when making the belt loop the bulge created by the passage of the blade is not seen, you are probably beyond the 300 μm depth. For this reason, a good benchmark to use is to pass the lamella blade while looking for the bulge of the blade beneath the sclera. If one can barely see the bulge of the blade beneath the sclera, but not visualize the blade itself, it will most likely be at the correct depth of 300 μm, the diamond blade supplied by Refocus Group Inc (formerly Presby Corp) is of such high quality that no force of the blade other than direct forward movement is necessary.

The blade does not have to be wiggled or moved in a fan-like fashion. If this motion were to be used, the entrance of the belt loop may be stretched, and implant stability may be compromised (Figure 15-24).

As seen in the diagram, the beveled tip of the lamella blade is designed in such a way that as one is making the belt loop, the bulge is not seen at the tip. Rather, it is seen approximately 0.50 mm behind that where the bevel begins to meet the full thickness of the lamella blade. For this reason, as one is preparing to exit the belt loop, one should anticipate the additional length of the blade. Approximately 0.50 to 0.75 mm prior to the exit, where the bulge is seen, the blade should be lifted slightly and the sclera depressed at the exit site so as to accommodate the blade coming out at the desired location. If one pulls up too early, the belt loop

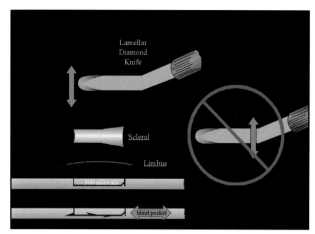

**Figure 15-24.** Proper and improper lamella diamond blade movement.

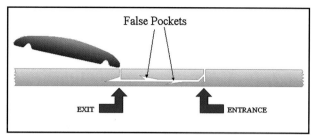

**Figure 15-25.** Implant approach for belt loop insertion.

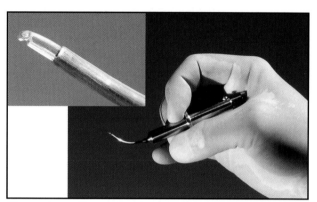

**Figure 15-26.** Proper hand position.

will be very thin at the exit site, and if one does not pull up in time, there will be an undercut as seen in the diagram (Figure 15-25).

If recognized by the surgeon, steps can be taken to avoid problems during SEB implant insertion. This will be discussed later. Furthermore, if one wishes to change the depth of the lamella blade as it passes in formation of the belt loop, one needs to slightly back the blade out. This can create various defects in the belt loop as illustrated in the diagram and ultimately affect implant insertion.

In thin sclera or very deep belt loops, it is not unusual to see a small amount of choroidal pigment coming from the sclerotomy site.

I have seen this on approximately 5 or 6 occasions, and there have been no consequences from this. However, when this is seen, one has to be aware that there is either very thin sclera or a defect in the scleral bed lying beneath the belt loop. It is of utmost importance to recognize this prior to placing the implant. Once the lamella blade has exited the sclerotomy site, one should make sure that the blade is fully passed through the exit sclerotomy in order to ensure a wide exit point for the future placement of the implant. Once the cutting portion of the blade is outside the scleral pocket, it may not be a bad idea to slightly wiggle the tip to widen ever so slightly at the exit point. This will facilitate implant placement in the next step. As one pulls the blade back out of the newly formed belt loop, one has to be sure that the globe is not intorted or extorted. In this situation, as the blade exits, the cutting portion could inadvertently widen the entrance point to the belt loop by cutting it. A suture will not help this situation, and the possibility of implant migration postoperatively will be increased.

During the formation of the belt loop, it is important for the assistant to constantly clear the surface sclera so the blade placement can be accurately assessed by direct visualization. Likewise, the exit site needs to be constantly visualized so one can direct the lamella blade when making the belt loop directly toward the exit site and not at an angle to it.

## Implant Insertion

The efficient way to proceed to the next step of implant insertion is by maintaining globe fixation, especially if good fixation is already established. The assistant will then hand the implant loaded in the implant inserter (Presby PY IN 6.1) or implant forceps to the surgeon (Figure 15-26).

It is important to decide at this point whether the implant should be placed upside down and then rotated or placed directly right side up through the belt loop. The following consideration should be made in making this decision.

If there is any difficulty in forming the belt loop, whether being excessively deep (especially if pigment is seen) or needing to change direction of the lamella blade during formation of the belt loop, one should opt for putting the implant in upside down.

As can be seen in the diagram, one must realize that when inserting the implant, if it is placed right side up, the leading nose of the implant has a tendency to want to project inwardly or toward the inner globe. This is due not only to the shape of the implant, but also because the tight scleral belt loop pushes down constantly on the implant as it is being inserted. If the scleral bed (the portion of sclera under the belt loop) is too thin, the implant will penetrate the underlying sclera and enter the suprachoroidal space. I have had this occur in my own hands and have seen it many times in first-time surgeons. It has been in my experience that no serious side effects whatsoever will occur from this. I am personally aware of 2 implants that have totally gone within this

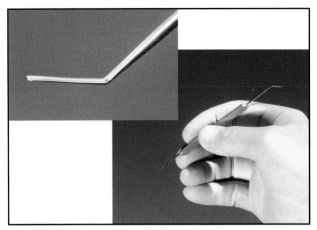

**Figure 15-27.** Spatula for checking belt loop integrity/patency.

suprachoroidal space and were left there. It has now been over 2 years with no significant sequelae occurring. Of course, the effect the implant has on scleral expansion is markedly decreased.

Yet another consideration to take into account regarding the insertion of the implant in the right side up position is the belt loop itself. This approach should be taken if the belt loop is particularly thin or if the entrance or exit sclerotomies are stretched out or enlarged. However, if the belt loop is particularly deep (thick) or there are undercuts or defects within the belt loop, the implant should be placed in upside down.

When inserting the implant right side up, it is easier to place the implant within the entrance point first, because it is traditionally a little wider and will allow for a little easier initial insertion. In order to get the insertion of the implant started, it has to be delivered at about a 45-degree angle and inserted into the sclerotomy and belt loop. This angle is maintained until the underside notch of the implant is reached (which is 0.75 mm from the end of the implant). At this point, the implant is pushed into the belt loop without advancing the inserter plunger. Once the portion of the implant that is exposed at the tip of the inserter is within the belt loop, the tip of the inserter should be angled up enough to prevent the tip of the implant from tearing the sclera at the base of the belt loop. Once this angle is maneuvered, the plunger of the inserter can begin to be advanced.

This maneuver will prevent the leading edge of the implant from damaging the scleral bed beneath or penetrating or tearing this portion of sclera. Of equal importance is the hand that is holding the fixation device. As the implant is being inserted, the fixation device held in the other hand applies an equal counter pressure—ie, as the implant is being inserted the fixation device is pushed toward the implant. This slightly puckers the sclerotomy exit opening provided

appropriate scleral depression of the fixation device is applied. The exit site of the sclerotomy will then pucker like a fishmouth and will allow an easier exit of the leading edge of the implant being inserted. If fixation is lost during this counter pressure maneuver, one can try refixating or even change to a different fixating device. Likewise, if one is using the twist pick (clockwise or counterclockwise), one must remember to apply the appropriate rotational force in order to maintain fixation on the sclera. By not applying this rotational force, one can inadvertently rotate the twist pick, and fixation will be lost. Another key point on using the twist pick is that one has to rotate the twist pick at least 360 degrees in order to achieve good scleral fixation.

The belt loop should be very tight, and it is often at this point just prior to the implant exiting the sclerotomy site that a lot of pressure needs to be exerted. Sometimes a slight wiggling of the implant will help and if one feels that the implant cannot be exited, the implant can be removed and inserted from the other direction or inserted upside down.

Often, exiting is difficult, because this exit site is always a little tighter than the entrance site when making the belt loop. Once the implant is inserted from the exit site as it approaches the original entrance to the belt loop, its advancement from the belt loop will be much easier. It is easier for 2 reasons. First, the entrance of the belt loop is a little larger because the entire length of the lamellar blade has been passed through this portion of the belt loop. Second, this portion of the belt loop has been stretched by the first attempt of the implant insertion.

When the implant is nearly ready to exit, but not quite, one can use the spatula (Presby PY SP 1.4) to depress the sclera and use the spatula as a ramp for the implant to exit over (Figure 15-27).

If the spatula is placed parallel to the belt loop, only very mild countertraction can be applied safely. If too much pressure is applied, the spatula will unexpectedly slip into the suprachoriodal space. For this reason, I place the spatula parallel to the sclerotomy and perpendicular to the belt loop. This will then allow the surgeon to exert as much counterpressure as is necessary. There is another helpful way to utilize the spatula. When making the belt loop or prior to placing the implant, it is often beneficial to insert the spatula all the way through the sclerotomy site and slightly depress in order to push back and compress the underlying scleral (scleral bed). This maneuver also verifies the belt loop space.

If the exit sclerotomy appears to be a little tight, the spatula can be used to slightly stretch this out thus making the exiting of the implant a little easier (Figure 15-28).

The following conditions should alert the surgeon as to the possibility of needing to place the implant in upside down. The advantage of placing the implant upside down is that the leading edge of the implant does not have a tendency to "submarine" into the suprachoroidal space, but rather it hugs the undersurface of the belt loop and allows for an easier exit. The disadvantage of upside-down insertion is that the belt loop is slightly stretched by rotating the implant back into its upright position. Submarineing of the implant can occur when inserted from either the entrance or exit side of the sclerotomy. The first indication for upside-down insertion is when the belt loop is particularly deep or if choroidal pigmentation is seen at either sclerotomy site.

Also, if during the belt loop formation there was a retraction of the lamella blade due to inadvertent swallowing and/or deepening of the belt loop, consider inserting the implant upside down. This implant insertion approach will avoid blind pockets (notches in the belt loop).

In addition, if there is an undercut past the end of the sclerotomy site, it would be avoided by placing the implant upside down. Furthermore, if there was any misdirection of the belt loop, it should also be placed upside-down. When inserting the implant upside-down, the position of the implant has to be greater than a 45-degree angle toward the entrance point of the sclerotomy in order to get the tip of the implant into the belt loop.

Once the implant is in past the notch on the implant, then the inserter can be angled back down parallel to the sclera, thus lifting the leading edge of the implant. This lift does not have to be done as much as when the implant is placed right-side-up.

Upside-down insertion avoids the leading edge of the implant digging into the sclera at the base of the belt loop (that portion of the belt loop just overlying the choroid). In this technique, the inserter with the implant loaded is positioned tip up as it is inserted through the belt loop. This insertion position will facilitate the exit of the implant out of the belt loop. In this manner the leading edge of the implant will not catch the scleral edge upon exiting. If difficulty is still encountered prior to implant exiting, counterpressure is needed in order to push the implant through the belt loop. It should be noted here that no viscoelastic or other lubricating material should be used to help the implant slide through the sclera, because whatever allows the implant to slide in easily will also allow the implant to slide out easily. To prevent postoperative subluxation, none of these lubricants should be considered. In addition, any viscoelastic agent underneath the conjunctiva causes a prolonged swelling and conjunctival edema and will prevent early adhesion of Tenon's and conjunctiva to the surface of the belt loop, which will help secure the implant in place. We learned this from experience, which again emphasizes the reason that I encourage surgeons starting out to refrain from making any changes.

Once the implant being inserted upside-down has exited and has equal portions extending out of both ends of the belt loop, the implant is now ready to be rotated.

There are 2 basic techniques for rotating a implant once it has been placed. The first technique that I developed was

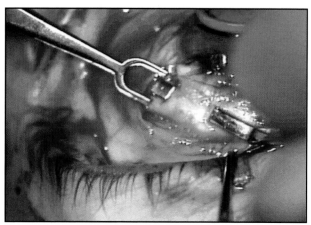

**Figure 15-28.** Spatula in the belt loop with 0.12 dual fixation forceps.

to use 0.12 Castroviejo forceps, which because of the angle of the tip allows the implant to be grasped across its width.

The surgeon should position his or her wrist and hand in such a fashion so as to anticipate the 180-degree rotation and allow this movement to be made in 1 smooth step. Often, due to poor exposure or other difficulties, this cannot be achieved, so a second 0.12 forceps can be used at the other end of the implant. Once the implant is rotated halfway, the other forceps is used to grab the opposite end of the implant and it is rotated the remaining 90 degrees. If the implant is not extended evenly on either side of the belt loop, the edge of the implant that is least prominent should be the one that is grasped by the forceps and rotated.

The reason for this is that, as one rotates with the forceps, it has a tendency to pull out the implant, and if one were to grab the edge of the implant that is projecting the most, the other end may fall back into the belt loop. If the surgeon uses the channeled forceps for SEB insertion, the implant can be rotated with these forceps as soon as the leading edge of the implant has exited the belt loop (Figure 15-29).

Because we believe that the accommodative effect may be proportional to the depth of the implant, the tendency for experienced surgeons is to place the implant deeper. The deeper the implant, the more likely it is that it will have to be put upside-down. Currently, I find myself placing many implants upside-down followed by rotation. Once the implant is in position, one has to make sure it is symmetrically exiting on either side of the belt loop (Figure 15-30).

This is particularly important, because the notches on the underside of the implant should be aligned with the edge of the sclerotomy site. This is the reason for the precise 4.0 mm width of the initial 4-prong marker. This allows the edge of the sclera to ride up into the notch and prevent the implant from subluxating.

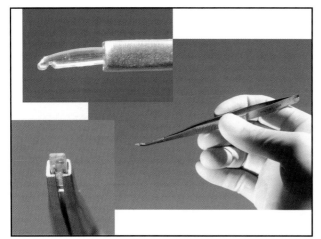

**Figure 15-29.** Channel forcep with implant loaded.

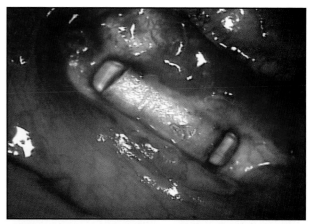

**Figure 15-30.** Properly positioned SEB implant in the belt loop.

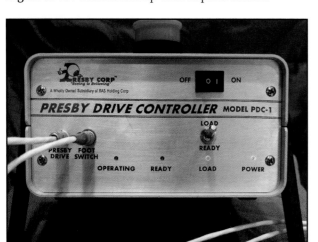

**Figure 15-31.** PresVIEW Drive control unit.

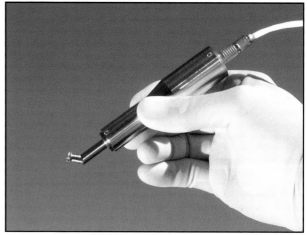

**Figure 15-32.** PresVIEW Drive with proper hand.

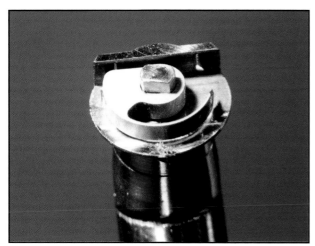

**Figure 15-33.** PresVIEW Drive top view with blade in place.

## PresVIEW Drive (Automated Belt Loop Maker)

The PresVIEW Drive is a highly sophisticated automated instrument designed to make the sclerotomy and belt loop in one single step. This instrument allows for greater uniformity and consistency among surgeons (Figures 15-31 through 34).

Numerous surgeons have been performing the SSP surgery worldwide and have found a variation of accommodation. Since these variations are consistent with the FDA Phase I Trials, further investigation was warranted. The findings revealed variability in the depth of the belt loop. A surgeon's natural instinct is to create a shallow belt loop. A lack of depth will result in a decrease in the gain of accommodation. This variable is eliminated through the development of the automatic belt loop maker called the PresVIEW Drive.

The PresVIEW Drive device has a rotating arcuate blade that passes through a slotted foot plate to make a belt loop 400 µm deep. The disposable blade advances to form the belt loop with foot pedal control. The control unit has a convenient abort button if progression of the blade needs to be stopped.

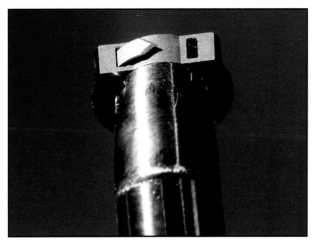

**Figure 15-34.** PresVIEW Drive underside view with partially advanced blade.

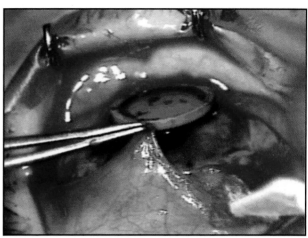

**Figure 15-35.** Pulling the conjunctiva over the SEB implant.

After completion of the belt loop, the PresVIEW Drive automatically senses the completed belt loop and retracts to the original position in preparation for the next belt loop. The speed and precision of belt loop formation with the PresVIEW Drive enables the surgeon to form all 4 belt loops consecutively.

It is apparent that the PresVIEW Drive will eliminate the need for the sclerotomy diamond blade and lamellar diamond blade in formation of the belt loop. Additionally the PresVIEW Drive has a limbal mark on its neck and the base plate is sized for a perfect belt loop length. These features eliminate the 4-prong marking step necessary during manual belt loop formation. Because scleral marks and visualization of the lamellar blade as it passes through the belt loop are not required, cautery is not necessary. Eliminating cautery saves time and decreases postoperative inflammation. Early clinical experience has demonstrated a marked improvement in postoperative recovery time using the PresVIEW Drive.

After the conjunctiva and tenons have been dissected, the PresVIEW Drive is placed on the sclera in the appropriate quadrant. The twist pick provides countertraction for stable and precise positioning while activating the PresVIEW Drive on the surface of the eye. When ready, the surgeon simply steps on the pedal to activate the PresVIEW Drive.

The ease of operation and handling of the PresVIEW Drive makes this an invaluable adjunct to SSP. The PresVIEW Drive replaces nearly half of the steps in the SSP procedure, reducing operating time by as much as 50%. The surgical time can be shortened even more if all 4 belt loops are made at once (avoiding passing the PresVIEW Drive back and forth to the scrub tech).

## Closing the Conjunctiva and Completion

After the implant is in position, the conjunctiva is pulled over the implant, the adjacent implant insertion is begun. Once both implants are placed inferiorly, the conjunctiva is then stretched over the implant and repositioned (Figure 15-35).

The 2 corners of the conjunctiva are then identified and a single 10-0 nylon suture is placed at the 6-o'clock position (12 o'clock for the superior conjunctiva) in a buried knot fashion taking a scleral bite to prevent the migration of conjunctiva.

Often if the conjunctiva is stretched or torn prior to placing the 10-0 nylon in the sclera, one should pull the conjunctiva and make sure the extreme aspects do provide sufficient coverage. This coverage should mean that the conjunctiva should be within 1.0 to 1.5 mm of its original insertion. If it is not, the suture bite should take a little extra conjunctiva and pull it toward the 6- or 12-o'clock position in order to pull it tighter. Only a single suture is necessary, and it has provided adequate coverage in all my cases.

Once the 2 inferior implants have been placed, the patient is then asked to look downward and the process is repeated. At this time, one may note that the quadrant mark may be worn or faded, and at this time, they should be remarked, and often the marker is not necessary. The pen itself may be enough to remark these quadrant marks.

## Postoperative

At the conclusion of the case, the pupil should be observed and if it is dilated or asymmetrical, 1% pilocarpine should be given to assure the pupil comes down and is round and symmetrical. If there is any oblique shape to the pupil, pilocarpine should be applied and the patient observed closely until the pupil is round.

The patient's eyes are patched only if there is a corneal abrasion. Otherwise, no patching is necessary. For the most part, the postoperative pain usually only requires extra strength acetaminophen, but there have been a few patients who have had more significant pain. Of course, if there is any corneal abrasion, I would hesitate putting on a collagen shield or contact lens, because this could migrate underneath the conjunctiva and prevent it from sealing down around the implant. Postoperative eye drops include antibiotic Ciloxan (Alcon, Fort Worth, Tex) and usually Flarex (Alcon) or other mild steroid is sufficient. For cases of marked inflammation postoperatively, one can change to a prednisone acetate 1% or even add Voltaren (CIBA Vision, Duluth, Ga). This is very rare, however, and most of the patients tolerate the postoperative irritation. The surgeon can often anticipate increased postoperative inflammation based on the presence of pigment from the belt loop or difficulty in implant insertion.

## REHABILITATION

SSP patients must undergo rehabilitative eye exercises to ensure optimal results. The ciliary muscle of these presbyopes has not been used for a number of years and requires physical therapy.

Before the exercises are started the quality and quantity of the tear film must be evaluated. During the first few weeks, the conjunctiva is swollen over the implants. This prevents the eyelids from spreading the tear adequately and artificial tears are necessary. Tears should be used every 2 hours and a bland ointment at bedtime. Sometimes punctal plugs are also necessary.

The accommodative exercise is called the push-up/push-out technique. The patient is given a reading card and told to hold it at 10 cm from their eyes. They are to focus on the smallest line they can see and then concentrate without squinting and see if they can see any letters on the next smaller line. This exercise is repeated as the patient slowly moves the near card away from their eyes while keeping the smaller line in focus until the near card is at arm's length. Then have the patient bring the near card slowly back up to 10 cm from his or her eyes while trying to keep the same line

in focus. Once the card is 10 cm from their eyes then they are instructed to try and see the next smaller line. This exercise should be done 6 to 8 times in each eye, 4 to 5 times a day.

Push-up exercises using a pencil or other nonaccommodative target will direct its affect more toward convergence than accommodation. The patient must focus on print while doing the eye exercises in order to increase ciliary muscle function. It has been found that it is better to start at near and move the target away, as described above, than to start with the target farther away and bring it close.

## OUTCOMES

The average preoperative amplitude of accommodation was 2.10 D, with a range of 1.30 to 3.10 D. Postoperatively, the patients had very impressive mean amplitude of accommodation of 5.90 D with a range of 1.80 to 11.10 D. The adjusted mean net gain of the amplitude of accommodation was 3.80 D. The postoperative gain in the amplitude of accommodation of the patients who had monocular surgery was nearly equal to the individual eyes of the patients who had binocular surgery. The binocular patients are more satisfied with their results.

The average time required for the patients to reach their maximum postoperative amplitude of accommodation is 1.5 months.

## REFERENCES

Cross WD, Zdenek GW. Surgical reversal of presbyopia. In: Agarwal S, et al, eds. *Refractive Surgery.* New Dehli, India: Jaypee Brothers. 2000;592-608.

Fukasaku H. Silcone expansion plug implant surgery for presbyopia. Presented at: American Society of Cataract and Refractive Surgery Symposium; May 21, 2000; Boston, Ma.

Schachar RA. Cause and treatment of presbyopia with a method for increasing the amplitude of accommodation. *Ann Ophthalmol.* 1992;24:445-452.

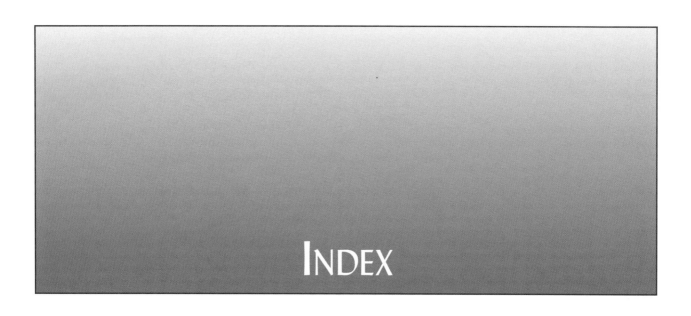

# INDEX

aberrometry, wavefront, in astigmatism, 152-154
accommodation. *See also* presbyopia
    IOLs for, 93-99, 261-265, 267-272
    terminology of, 261
accommodative esotropia, in hyperopia, surgical treatment
    of, 207-209
acetazolamide, for uveitis, after cataract surgery, 70
adhesions, iris, cataract surgery in, in pseudoexfoliation syn-
    drome, 118-119
against-the-rule astigmatism, 49, 52, 54
alcohol, for epithelial removal, in photorefractive keratecto-
    my, 248
Allergan Medical Optics teledioptric implants, 140, 145-146
ALRI (anterior limbal relaxing incisions), for astigmatism,
    11, 12-13, 161-163
amblyopia, with congenital cataract, 24, 25
anesthesia. *See specific procedures*
angiography, fluorescein, in uveitis, 64
angle-supported (Baikoff) phakic lens, 221
aniridia, cataract surgery in, 3-10
anterior capsule, management of, in congenital cataract, 25-28
anterior limbal relaxing incisions (ALRI), for astigmatism,
    11, 12-13, 161-163
anterior vitrectomy, in dislocated lens removal, 44
arcuate incisions, for astigmatism correction, 48, 51, 53
Array multifocal IOL, 101-108, 267-268, 270

Artisan phakic lens, 212-213, 217-222
aspiration, in cataract surgery, in uveitis, 66-68
ASSORT program, for astigmatism treatment planning,
    154-157
astigmatism, corneal. *See* corneal astigmatism
astigmatomes, 49, 54

Baikoff angle-supported phakic lens, 221
band keratopathy, in uveitis, cataract surgery in, 65
Bechert Rotator, in phacoemulsification, 123
belt loop formation, in presbyopia surgery, 279-282, 285-286
betamethasone, subconjunctival, after pediatric cataract sur-
    gery, 30
bioptics
    in cataract surgery, 11-22, 177-180
        anterior corneal relaxing incisions in, 12-13
        complications of, 19-20
        definition of, 20-21, 177
        equipment for, 16
        measurement for, 13-14
        options for, 11, 21-22
        preoperative conditions and, 16-18
        preoperative marking for, 14-15
        technique for, 15-16
        toric IOLs in. *See* toric intraocular lenses
    pseudophakic, 179-180

blades
  for astigmatism correction, 15-16, 49, 53-56
  in Intacs procedure, 241
  in presbyopia surgery, 279, 281-282

can-opener capsulorrhexis, 26
Canrobert "C" procedure, for astigmatism, 53
capsular tension rings, in cataract surgery, in zonular dialy-
      ses, 36-41
capsule
  anterior, management of, in congenital cataract, 25-28
  posterior. *See* posterior capsule
capsule retraction syndrome, after cataract surgery, in
      uveitis, 72
capsulorrhexis
  in aniridia, 6-7
  can-opener, 26
  in congenital cataract, 25-29
  continuous curvilinear. *See* continuous curvilinear capsu-
        lorrhexis
  vitrector, 26
  in zonular dialyses, 37-38
catadioptric posterior chamber implants, 140
cataract formation, after phakic lens implantation,
      223-224, 235
cataract surgery
  accommodating lens in, 93-99, 261-265, 267-272
  in aniridia, 3-10
  bioptics in, 11-22, 177-180
  in congenital cataract, 23-34
  in corneal astigmatism. *See* corneal astigmatism
  in dislocated and subluxated lenses, 43-46
  extracapsular, in uveitis, 66-68
  in glaucoma. *See* glaucoma, cataract surgery in
  in hypermature cataract, 109-112
  in hyperopia, 11-22, 192
  implant malposition after, 73-83, 127-128
  intracapsular, in uveitis, 66
  intraocular lens exchange and, 85-87
      for malposition, 80-81
      multifocal, 103
  laser, 89-92
  multifocal lens in, 101-108, 267-268
  in myopia, bioptics in, 11-22
  piggyback intraocular lens implantation in, 133-137, 170
  PRELEX (*PRE*sbyopic *L*ens *EX*change) procedure,
        268-272
  in pseudoexfoliation syndrome, 113-132
  telescopic intraocular lens in, 139-147
  in uveitis, 63-72
  in zonular dialyses, 35-42, 76, 128
CCC. *See* continuous curvilinear capsulorrhexis
CCI (clear-corneal incision)
  for astigmatism correction, 49, 53, 54

  for cataract surgery, in pseudoexfoliation syndrome, 117
children, cataract surgery in, 23-34
Choyce anterior chamber intraocular implant, 140
CIBA-Medennium phakic refractive lens, 228-236
  for astigmatism, 233-234
  complications of, 234-235
  evaluation for, 230
  postoperative management of, 233
  properties of, 228-230
  technique for, 230-233
Cionni modified capsular tension rings, in cataract surgery,
      in zonular dialyses, 36-41
claws, on Artisan phakic lens, 212-213, 217-222
clear-corneal incision
  for astigmatism correction, 49, 53, 54
  for cataract surgery, in pseudoexfoliation syndrome, 117
computer-assisted videokeratography, in astigmatism, 153
conductive thermal keratoplasty
  in bioptic procedures, 22
  for hyperopia, 181-185
congenital conditions, cataract surgery in, 23-34
  aniridia, 3-10
  indications for, 25
  lenses for, 31-32
  in neonates, 30
  preoperative evaluation in, 23-25
  technique for, 25-31
  timing of, 25
  for unilateral vs. bilateral cataracts, 24-25
contact lens, implantable, for cataract with astigmatism, 56-58
continuous curvilinear capsulorrhexis
  anterior, 26-28
  in lens malposition prevention, 74-76
  posterior, 28-29
  in pseudoexfoliation syndrome, 119-121
contrast sensitivity, with multifocal IOL, 102-103
cornea. *See also subjects starting with* kera-
  anatomy of, 187-189
  decompensation of, after phakic lens implantation, 224
  edema of, in phakic lens implantation, 234
  erosions of, after corneal refractive surgery, 200-201
  haze on, in photorefractive keratectomy, 250
  rings in, 11, 22, 237-244
  surface ablation of, in bioptic procedures, 21
corneal astigmatism, 47-61
  against-the-rule, 49, 52, 54
  with cataract
    bioptic correction of. *See* bioptics
    incisional correction of, 12-20, 48-55
    intraocular correction of, 55-60, 135-136, 165-170
    reduction of, 161-163
    six-step management system for, 59-60
  classification of, 47-48
  after corneal refractive surgery, 199-200

irregular, 151, 158-159
measurement of, 152-153
optical, 152-153
phakic lenses for, 233-234
PRELEX (*PRE*sbyopic *L*ens *EX*change) procedure for, 271
regular, 151
residual, 151, 154-156
shape-related, 153
surgical treatment of, 153-157
three-dimensional view of, 161
types of, 151
with-the-rule, 52, 54
cortex, management of, in pseudoexfoliation syndrome, 124
corticosteroids, for uveitis, 65
Crystal keratome, in cataract surgery, in pseudoexfoliation syndrome, 118
Crystalens accommodative IOL, 93-99
cycloplegics, after cataract surgery, in uveitis, 70
cystoid macular edema, in cataract surgery, in aniridia, 8

debridement, in photorefractive keratectomy, 248
decentration
    in corneal procedures
        LASIK, 253
        photorefractive keratectomy, 250
    of intraocular lenses. *See* intraocular lens(es), malposition of
dexamethasone
    after pediatric cataract surgery, 30
    for uveitis, 65
diamond blades/knives, for astigmatism correction, 15-16, 49, 53-56
dislocation, of intraocular lenses. *See* intraocular lens(es), malposition of
Dodick Photolysis system, for cataract extraction, 89-92
dry eye
    corneal incisions in, 17
    hyperopia with, surgical treatment of, 191

ectasia
    after corneal refractive surgery, 201
    Intacs procedure in, 243-244
edema, corneal, in phakic lens implantation, 234
emmetropia, refractive lens exchange in, 106
emulsification. *See* phacoemulsification
endocapsular rings, for aniridia, 4-9
epiphora, after corneal refractive surgery, 199
epithelium
    delayed healing of, in photorefractive keratectomy, 249
    ingrowth of
        after corneal refractive surgery, 200
        after LASIK, 254-255
    loss of
        in LASIK, 253
        in pseudoexfoliation syndrome, 128

removal of, in photorefractive keratectomy, 248-248
esotropia, accommodative, in hyperopia, surgical treatment of, 207-209
exchange, of intraocular lenses, 85-87
    for malposition, 80-81
    multifocal, 103
    presbyopic, 267-272
excimer laser photorefractive keratectomy. *See* photorefractive keratectomy (PRK)
explantation, of intraocular lenses, 85, 211
extracapsular cataract surgery, for uveitis, 66-68
EyeSys corneal topographical system, 13-14

Feaster diamond blades, for astigmatism correction, 49, 55
flap complications
    in LASEK, 257
    in LASIK, 253-255
fluorescein angiography, in uveitis, 64
foreign body sensation, after corneal refractive surgery, 198-199
Fyodorov technique, for astigmatism correction, 48

Galilean telescope. *See* telescopic intraocular lenses
genetic factors, in congenital cataract, 24-25
Gills technique, for astigmatism correction, 48, 51, 52
glare disability
    after cataract surgery, in aniridia, 9
    after corneal refractive surgery, 199
glaucoma
    cataract surgery in
        aniridia, 9
        phacolytic phacomorphic, 109-112
        with pseudoexfoliation syndrome, 114
        uveitis, 66
    after corneal refractive surgery, 201
    after phakic lens implantation, 223-224
guided trephine system, for astigmatism correction, 49, 54, 55

Hanna arcitome, 49
Helmholtz theory, of accommodation, 94
herpes virus infections, keratouveitis in, cataract surgery in, 65
HumanOptics accommodative IOL, 261-265
hydrodissection, in cataract surgery
    in pseudoexfoliation syndrome, 121-122
    in zonular dialyses, 38
hydroxypropyl methylcellulose, in phakic lens implantation, 217-221
hyperopia
    with accommodative esotropia and/or nystagmus, 207-209
    bioptic correction of. *See* bioptics
    conductive thermal keratoplasty for, 181-185
    LASEK for, 187-205
        complications of, 198-201

contraindications for, 189
corneal anatomic and physiologic considerations in, 187-189
indications for, 189
outcomes of, 201-203
patient selection for, 189-192
postoperative management of, 193-198
preoperative evaluation for, 189-190
techniques for, 192-193
LASIK for, 187-205
complications of, 198-201
contraindications for, 189
corneal anatomic and physiologic considerations in, 187-189
indications for, 189
outcomes of, 201-203
patient selection for, 189-192
postoperative management of, 193-198
preoperative evaluation for, 189-190
techniques for, 192-193
multifocal IOLs for, 101-108
phakic lenses for. *See* phakic intraocular lenses
photorefractive keratectomy for, 187-205
complications of, 198-201
contraindications for, 189
corneal anatomic and physiologic considerations in, 187-189
indications for, 189
outcomes of, 201-203
patient selection for, 189-192
postoperative management of, 193-198
preoperative evaluation for, 189-190
techniques for, 192-193
piggyback IOLs for, 133-137
PRELEX procedure for, 269
after radial keratotomy, 171-175
hypertension, ocular. *See* intraocular pressure, increased
hyphema, after phakic lens implantation, 223
hypotony, in cataract surgery
in aniridia, 8
in uveitis, 66

ICRs (intracorneal rings), 11, 22, 237-244
implantable contact lens, for cataract with astigmatism, 56-58
implantable miniaturized telescopic intraocular lenses, 140-141, 143-144, 146
incisional correction, of corneal astigmatism with cataract, 48-55
bioptics with, 12-20
complications of, 19-20
history of, 48
instrumentation for, 16, 49, 54-56
marking for, 14-15

measurement for, 13-14
planning for, 48-53
preoperative conditions and, 16-18
indocyanine green, for capsulorrhexis, in congenital cataract, 26-27
indomethacin, for uveitis, 65
inflammation, in uveitis, control of, 65
Intacs procedure, 237-244
intracapsular cataract surgery, for uveitis, 66
intracorneal rings (ICRs), 11
in bioptic procedures, 22
Intacs system, 237-244
intralenticular opacification, in piggyback IOL use, 136
intraocular lens(es)
accommodating, 93-99, 261-265, 267-272
in anterior chamber, 86
for astigmatism, 19-21, 55-60, 161-163
exchange of, 85-87
for malposition, 80-81
multifocal, 103
presbyopic, 267-272
explantation of, 85, 211
foldable, explanation of, 80
for hyperopia, 101-108, 133-137, 173-174
iris fixation of, 79, 86
malposition of, 73-83
damage control and, 75-78
etiology of, 74
phakic, 235
prevention of, 74-75
in pseudoexfoliation syndrome, 127-128
symptoms of, 73
treatment of, 78-81, 85-87
multifocal, 101-108, 267-268
for myopia, 139-147, 173-174
for pediatric patients, 31-32
phakic. *See* phakic intraocular lenses
piggyback, 133-137, 170
posterior support of, in zonular dialyses, 36-40
power calculation for, 214
with prosthetic iris, 4-9
pseudoaccommodative, 267-272
for pseudoexfoliation syndrome, 127-128
removal of, in uveitis, 72
scleral fixation of, 86-87
second, 81
telescopic, 139-147
toric. *See* toric intraocular lenses
for uveitis, 67-68, 70, 72
intraocular pressure, increased. *See also* glaucoma
in hyperopia, 191-192
in phakic lens implantation, 234
after photorefractive keratectomy, 250
in pseudoexfoliation syndrome, 128

IOLs. *See* intraocular lens(es)

iridectomy, in phakic lens implantation, 217, 230-231

iridotomy

in glaucoma, in cataract surgery, 66

in uveitis, 69-70

iris

absence of (aniridia), cataract surgery in, 3-10

adhesions of, cataract surgery in, in pseudoexfoliation syndrome, 118-119

forward position of, in phacomorphic glaucoma, 111-112

IOL fixation to, 79, 86

phakic lens anchored to, 213-214, 217-222

iris bombé, after cataract surgery, in uveitis, 71

iris capture, after cataract surgery, in uveitis, 71

irregular astigmatism, 151, 158-159

irrigation, in cataract surgery, in uveitis, 66-68

ischemic optic neuropathy, after corneal refractive surgery, 201

Kenalog, after vitreous removal, 40-41

keratectomy

photorefractive. *See* photorefractive keratectomy (PRK)

phototherapeutic, after radial keratotomy, 173

keratitis

after corneal refractive surgery, 199, 200

diffuse lamellar, after LASIK, 254

after photorefractive keratectomy, 250

keratoconus

hyperopia in, surgical treatment of, 191

Intacs procedure in, 243-244

keratometry

in astigmatism, 153-154

for toric IOLs, 168-169

keratopathy

band, in uveitis, cataract surgery in, 65

punctate epithelial, after LASIK, 254

keratoplasty

conductive, 22, 181-185

laser thermal, 173, 183-184

thermal, 22, 181-185

keratopyramis phenomenon, in keratotomy, 20

keratotomy

astigmatic, 48-55, 233-234

radial, 21-22, 171-175

KeraVision Intacs, 238-244

knives. *See* blades

Kozoil-Peyman teledioptric posterior chamber intraocular lens, 140, 143, 145-146

Krumeich Guided Trephine System, for astigmatism correction, 49, 54, 55

LASEK (laser-assisted epithelial keratomileusis), 11

for astigmatism, 153-159

in bioptic procedures, 21

for hyperopia, 187-205

with accommodative esotropia and/or nystagmus, 207-209

for myopia, 256-257

laser(s). *See also* LASEK; LASIK

in astigmatism correction, 234

in cataract surgery, 89-92

in glaucoma, 66

in phakic lens implantation, 231

in photorefractive keratectomy. *See* photorefractive keratectomy (PRK)

laser thermal keratoplasty (LTK)

vs. conductive keratoplasty, 183-184

after radial keratotomy, 173

LASIK (laser-assisted in-situ keratomileusis)

for astigmatism, 153-159

in bioptic procedures, 21, 177-180

complications of, 253-255

vs. conductive keratoplasty, 183-184

for hyperopia, 187-205

with accommodative esotropia and/or nystagmus, 207-209

limitations of, 212

for myopia, 250-256

after radial keratotomy, 172

lasso technique, after radial keratotomy, 174

lens (artificial), intraocular. *See* intraocular lens(es)

lens (contact), implantable, for cataract with astigmatism, 56-58

lens (natural)

dislocated or subluxated, cataract with, 43-46

removal of, in congenital cataract, 28

subluxation of, in zonular dialyses, 35-37

lens particle glaucoma, cataract surgery in, 110-111

lens protein glaucoma, cataract surgery in, 109-110

lensectomy, 173-174. *See also* cataract surgery; intraocular lens(es)

macular degeneration, age-related, telescopic IOLs for, 139-147

malposition, of intraocular lenses. *See* intraocular lens(es), malposition of

manifest refraction, in astigmatism, 152

Marfan syndrome, cataract surgery in, 35-37

Martin's Nasal Corneal Relaxing Nomogram, 12

Mendez axis gauge, for astigmatism correction, 15, 55, 56, 58

microkeratomes, in LASIK, 251-252

miotics, for malpositioned lens, 79

modified capsular tension rings, in cataract surgery, in zonular dialyses, 36-41

monovision techniques, for presbyopia, 267

Morcher prosthetic iris, 4-9

multifocal intraocular lenses, 101-108, 267-268

mydriatics, after cataract surgery, in uveitis, 70

myopia

anatomic considerations in, 245

bioptic correction of. *See* bioptics

Intacs procedure for, 237-244

LASEK for, 256-257

LASIK for, 250-256

phakic lenses for. *See* phakic intraocular lenses

photorefractive keratectomy for, 246-250

PRELEX procedure for, 270-271

after radial keratotomy, 171-175

telescopic IOLs for, 139-147

Nasal Corneal Relaxing Nomogram, 12

neonates, cataract surgery in, 30

Nichamin technique, for astigmatism correction, 48, 52

Nidek intraocular lens, for cataract with astigmatism, 56

nomograms, for astigmatism correction, 12, 13, 48, 50-54

nystagmus, in hyperopia, surgical treatment of, 207-209

ocular residual astigmatism, in planning, 154-156

Oliveira technique, for astigmatism correction, 48

opacification, intralenticular, in piggyback IOL use, 136

Ophtec prosthetic iris, 4, 7

optical astigmatism, 152-153

pain

after corneal refractive surgery, 198

in photorefractive keratectomy, 249

in uveitis, 65

pars plana vitrectomy, in dislocated lens removal, 45-46

pediatric patients, cataract surgery in, 23-34

phacoanaphylactic glaucoma, cataract surgery in, 112

phacoemulsification, in cataract surgery

in pseudoexfoliation syndrome, 122-124

in uveitis, 66-69

in zonular dialyses, 38

phacolytic glaucoma, cataract surgery in, 109-112

phacomorphic glaucoma, cataract surgery in, 111-112

phakic intraocular lenses, 211-236

alternatives to, 222

anatomic considerations in, 213-214

for astigmatism, 233-234

CIBA-Medennium, 227-236

complications of, 222-224, 234-235

contraindications for, 215

evaluation for, 211-213

history of, 227-228

indications for, 214-215

with LASIK, 177-180

lens power calculation in, 214

outcomes of, 225

patient selection for, 229-230

pitfalls in, 222

postoperative management in, 222, 233

preoperative considerations in, 216

properties of, 228-229

after radial keratotomy, 174

rehabilitation in, 225

technique for, 217-222, 230-233

teledioptric, 141, 144

types of, 212, 227-228

photic phenomena, with multifocal IOL, 103

photophobia

after corneal refractive surgery, 199

in uveitis, 65

photorefractive keratectomy (PRK)

for astigmatism, 153-159

vs. conductive keratoplasty, 183-184

for hyperopia, 187-205

for myopia, 246-250

after radial keratotomy, 172-173

phototherapeutic keratectomy, after radial keratotomy, 173

piggyback intraocular lenses, 133-137, 170

pigment dispersion syndrome, vs. pseudoexfoliation syndrome, 114

pigment disturbance, after phakic lens implantation, 222

pigment epithelial sheet growth, after phakic lens implantation, 224

polymethylmethacrylate lens, for cataract with astigmatism, 56-58

polymethylmethacrylate rings

in cataract surgery, in zonular dialyses, 36-38

in Intacs procedure, 237-244

posterior capsule

accommodative IOL effects on, 97

management of

in congenital cataract, 28-29

in pseudoexfoliation syndrome, 124-125

opacity of, after cataract surgery, in uveitis, 72

posterior chamber

intraocular lenses for, accommodative, 261-265

phakic lens implantation in, 221-222

posterior optic capture technique, in pediatric cataract surgery, 31-32

posterior synechiae, after cataract surgery, in uveitis, 71

potential acuity meter, in uveitis, 64

prednisone, for uveitis, 65

PRELEX (*PRE*sbyopic *L*ens *EX*change) procedure, 268-272

presbyopia

IOLS for

accommodating, 93-99, 261-265, 267-272

exchange of, 267-272

multifocal, 101-108, 267-268

surgical reversal of, 273-287

anatomic considerations in, 273-274

contraindications for, 275

indications for, 275

preoperative evaluation for, 274-275
rehabilitation in, 287
techniques for, 276-287
PresVIEW Drive unit, 277, 285-286
PRK. *See* photorefractive keratectomy (PRK)
prolate corneal configuration, maintenance of, in Intacs procedure, 237-244
prostheses, iris, 4-9
pseudoaccommodative IOLs, 267-272
pseudoexfoliation syndrome, cataract surgery in, 113-132
　　complications of, 127-128
　　indications for, 115
　　pathophysiology of, 113-115
　　postoperative management in, 126-127
　　procedure for, 116-126
　　technique for, 115-116
pseudophakic accommodation, 261
pseudophakic bioptics, 179-180
pseudophakic pseudoaccommodation, 261
pterygia, corneal incisions in, 17-18
ptosis, after corneal refractive surgery, 201
pupil
　　eccentric, in hyperopia, 191
　　ovalization of, after phakic lens implantation, 223
　　size of, in hyperopia, 191
　　small, cataract surgery in, 118-119
pupillary block, after phakic lens implantation, 234

radial keratotomy (RK)
　　in bioptic procedures, 21-22
　　refractive error correction after, 171-175
Rand-Stein Analgesia Protocol, for cataract surgery, 115-117
Raut technique, for laser cataract extraction, 91
Refractec corneal shaper system, 182-183
refractive errors. *See also* hyperopia; myopia
　　after corneal refractive surgery, 199
　　in IOL exchange, 106
refractive lensectomy, after radial keratotomy, 173-174
refractive surgery. *See also* LASEK; LASIK; photorefractive keratectomy
　　accommodating IOLs for, 93-99, 261-265, 267-272
　　for astigmatism. *See* corneal astigmatism
　　bioptics and. *See* bioptics
　　Intacs procedure, 237-244
　　IOLs for. *See* toric intraocular lenses
　　lensectomy, 173-174. *See also* cataract surgery; intraocular lens(es)
　　phakic lens implantation. *See* phakic intraocular lenses
　　radial keratotomy, 21-22, 171-175
　　reversible, 237-244
　　scleral implants, 273-287
　　thermal keratoplasty, 22, 181-185
regular astigmatism, 151
residual astigmatism, 151, 156

retinal detachment
　　after corneal refractive surgery, 201
　　in dislocated lens interventions, 43-46
　　in hyperopia, 192
rings
　　capsular tension, in cataract surgery, in zonular dialyses, 36-41
　　intracorneal, 11, 22, 237-244
RK (radial keratotomy), 21-22, 171-175
rotation, of intraocular lens
　　in malposition, 79
　　toric, 58-59, 167-170

sands of Sahara, after LASIK, 254
scleral fixation, of IOL, 86-87
scleral spacing procedure. *See* presbyopia, surgical reversal of
scleral-pocket incision, for astigmatism correction, 49, 53
STAAR intraocular lens, for cataract with astigmatism, 19-21, 56-58
striae, after LASIK, 254
synechiae, posterior, after cataract surgery, in uveitis, 71

T cuts, for astigmatism correction, 48, 50
target induced astigmatism vector, in planning, 156, 158
telescopic intraocular lenses, 139-147
　　anatomic considerations in, 139-141
　　anterior chamber high-minus, 139
　　catadioptric posterior chamber, 140
　　complications of, 144-145
　　contraindications for, 143
　　evaluation for, 141-142
　　implantable miniaturized, 140-141, 143-144, 146
　　indications for, 142-143
　　outcomes of, 145-146
　　phakic teledioptric, 141, 144
　　posterior chamber high-minus, 139-140
　　rehabilitation with, 145
　　techniques for, 143-144
　　teledioptric posterior chamber, 140, 143, 145-146
Terry astigmatome, 49, 54
thermal keratoplasty
　　in bioptic procedures, 22
　　conductive, 22, 181-185
　　laser, 173, 183-184
Thornton technique and nomograms, for astigmatism correction, 48, 50-51
topography
　　corneal, in astigmatism, 153, 154
　　for toric IOLs, 169
toric intraocular lenses, 19, 56-59, 165-170
　　axis stabilization of, 167, 169
　　clinical results with, 166-167
　　design of, 165-166
　　enhanced results with, 168-170

optic reversal with, 167-168
piggyback, for high astigmatism, 135-136, 170
preoperative considerations in, 166
types of, 166
toxoplasmosis, retinochoroiditis in, cataract surgery in, 65-66
trauma
 aniridia in, cataract surgery in, 3-10
 zonular dialyses in, 35
triamcinolone
 for uveitis, 65
 for vitreous removal, 40-41
trimethoprim-sulfamethoxazole, for toxoplasmosis, 65-66

ultrasonography, in uveitis, 64
ultrasound biomicroscopy, in uveitis, 64
uveitis
 cataract surgery in, 63-72
 after phakic lens implantation, 222-223

Vannas scissors, for capsulorrhexis, 27
varicella zoster keratouveitis, cataract surgery in, 65
vector planning, for astigmatism correction, 154-157
vestibuloocular conflict, with telescopic IOL, 144-145
videokeratography, computer-assisted, in astigmatism, 153
viscoelastic injection
 in cataract surgery, in zonular dialyses, 38
 retention of, after phakic lens implantation, 234

visual acuity
 after cataract surgery, in aniridia, 9
 with congenital cataract, 24
 after corneal refractive surgery, 199
 after photorefractive keratectomy, 249
 with toric IOLs, 167
vitrectomy, in cataract surgery
 anterior
  in congenital cataract, 28-29
  in dislocated lens removal, 44
 pars plana, 45-46
 posterior, 28, 68-69
 in uveitis, 68-69
vitrector capsulorrhexis, 26
vitreous, removal of, in cataract surgery, in zonular dialyses, 40-41

Wallace LRI kit, 162
wavefront aberrometry, in astigmatism, 152-154
Wehner technique, for laser cataract extraction, 91
with-the-rule corneal astigmatism, 52, 54

Zerdab technique, for laser cataract extraction, 91
zonular dialyses, cataract surgery with, 35-42, 76, 128

# Build Your Library

Along with this title, we publish numerous products on a variety of topics. We are sure that you will find the below titles to be an essential addition to your library. Order your copies today or contact us for a copy of our latest catalog for additional product information.

## MASTER TECHNIQUES IN CATARACT AND REFRACTIVE SURGERY

*F. Hampton Roy, MD, FACS and Carlos Walter Arzabe, MD*

320 pp., Hard Cover, 2004, ISBN 1-55642-696-8, Order #66968, **$174.95**

*Master Techniques in Cataract and Refractive Surgery* combines the wisdom of cataract surgery with the progressiveness of refractive surgery. This text paves the way for today's surgeon to keep pace with all of the newest surgical techniques and technologies available. Each chapter covers indications, contraindications, detailed surgery, complications, results and references. Covering the latest procedures, as well as those that will soon emerge, this all-inclusive and comprehensive text is a necessity for all surgeons.

## PHACOEMULSIFICATION: PRINCIPLES AND TECHNIQUES, SECOND EDITION

*Lucio Buratto, MD; Liliana Werner, MD, PhD; Maurizio Zanini, MD; and David J. Apple, MD*

768 pp., Hard Cover, 2003, ISBN 1-55642-604-6, Order #66046, **$234.95**

*Phacoemulsification: Principles and Techniques, Second Edition* is perfect for the surgeon interested in learning the concepts, developing skills, and preparing for the actual surgical procedure. This comprehensive resource contains a detailed description of the basic technique of phacoemulsification and the special techniques devised by Dr. Buratto and a group of highly acclaimed international surgeons when encountering unusual circumstances.

## CUSTOM LASIK: SURGICAL TECHNIQUES AND COMPLICATIONS

*Lucio Buratto, MD and Stephen F. Brint, MD*

816 pp., Hard Cover, 2003, ISBN 1-55642-606-2, Order #66062, **$234.95**

The collaboration of Drs. Buratto and Brint, along with a team of international surgeons, has produced a complete text specifically to improve the quality of vision. Topics include the latest in wavefront technology, new microkeratome instruments, and the most recent surgical procedures, in addition to various complex cases and complications. With over **1,000** color illustrations demonstrating the various procedures and concepts, readers are able to develop a more thorough understanding of LASIK.

## Contact Us

SLACK Incorporated, Professional Book Division
6900 Grove Road, Thorofare, NJ 08086
1-800-257-8290/1-856-848-1000, Fax: 1-856-853-5991
orders@slackinc.com or www.slackbooks.com/eyecare

---

# ORDER FORM

| QUANTITY | TITLE | ORDER # | PRICE |
|---|---|---|---|
| | Master Techniques in Cataract and Refractive Surgery | 66968 | $174.95 |
| | Phacoemulsification: Principles and Techniques, Second Edition | 66046 | $234.95 |
| | Custom LASIK: Surgical Techniques and Complications | 66062 | $234.95 |
| | | Subtotal | $ |
| | | Applicable state and local tax will be added to your purchase | $ |
| | | Handling | $5.00 |
| | | Total | $ |

Name: _____

Address: _____

City: _____ State: _____ Zip: _____

Phone: _____ Fax: _____

Email: _____

- Check enclosed (Payable to SLACK Incorporated)_____

- Charge my: ___ ___ VISA ___ MasterCard

Account #: _____

Exp. date: _____ Signature: _____

**NOTE:** *Prices are subject to change without notice.*
*Shipping charges will apply.*
*Shipping and handling charges are non-refundable.*

**CODE: 328**